Detection and Diagnosis of
Early Gastric Cancer
Using Conventional Endoscopy

■ **Supervising Editor**

Junko Fujisaki Director, Gastroenterological Medicine Department, Cancer Institute Hospital of JFCR

■ **Authors**

Toshiaki Hirasawa Head, Upper GI Medicine Department, Cancer Institute Hospital of JFCR

Hiroshi Kawachi Head, Department of Pathology, Cancer Institute Hospital of JFCR

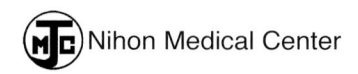 Nihon Medical Center

Detection and Diagnosis of Early Gastric Cancer
Using Conventional Endoscopy

Supervising Editor   Junko Fujisaki

Authors   Toshiaki Hirasawa

Hiroshi Kawachi

Copyright ⓒ 2019 by Nihon Medical Center, Inc.

1-64 Kanda-jinbo-cho, Chiyoda-ku, Tokyo 101-0051, Japan

Japanese edition published in Tokyo in 2016 by Nihon Medical Center, Inc.

English Translation   Atsushi Chiba

ISBN: 978-4-88875-314-2

通常内視鏡観察による
早期胃癌の拾い上げと診断〔英語版〕

2019 年 5 月 20 日　第 1 版 1 刷発行

監　修　藤崎　順子
著　者　平澤　俊明／河内　　洋
発行者　増永　和也
発行所　株式会社日本メディカルセンター
　　　　東京都千代田区神田神保町 1-64（神保町協和ビル）
　　　　〒101-0051　TEL 03（3291）3901 ㈹
印刷所　株式会社アイワード

ISBN978-4-88875-314-2

ⓒ2019　乱丁・落丁は，お取り替えいたします.

Preface

This book originated when Dr. Toshiaki Hirasawa, one of the coauthors of this book, sent out quiz-style emails to residents and medical staff at Cancer Institute Hospital of JFCR. The email quiz had been developed as a teaching tool for use in resident training. A series of slides were attached that showed images of various unusual cases Dr. Hirasawa had worked with, as well as cases where lesions were missed. In the first email distribution, the slides were not accompanied by the associated diagnoses. Instead the recipients were left to examine the images and come to a diagnosis on their own. The actual diagnoses were distributed a few days later. The clinical cases were all very instructive; they included typical cases, difficult-to-diagnose cases, cases where lesions were missed, and so on. The results were very positive. We staff doctors also found them beneficial.

In fact the emails proved so informative that Dr. Masahiro Igarashi, who was Director of the Department of Gastroenterology at the time, thought that it would be a good idea to turn the emails into a series of articles for a Japanese journal called Clinical Gastroenterology. The articles turned into a long-running serial, appearing in every issue and were subsequently collected and revised for inclusion in this volume.

The Cancer Institute Hospital of JFCR is a high-volume center, performing ESD for early cancer on almost 500 cases annually. All the cases are treated only after they have been examined at conferences. In fact, when surgeries are added in, it would be possible for a physician to study close to 1,000 cases of gastric cancer a year simply by attending the conferences. This book can be regarded as a comprehensive compilation of clinical cases that are experienced every day at the Cancer Institute Hospital of JFCR.

This book is so helpful, so packed with invaluable information, that readers will immediately find themselves looking at endoscopic images in a whole new way, starting with the very next endoscopy they perform. I was fortunate to have the opportunity to review all the clinical cases when they were written up for Clinical Gastroenterology. The data and the conclusions were so impressive and convincing that I was literally nodding non-stop while I looked over the material. In this book, you will find a wealth of practical information, including tips on detecting lesions, how to use endoscopes, and details on actual practice.

When we look at the clinical cases introduced in this book, we cannot avoid noticing that there are doctors today who are fully skilled in endoscopic submucosal detection (ESD), yet are unable to make an accurate diagnosis. On the other hand, there are doctors who have technical skill of ESD, yet totally incapable of finding and diagnosing them. This book attempts to solve these problems, making it a must-have for anyone who wants to master everything from detection to diagnosis using conventional endoscopy, which in turn is prerequisite that must be mastered before using magnifying endoscopy.

I have been watching as Dr. Hirasawa devoted all his energy to the creation of this book, so I cannot help feeling even more impressed by the result. As I have already mentioned, this extraordinary project had its genesis in our everyday work. Now it has turned into a single complete book. I hope that all doctors — whether they are just starting out or have years of experience — will find it helpful in their daily practice.

Finally, I would just like to congratulate Dr. Hirasawa on the completion of this book.

October 2016

Junko Fujisaki

Gastroenterological Medicine Department,

Cancer Institute Hospital of JFCR

And this book have just tranlated in English. I would like the doctors doing ESD all over the world to read this book.

March 2019

Junko Fujisaki

Introduction

In Japan, gastric cancer ranks third in deaths from malignant tumors. Every year about 130,000 people are diagnosed with this disease and 50,000 die from it. Ironically, gastric cancer can be completely cured if it is detected early enough — with a Stage I 5-year survival rate of more than 95%. Moreover, when treated and resected endoscopically, there is no difference between the patient's postoperative quality of life and what they experienced before the operation. In short, then, this is a highly treatable cancer with an excellent prognosis and assured QOL as long as it is detected and treated early. Unfortunately, the opposite is true if it is not found until it is already well advanced. In this case, the prognosis is poor, with a 5-year survival rate for Stage IV of less than 10%. Inevitably, whenever we encounter a patient with advanced gastric cancer, our first thought is "if only we could have caught it sooner."

For many years now, the standard population-based screening for gastric cancer in Japan has been a stomach X-ray examination. It was not until 2015 that the National Cancer Center Japan announced the 2014 revision of the Japanese guidelines for gastric cancer screening which accepted that there was sufficient evidence to show that screening using upper gastrointestinal endoscopy could be effective in decreasing the mortality rate of gastric cancer and should be recommended for population-based and opportunistic screening. In response to this, Japan's Ministry of Health, Labour and Welfare revised "Guidelines for Health Education for Cancer Prevention and Cancer Screening" in 2016 and advised that gastric cancer screening shall be conducted using either gastric X-ray examination or upper GI endoscopy.

From the perspective of those of us who are engaged in the diagnosis and treatment of gastric cancer, there is no denying that the introduction of screening using upper GI endoscopy is a little too late. At any rate, it is obvious that opportunistic screening for gastric cancer will shift from X-ray to endoscopy, escalating the already growing demand for endoscopy.

The downside of using upper GI endoscopic examinations to screen for cancer is the enormous disparity in skill levels. This is critical as it can literally mean the difference between life and death. For example, every year at the Cancer Institute Hospital of JFCR, doctors who have completed their senior residency in gastroenterology come to us for training in endoscopy. However, even when they have achieved a satisfactory level of skill in endoscopy, there is still a clear difference between their ability to detect cancer and that of our experienced staff, underscoring once again just how profoundly difficult it is to diagnose gastric cancer against a background of chronic gastritis. The background mucosa exhibits a coarse, irregular appearance due to atrophy and intestinal metaplasia, and the color tones range from redness to fading. Gastric cancers lurking behind the mucosa do not necessarily manifest as textbook-like, typical images; none looks like another.

Over the years, many books have been published on the subject of gastrointestinal endoscopy. Recently there has been a surge in books that cover leading-edge fields such as image enhanced endoscopy (IEE), which includes NBI and magnifying endoscopy. It is certain that NBI magnifying observation wields great strength in qualitative diagnosis such as differentiation between gastritis and gastric cancer. Nonetheless, in order to perform NBI magnifying observation in all areas of chronic gastritis, there will never be enough time for examination. Diagnosis of gastric cancer starts with detection of cancer with conventional endoscopy and dye-spraying chromoendoscopy. Up until now, there have been virtually no books specializing in detection of gastric cancer with conventional endoscopy — which is the most fundamental aspect of all the basics.

From June 2015 to May 2016, we published a series of articles entitled "Where's the Gastric Cancer?" in Clinical Gastroenterology, a monthly journal published by Nihon Medical Center. Illustrated with images from our cases and structured in standard Q&A style, these articles focused on showing readers how to detect gastric cancer using conventional endoscopy. The series was widely praised by our colleagues, and we decided to compile the collected articles into a single volume.

While we were putting the book together, the number of clinical cases worthy of inclusion continued to grow. In addition to an introductory chapter that provides an overview of normal gastric mucosa and gastritis, as well as describing the classification and clinical characteristics of gastric cancer, we included a new chapter that explains how to find gastric cancer, as well as detailing the basic knowledge needed in order to detect gastric cancer. We also added sections devoted to *H. pylori*-uninfected gastric cancer and gastric adenocarcinoma of fundic gland type — both of which are expected to become more prevalent in the future. Most importantly, we included as many pictures as possible throughout the book, and always made sure that everything we wrote was clear and understandable so that even beginners would quickly grasp the details. Images of gastric cancer and adenoma from more than 100 clinical cases are included in this book, making it one of the most comprehensive available.

In the Q&A-style sections, we use the actual endoscopic images captured at the time the lesions were detected. These best represent the lesions in their original state. After biopsy, the shapes and color tones of the lesions change due to biopsy scars and regenerated epithelium, so they look different. Moreover, unlike cases which have been subject to detailed examination, many of the cases in this book have been subject only to cursory examination, meaning that the number of pictures taken is not yet sufficient and no NBI magnifying images are available. The point is that this book focuses on detection of lesions, not on diagnosis or treatment.

We sincerely hope that this book will be widely read by doctors engaged in endoscopic diagnosis and treatment of gastric cancer and that it will help them detect gastric cancers early enough for recovery to be possible — in other words, at a point where endoscopic resection is still possible and the lives of many patients can be saved.

October 2016

Toshiaki Hirasawa
Hiroshi Kawachi

Contents

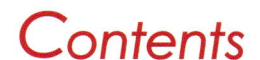

Chapter III | Where's the Gastric Cancer? — Detection and diagnosis

Chapter IV　Did You Find the Gastric Cancer? — Answers and Diagnoses

Side Note

Frequent abbreviation list

EGJ	esophagogastric junction
ESD	endoscopic submucosal dissection
GERD	gastroesophageal reflux disease
LECS	laparoscopy and endoscopy cooperative surgery
MALT	mucosa-associated lymphoid tissue
muc	mucinous adenocarcinoma
NBI	Narrow Band Imaging
NEC	neuroendocrine carcinoma
NET	neuroendocrine tumor
pap	papillary adenocarcinoma
por	poorly differentiated adenocarcinoma
por1	solid type
por2	non-solid type
PPI	proton pump inhibitor
RAC	regular arrangement of collecting venules
SCJ	squamocolumnar junction
sig	signet-ring cell carcinoma
SMT	submucosal tumor
SSBE	short segment Barrett's esophagus
tub	tubular adenocarcinoma
tub1	well differentiated
tub2	moderately differentiated
UL	ulcer/ulcer scar
WGA	white globe appearance
WOS	white opaque substance

Cover photo

① p.153, ② p.93, ③ p.72, ④ p.137, ⑤ p.99, ⑥ p.77, ⑦ p.137, ⑧ p.67, ⑨ p.104, ⑩ p.109, ⑪ p.49, ⑫ p.54, ⑬ p.117, ⑭ p.55, ⑮ p.56, ⑯ p.38, ⑰ p.55, ⑱ ⑲ p.134, ⑳ ㉑ p.56, ㉒ ㉓ p.53, ㉔ p.115, ㉕ p.202, ㉖ p.203, ㉗ p.203, ㉘ ㉙ p.59, ㉚ ㉛ p.41, ㉜ p.158, ㉝ p.120

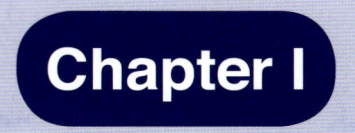

Basic Knowledge in Gastric Cancer Detection

1 Normal gastric mucosa and gastritis

- Gastric cancer is hidden in gastritis. Understanding gastritis is required in order to detect gastric cancer. In this section, we compare and discuss images of gastritis and of the normal stomach.

2 Classification of gastric cancer and clinical characteristics

- Understanding how gastric cancer develops makes it easier to understand the characteristics of gastric cancer.

1 Normal gastric mucosa and gastritis

Understanding the background mucosa of gastric cancer

- The fundic glands of normal gastric mucosa look different depending on the region, so endoscopic images look different as well. In many cases, findings of chronic gastritis — which can often lead to gastric cancer — also differ significantly from one another, manifesting in a wide variety of morphologies. Similarly, the background mucosa itself also differs widely in terms of histology, morphology, and color tone — all of which must be evaluated in order to assess the risk of gastric cancer. This variability makes early detection of gastric cancer difficult. It is the complete opposite of cancers where tumors are set against a background in which there is no inflammation — such as colorectal cancer — and so are relatively easy to detect.
- As the first step to detecting gastric cancer is accurate evaluation of gastritis, we are first going to discuss normal gastric mucosa and gastritis before moving on to gastric cancer.

I Normal gastric mucosa (*Helicobacter pylori* [*H. pylori*]-uninfected)

A normal stomach is one free from *H. pylori* infection and with no history of *H. pylori* infection (*H. pylori*-uninfected). Somewhere between one-third and two-thirds of the surface layer of a normal stomach's mucosa is covered with foveolar epithelium to prevent the gastric acid from causing autolysis. The proper gastric glands are found beneath the foveolar epithelium. The border between the foveolar epithelium and the proper gastric glands is called the neck of glands. It is a proliferative zone where active cell division takes place (**Fig. 1**).

Normal *H. pylori*-uninfected gastric mucosa is divided into three regions that correspond to the distribution of proper gastric glands (**Fig. 2**). Pyloric glands are distributed from the prepyloric region to the antrum, fundic glands are distributed from the body to the fornix, and cardiac glands are distributed in the vicinity of the esophagogastric (EG) junction. The fundic glands are composed of parietal cells that secrete acid, chief cells that secrete pepsinogen I — a proteolytic enzyme that is a precursor of pepsin, mucous neck cells that secrete mucus, and a small number of endocrine cells. The pyloric and cardiac glands are composed of mucous cells and endocrine cells. Gastrin — a gastrointestinal hormone — is secreted by G cells in the pyloric glands.

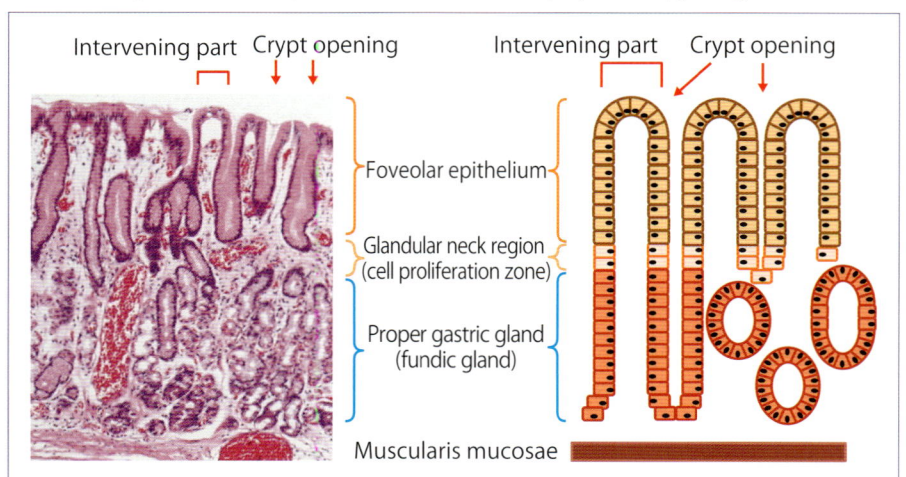

Intervening part Crypt opening   Intervening part   Crypt opening

Foveolar epithelium

Glandular neck region
(cell proliferation zone)

Proper gastric gland
(fundic gland)

Muscularis mucosae

Fig. 1 Normal gastric mucosa (fundic gland region)

Normal gastric mucosa is shown in the histopathological image on the right and diagram on the left. Active proliferation of cells is occurring in the neck of gland. There are two types of cells: one type differentiates upwards into the foveolar epithelium and the other differentiates downwards into the proper gastric glands.

Endoscopic images of a normal fundic gland region show mucosa that is uniformly reddish orange and glossy. The surface is smooth, with no signs of irregularity or unevenness. The folds in the body are narrow and straight, with no tortuosity or swelling visible (**Fig. 3**). The most characteristic finding is the presence of countless small erythematous spots known as a "regular arrangement of collecting venules" or RAC. From a distance, RAC looks like innumerable regularly arranged minute red points. However, when viewed up close, those minute points appear to be starfish-like venules[1] (**Fig. 4**). Histologically, RAC is a group of collecting venules present below the mucosal epithelium (**Fig. 5**). Magnifying endoscopy shows reticular true capillaries that surround crypt openings. The collecting venules where those capillaries merge — that is to say, RAC — can also be confirmed with magnifying endoscopy (**Fig. 6**).

Atrophy of gastric mucosa causes RAC to disappear, so it can be a good barometer for normal mucosa without atrophy. When RAC is observed throughout the body, it is diagnosed as RAC-positive. RAC-positive cases can be diagnosed as *H. pylori*-uninfected with diagnostic accuracy of 95%[1]. Since RAC is observed in the upper and middle gastric body in atrophic cases with a degree of C-1 or so, we recommend observation from the region of the angulus to the lesser curvature of the lower body when assessing whether or not a case is RAC positive[2].

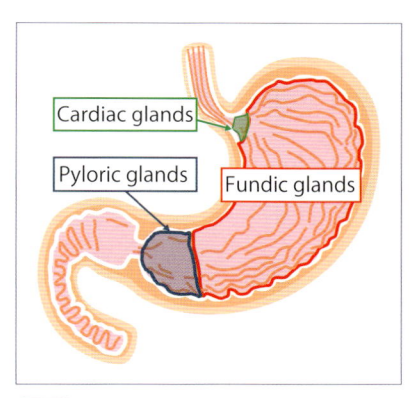

Fig. 2 Normal distribution of proper gastric glands

In a normal stomach without atrophy, pyloric glands are distributed from the prepyloric region to the antrum, fundic glands are distributed from the body to the fornix, and cardiac glands are distributed around the cardia.

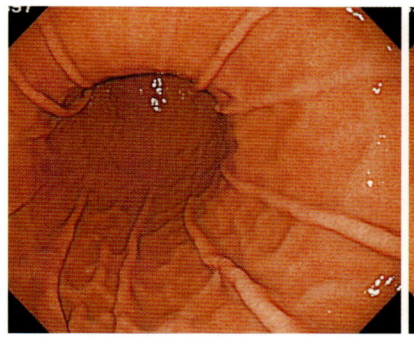

Fig. 3 Normal fundic gland region

The mucosa is smooth and glossy. The folds are narrow and almost straight. There is no sign of either swelling or tortuosity. A fundic gland polyp can be seen.

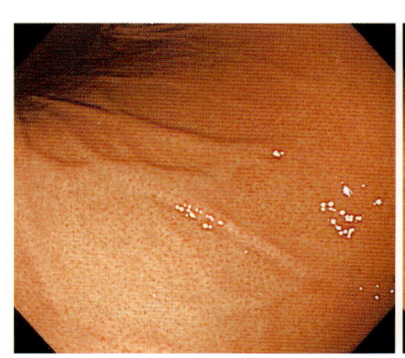

Fig. 4 RAC

In the distant view(left), RAC is visible as numerous minute red points; however, those small points turn out to be minute vessels when viewed from up close(right).

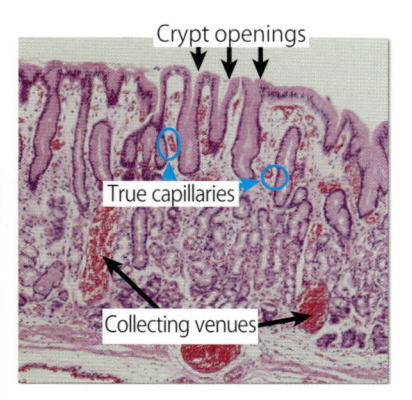

Fig. 5 Histological image of collecting venules

True capillaries have developed around the crypt openings in the shallow layer of the mucosa, while in the deeper layer the capillaries have merged to form collecting venules.

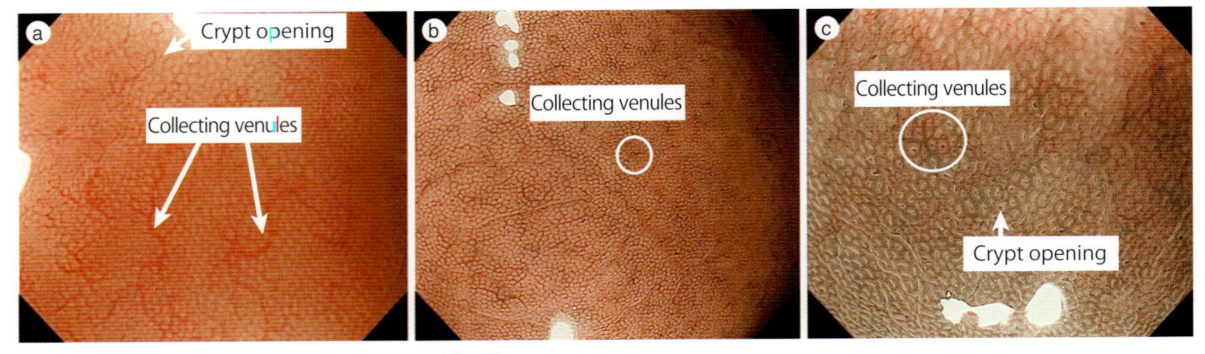

Fig. 6 Magnified images of RAC

a : White-light imaging (WLI). WLI magnifying observation confirms that reticular true capillaries surround the round-shaped crypt openings and those capillaries have merged to form collecting venules. Although it is difficult to confirm with WLI, the small dots in the center of the reticulated true capillaries are the crypt openings.

b, c : Narrow Band Imaging (NBI). NBI observation with low magnification (b) confirms that the reticular true capillaries and tortuous collecting venules are regularly arranged. The crypt openings are clearly visible at high magnification (c).

② Pyloric gland region

As in the fundic gland region, the mucosa in the pyloric gland region is smooth and glossy. The most noticeable difference is that RAC is not visible because collecting venules have not developed in the pyloric region[3]. In some cases, however, RAC may be observed on the proximal side of the antrum since the fundic glands are often present in this area[2]. As for the distribution ranges of pyloric glands, they can vary significantly from one individual to another. Consequently, in some cases, RAC may be observed across a wide range even in the antrum, while in other cases it may not be seen at all. Additionally, fine branching vessels may be observed in the pyloric gland region (**Fig. 7**).

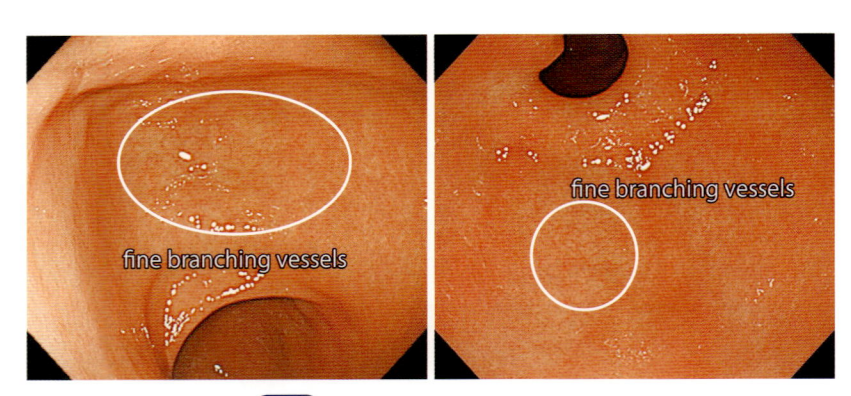

Fig. 7 Normal pyloric gland region

A normal pyloric gland region is glossy and exhibits a smooth mucosal surface. RAC is not visible. In some areas, fine branching vessels can be seen, but these should not be mistaken for atrophy.

③ Cardiac gland region

In a normal *H. pylori*-uninfected stomach, cardiac gland mucosa extends a few millimeters from the EG junction (**Fig. 8**). When *H. pylori* infection is present, the cardiac gland mucosa extends towards the distal side[4), 5)].

Pitfall to be avoided

Be careful not to misdiagnose a normal pyloric region as atrophic

- As a result of differences in color between fundic gland and pyloric gland regions, as well as presence/absence of RAC and fine branching vessels, a normal pyloric region may be mistaken as atrophic. Typically, changes induced by chronic gastritis caused by *H. pylori* infection occur first in the antrum. It can be difficult, however, to make an endoscopic evaluation of whether it is normal or atrophic gastritis.

- The color of a normal pyloric gland region is slightly more yellowish-red than a fundic gland region. Due to the presence of fine branching vessels, the region may look atrophic at first glance. However, since the mucosal surface is glossy and smooth, it should be diagnosed as a normal pyloric gland region. This case had been misdiagnosed as C–1 atrophy.

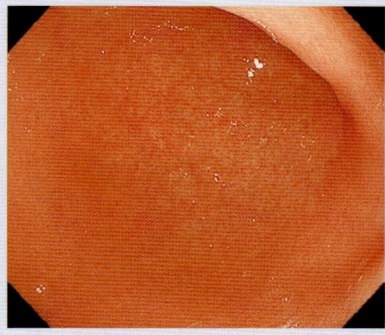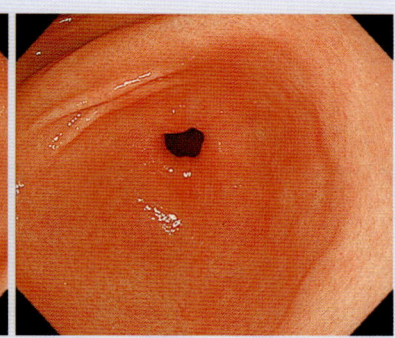

Compare!   Magnifying endoscopic finding with NBI of nomal fundic gland and pyloric gland regions

- The findings of the fundic gland region and pyloric gland region are completely different in NBI magnifying observation as well. Reticular true capillaries and starfish-like collecting venules are arranged regularly in the fundic gland region while coiled vessels are recognized inside ridged and tubular patterns of mucosa.

- The reason why such a difference in findings occurs is because of the different roles played by the fundic gland and pyloric gland. The main role of the fundic gland is secretion of acid and pepsin to help digest food whereas the pyloric gland is a mucous gland and does not secrete digestive fluid. The pyloric gland's role is to perform rapid peristalsis to push food through a small exit called the pyloric ring into the duodenum after food has been accumulated and mixed in the stomach. In other words, the pyloric gland region in the antrum is designed so that the mucosa stretches and contracts — just like a bellows — to perform peristalsis.

- In NBI magnifying observation, completely different findings are also exhibited in the fundic gland region (left) and the pyloric gland region (right).

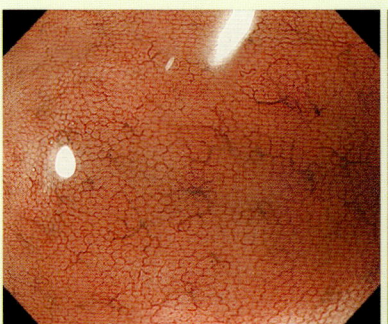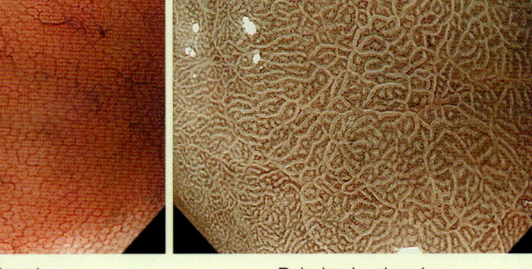

Fundic gland region   Pyloric gland region

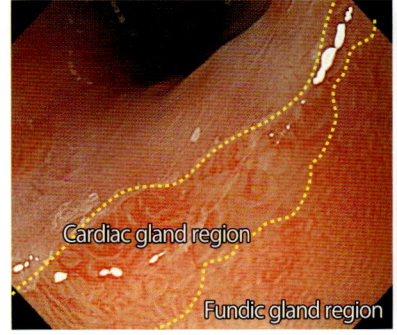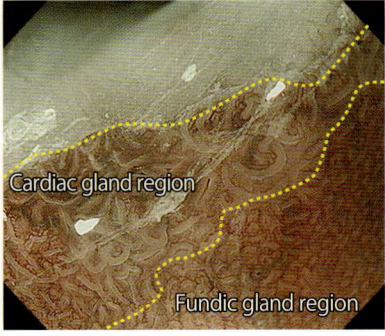

WLI, medium magnification   NBI, medium magnification

Fig. 8 Normal cardiac gland region

In a zone 1 to 2 mm from the EG junction, ridged and tubular mucosal patterns can be seen. This narrow zone corresponds to the cardiac gland region.

1) Fundic gland polyps (Figs. 9 & 10)

These are protruded polyps ranging in size from roughly 2 to 5 mm. They are present in multiple locations throughout the region from the body to the fornix where fundic glands are distributed. The originating points of the elevations form the margins of the polyps. The surfaces of the polyps have the same color tones and mucosal patterns as the surrounding fundic glands. When the surface is viewed up close, dilated capillaries are sometimes seen. Histologically, cystically dilated glands, hyperplasia of the fundic glands and misplacement of the foveolar epithelium are recognized. These findings disappear when the background mucosa is atrophied.

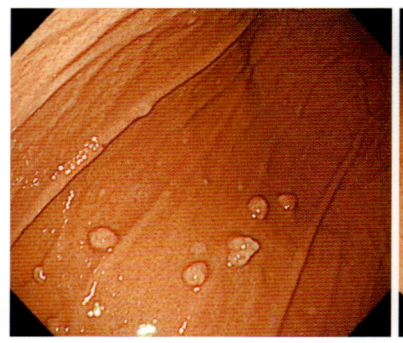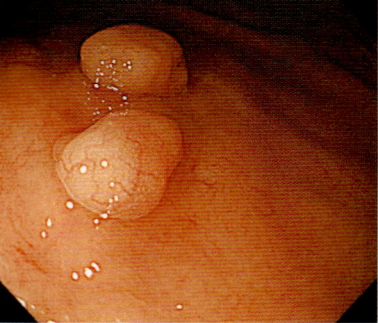

Fig. 9 Fundic gland polyps ①

Against the non-atrophic background mucosa, protruded polyps occur in multiple locations. They have the same color tones and mucosal patterns as the surroundings. The margins of the polyps are completely circumferential and are very clear. When observed from up close, dilated capillaries can be seen on some of the polyps.

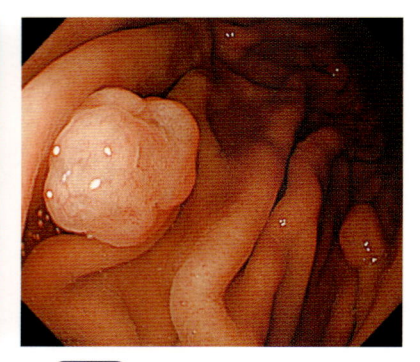

Fig. 10 Fundic gland polyps ②

When a proton pump inhibitor (PPI) has been taken for a long period, fundic gland polyps may occur in multiple locations and their sizes may increase.

2) Attachment of hematin (Fig. 11)

Hematin is old dark-red blood attached to the gastric mucosa. It is one of findings in *H. pylori*-uninfected cases, but can also be seen after eradication[6), 7)]. The region where hematin had been attached was washed and then observed, but neither erosion nor inflammation was found. It was hypothesized that the blood exuded from normal crypts. While hematin attachment is often accompanied by erosion, hematin attachment not caused by inflammation is also sometimes observed in *H. pylori*-uninfected cases.

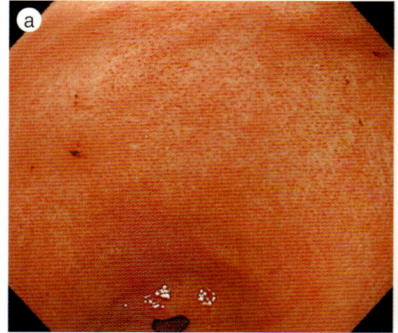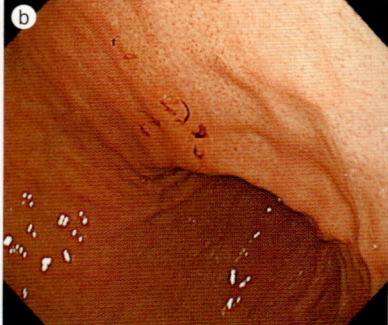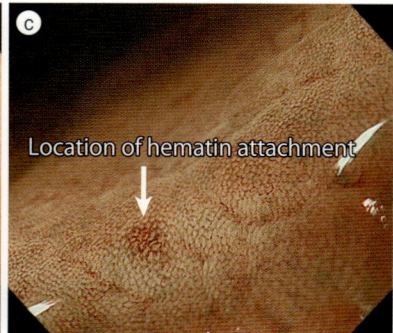

Location of hematin attachment

Fig. 11 Hematin attachment

a, b : Hematin is attached here and there on the non-atrophic mucosa.

c : When the hematin has been washed off and then the area where the hematin was attached is observed with magnifying endoscopy with NBI, normal round crypt openings can be seen. No findings such as erosion present.

3) Red streaks (Fig. 12)

A reddish band that runs longitudinally in the antrum and body along the long axis of the stomach is called a red streak. Red streaks are often seen on the lesser curvature side, but may also be seen all around the circumference. The redness ranges from pale to vivid red and may occasionally be accompanied by erosion and hematin attachment. This finding is typical of *H. pylori*-uninfected stomachs, but may also be seen in infected stomachs after eradication. There are no specific histological findings. When the stomach is deaerated, red streaks correspond with the crests of the folds. It is believed that these streaks are generated when the stomach is contracted and the crests of the folds come into contact with gastric juice. In other words, red streaks are generated when the crests of folds are stimulated chemically and mechanically[3), 9)].

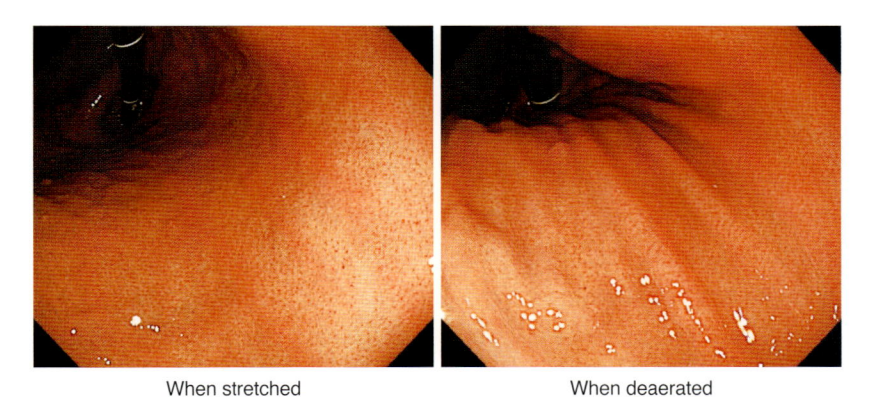

When stretched   When deaerated

Fig. 12 Red streaks

The background is RAC-positive fundic gland mucosa without atrophy. Red strips running longitudinally along the lesser curvature of the body can be seen; these are red streaks. When deaerated, the red streaks correspond with the crests of folds.

4) Raised erosion (Figs. 13 & 14)

A raised erosion is an elevation that is eroded on the top and occurs in multiple locations in the antrum. It is also called a verrucous erosion or an "octopus-sucker" erosion. It tends to run longitudinally and assumes various morphologies including polypous, eruciform, clavate, and moniliform. Raised erosions usually occur in multiple locations, but may occur in just a single location. Histopathologically, erosion is recognized on the crests and edema and hyperplasia are recognized in the surrounding proper gastric glands.

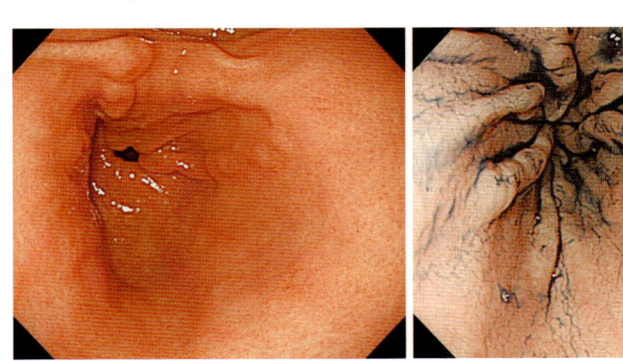

Fig. 13 Raised erosion ①

This raised erosion runs radially in the antrum. Gently sloping, edematous elevations occur in multiple locations. If the erosion is likened to suction cups, it looks like octopus tentacles. That is why it is also called "octopus-sucker" erosion.

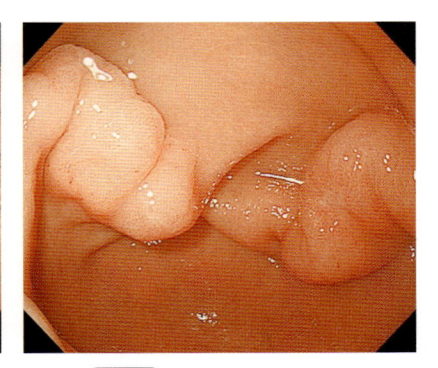

Fig. 14 Raised erosion ②

This raised erosion adheres in the long-axis direction and forms a shape like a string of beads. Conspicuous elevations like this occur in some cases.

Ⅱ   *H. pylori*-infected gastritis (*H. pylori* current infection and past infection)

H. pylori-infected gastritis can refer to both a current infection and one which has been eradicated (past infection). Depending on the infection duration and differences in individual reactions, *H. pylori*-infected gastritis can yield various findings. There are also different findings between current and past infections.

❶ Findings often seen in *H. pylori* current infection

Histopathologically, gastric mucosa that is currently infected with *H. pylori* displays lymphocyte and neutrophil infiltration, which leads to chronic changes including atrophy of proper gastric glands and intestinal metaplasia. Endoscopic findings include atrophy, intestinal metaplasia, spotty redness, diffuse redness, enlarged/tortuous folds, sticky mucus, mucosal swelling, hyperplastic polyps, nodular gastritis, xanthoma, etc[10), 11)].

1) Atrophy

Atrophy is a condition in which the proper gastric glands have been destroyed or are absent as a result of the inflammation caused by *H. pylori* infection. In the endoscopic findings, small yellowish-white dots are observed in the region from the antrum to the lesser curvature of the angulus. Eventually, the dots fade, forming patches that ultimately merge into an atrophic area. As atrophy progresses, the destruction of the proper gastric glands becomes more pronounced and the mucosa starts thinning. As a result, submucosal vascular patterns become visible.

① Diagnosis of the extent of atrophy (Figs. 15–17)

Atrophy starts from the pyloric gland region and extends from the lesser curvature of the body towards the proximal side and greater curvature side. Kimura and Takemoto classified atrophy that does not go beyond the cardia as "closed," and atrophy that goes beyond the cardia and advances as far as the greater curvature side as "open." The closed type is subclassified into C-1, C-2, and C3 depending on the extent of atrophy, while the open type is subclassified into O-1, O-2, and O-3[12)].

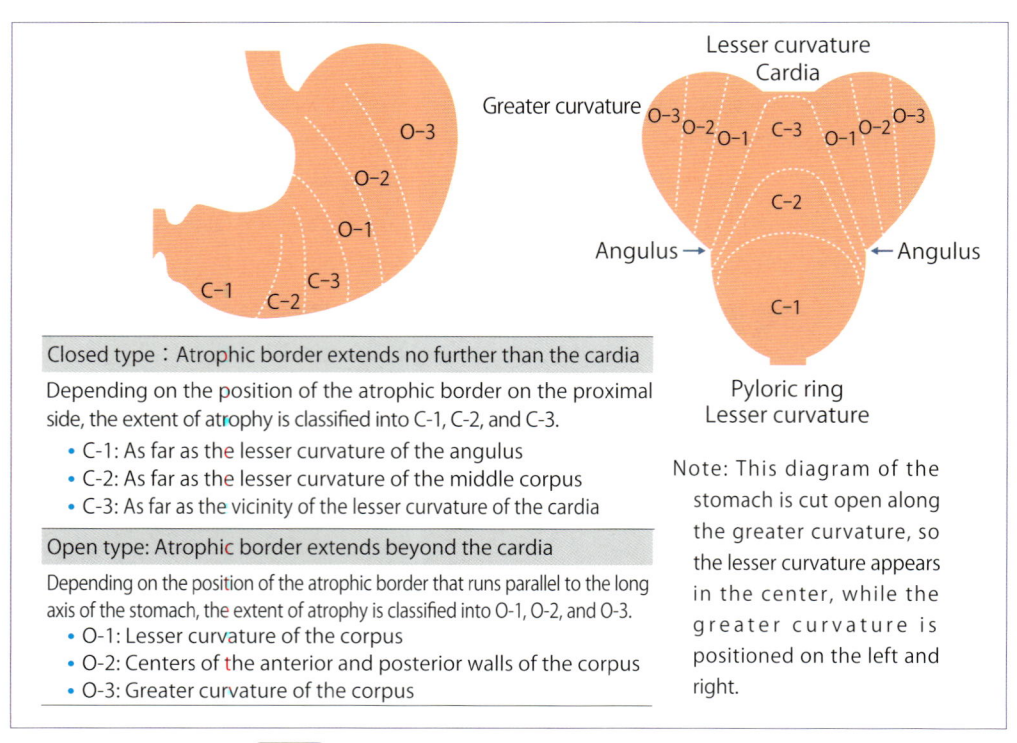

Closed type : Atrophic border extends no further than the cardia

Depending on the position of the atrophic border on the proximal side, the extent of atrophy is classified into C-1, C-2, and C-3.
- C-1: As far as the lesser curvature of the angulus
- C-2: As far as the lesser curvature of the middle corpus
- C-3: As far as the vicinity of the lesser curvature of the cardia

Open type: Atrophic border extends beyond the cardia

Depending on the position of the atrophic border that runs parallel to the long axis of the stomach, the extent of atrophy is classified into O-1, O-2, and O-3.
- O-1: Lesser curvature of the corpus
- O-2: Centers of the anterior and posterior walls of the corpus
- O-3: Greater curvature of the corpus

Note: This diagram of the stomach is cut open along the greater curvature, so the lesser curvature appears in the center, while the greater curvature is positioned on the left and right.

Fig. 15 Kimura-Takemoto Classification of atrophy
[Created based on: Kimura K, Takemoto T. Endoscopy. 1969; 1 (3): 87–97[12)]]

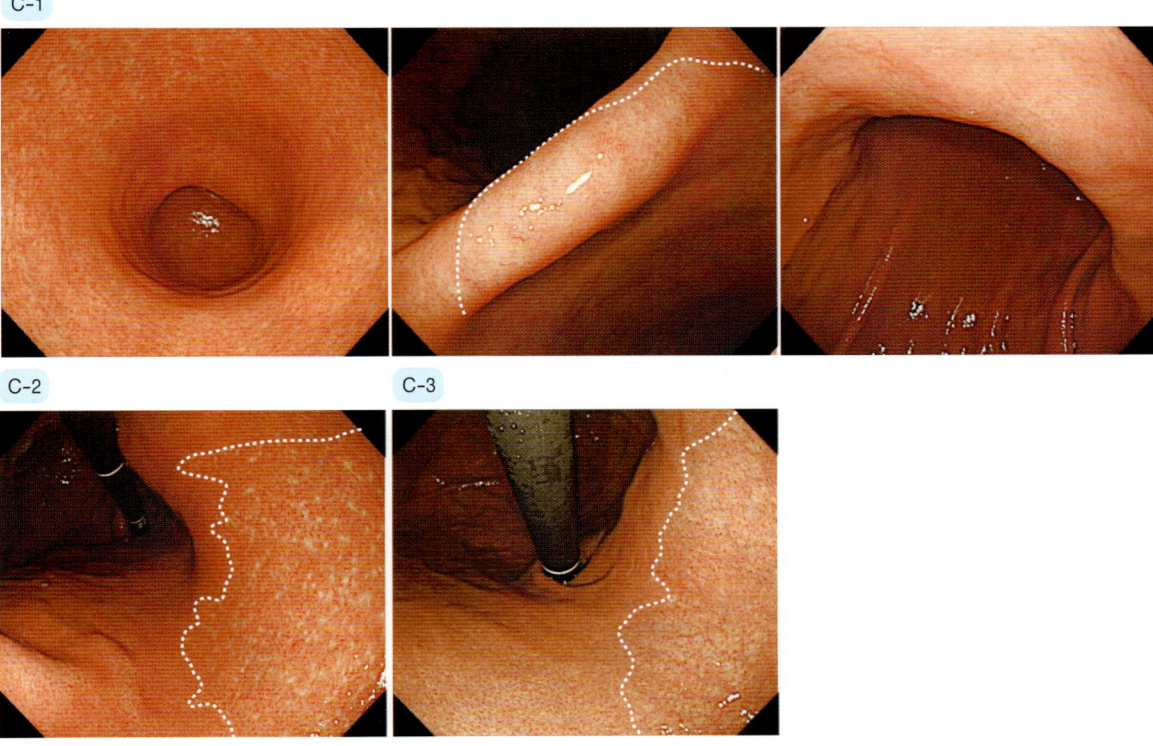

Fig. 16 Kimura-Takemoto Classification: Closed type

C-1 : Small yellowish-white patches occur in multiple locations in the antrum and angulus. Vascular patterns are not visible. The border between atrophic mucosa and non-atrophic mucosa is indicated by a dotted line. The atrophic border is on the angulus, and the atrophy has not advanced into the lesser curvature of the lower body.

C-2 : Small dotted, patchy faded coloring has advanced into the lesser curvature of the middle body. The faded coloring does not always advance in a linear fashion – sometimes it looks as though eaten by worms.

C-3 : The patchy faded areas merge, forming a relatively flat surface. Vascular patterns are slightly visible. The atrophy has not reached the cardia.

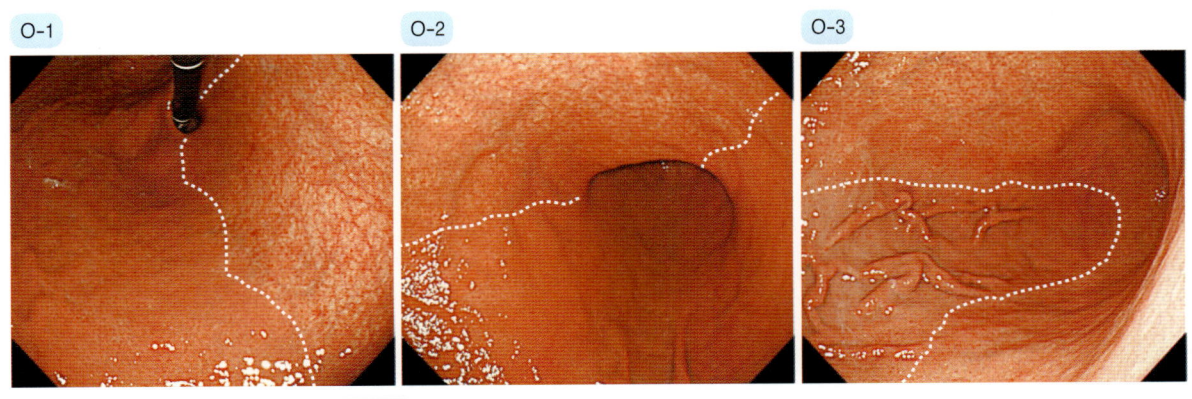

Fig. 17 Kimura-Takemoto Classification: Open type

O-1 : The atrophic border runs along the lesser curvature of the body and has reached the cardia. Vascular patterns are prominent, and fading has intensified.

O-2 : The atrophic border is located on the anterior and posterior walls. Fading and fine vascular patterns can be seen in the atrophic area.

O-3 : The atrophic border is located on the greater curvature of the body. Folds are absent in the atrophic area, but can be seen in the non-atrophic area.

② Diagnosis of the degree of atrophy

To evaluate the degree of atrophy, observe the lower body while it is extended[13].

- **Low-degree atrophy** : Faded patches are observed on the mucosa (**Fig. 18**).
- **Medium-degree atrophy** : Fine vascular patterns are observed (**Fig. 19**).
- **High-degree atrophy** : Clear, reticulated vascular patterns are observed (**Fig. 20**).

Vascular patterns look different depending on the amount of insufflation. Be sure to make your evaluation while the mucosa is stretched. The extent and degree of atrophy often correlate with each other.

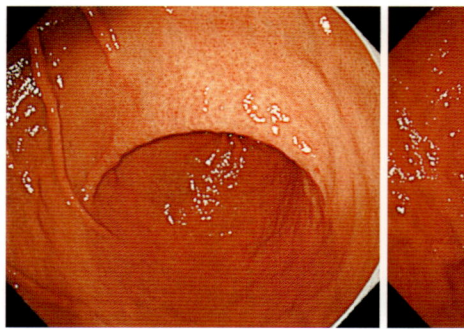
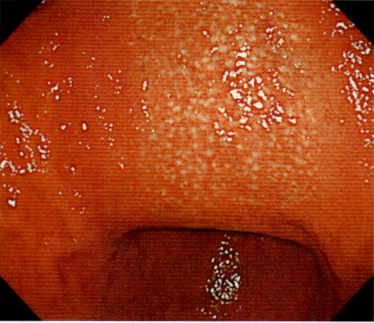

Fig. 18 Low-degree atrophy

Faded spotty, patchy depressions are observed. Eventually, they merge into larger patches. Initially, the patches are yellowish white, but as the mucosa gets thinner, the fading increases. No vascular patterns are observed.

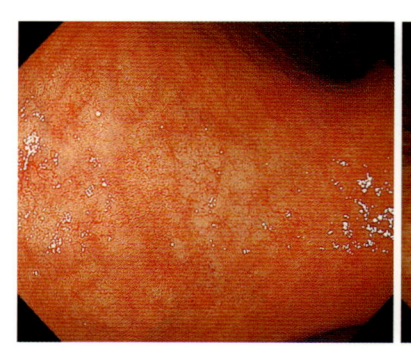
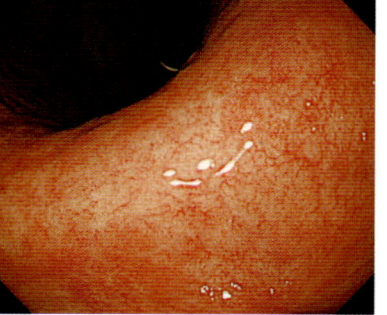

Fig. 19 Medium-degree atrophy

Fine vascular patterns are visible within areas of patchy, planar fading. This is due to the thinning of the mucosa, which allows the submucosal vessels to become visible.

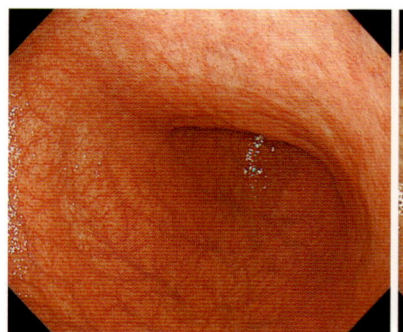
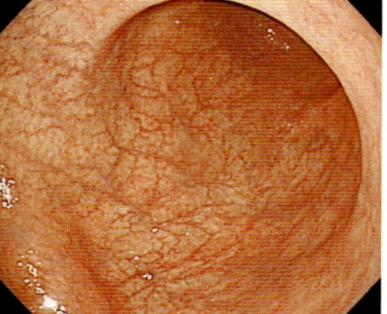

Fig. 20 High-degree atrophy

The entire mucosa appears faded. Reticulated and fine branched vascular patterns are visible.

2) Intestinal metaplasia

Intestinal metaplasia is a condition in which gastric foveolar epithelium is replaced by epithelium that resembles intestinal epithelium. It emerges during chronic gastritis and is usually observed across a wide area in atrophic gastritis.

In histological observation, goblet cells containing mucus are observed in cytoplasms. In some cases, absorptive cells with brush borders and Paneth cells with eosinophilic granules may also be observed (in the case of complete-type intestinal metaplasia) (**Fig. 21**).

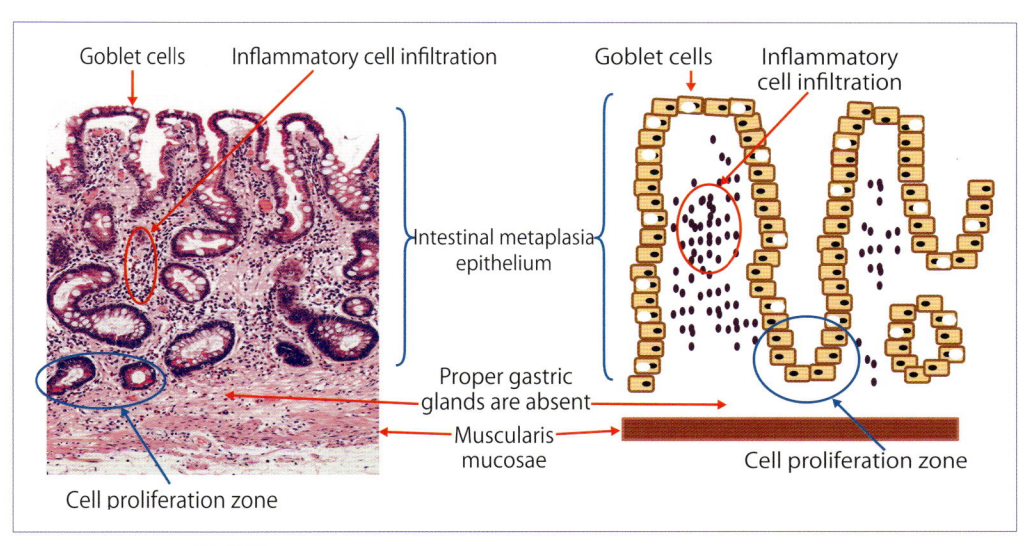

Fig. 21 Histological images of atrophy and intestinal metaplasia

The proper gastric glands have disappeared, and the foveolar epithelium has been replaced with intestinal metaplastic epithelium. Multiple goblet cells containing mucus occur in the cytoplasm. Cryptic openings are absent and a villous structure is observed. Inflammatory cell infiltration is prominent and diffused throughout the lamina propria mucosae. The cell proliferation zone is located at the bottom of the glands near the muscularis mucosae.

Pitfall to be avoided

Is this atrophy ?

- Even with normal mucosa, excessive stretching by insufflation can cause fine branched vascular patterns in the submucosa to be visible. This is especially likely in the fornix where the thin mucosa makes vascular patterns easier to see. This finding — visible vascular patterns in the fornix — can easily be mistaken for atrophy.

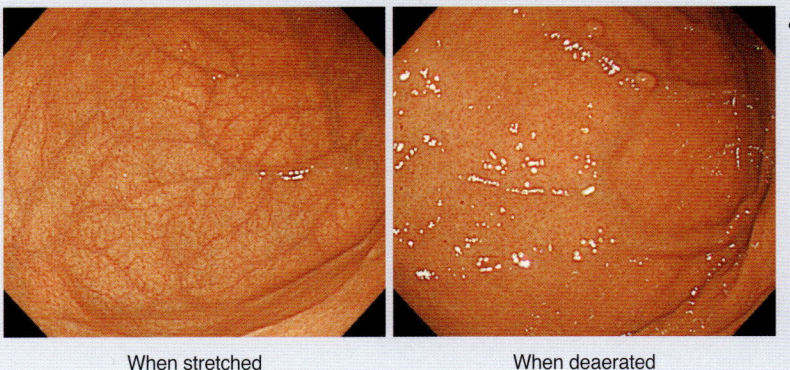

When stretched   When deaerated

- The photos are of an *H. pylori*-uninfected case and show the greater curvature of the fornix in a stretched condition and in a deaerated condition. The mucosa in the fornix is thin; when it is stretched by insufflation, submucosal vascular patterns become visible. The RAC is not clear when the fornix is stretched, but emerges when it is deaerated.

In endoscopic observation, intestinal metaplasia is observed as grayish-white flat elevations in various sizes or slightly hyperplastic grayish-white mucosa (Fig 22 & 23). The elevations can be seen clearly in indigocarmine chromoendoscopy and NBI endoscopy. As intestinal metaplasia progresses, the vascular patterns visible in gastric atrophy become harder to see. The grayish-white mucosa is a clear endoscopic indicator of intestinal metaplasia. However, although the specificity is high, the sensitivity is substantially low[14].

In addition to the grayish-white mucosa that can be confirmed in endoscopy, there are many histopathological findings for intestinal metaplasia including villous appearance[15] that can be confirmed in conventional close-up observation (**Fig. 24**) and light blue crests (LBCs)[16] that can be confirmed in NBI magnifying observation (**Fig. 25**). These findings are high in both sensitivity and specificity. While it is difficult to use endoscopy to fully diagnose all intestinal metaplasia, it is also important to be aware of the fact that intestinal metaplasia can also be accompanied by redness.

It is also important to point out that where intestinal metaplasia is present, the mucosal environment is not suitable for the survival of *H. pylori*, resulting in a sharp decrease in the number of bacteria[17].

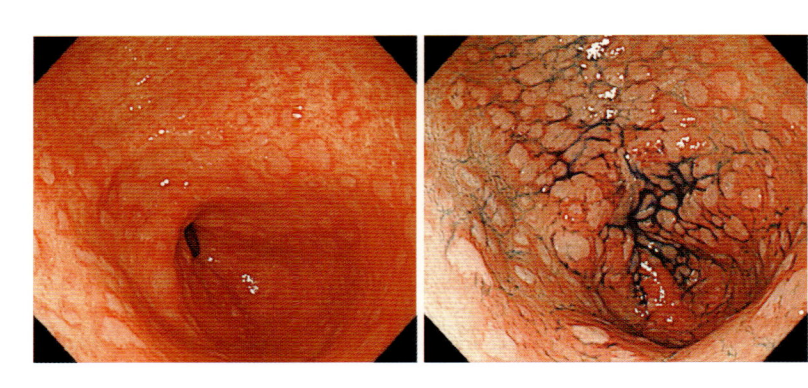

Fig. 22 Intestinal metaplasia ① : Grayish-white

Multiple flat elevations in a grayish-white color are present. Their shapes and sizes are not uniform.

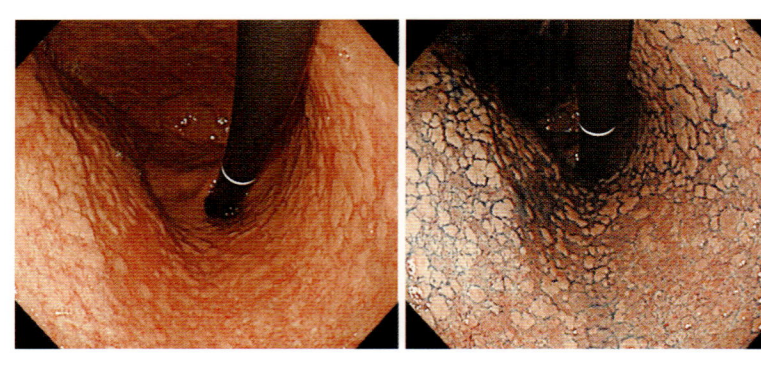

Fig. 23 Intestinal metaplasia ② : Grayish-white

Slightly hyperplastic grayish-white mucosa expands, creating a map-like shape.

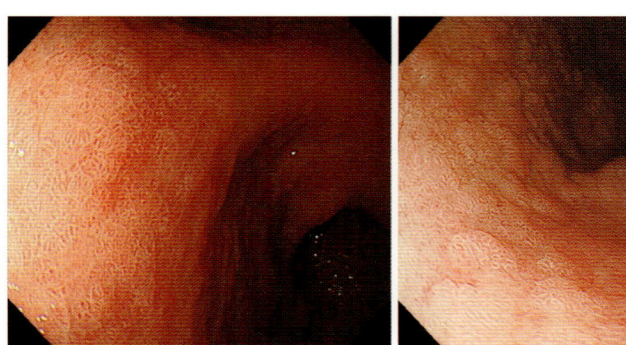

Fig. 24 Intestinal metaplasia ③ : Villous appearance

When viewed up close, the mucosa exhibits pattern with a villous structure.

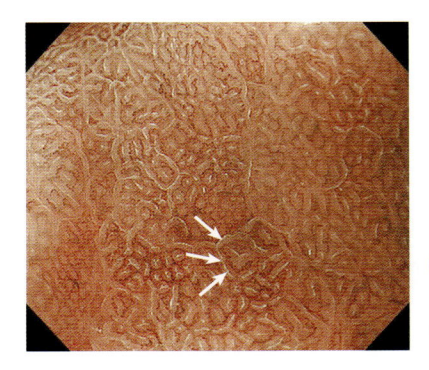

Fig. 25 Intestinal metaplasia ④ : light blue crest

In NBI magnifying observation, pale edges can be seen on the periphery of epithelium, and these are called light blue crest (LBCs).

Pitfall to be avoided

Intestinal metaplasia and atrophic areas

- When intestinal metaplasia emerges, the mucosa thickens and turns grayish-white. The vascular patterns apparent in gastric atrophy are no longer clear. Because intestinal metaplasia is accompanied by atrophy, the extent of intestinal metaplasia coincides with the atrophic area.
- The grayish-white mucosa caused by intestinal metaplasia spreads throughout the body. No vascular patterns are visible.

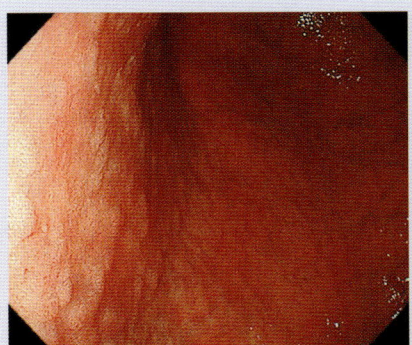
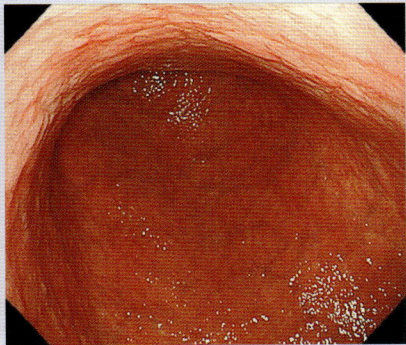

ble. Villous appearance can be observed when viewed up close. The region where intestinal metaplasia is present should also be considered atrophic. The degree of atrophy is O-3. If only the extent of fading and vascular patterns is examined, it is possible to incorrectly diagnose the actual extent of atrophy.

3) Spotty redness (Fig. 26)

Observed on the fundic mucosa, spotty redness is composed of small, dot-like erythema that occurs in multiple locations. It frequently occurs in the fornix and upper body and is usually seen in cases with a current *H. pylori* infection. Eradication often results in the reduction and rapid disappearance of spotty redness[8), 18)–20)].

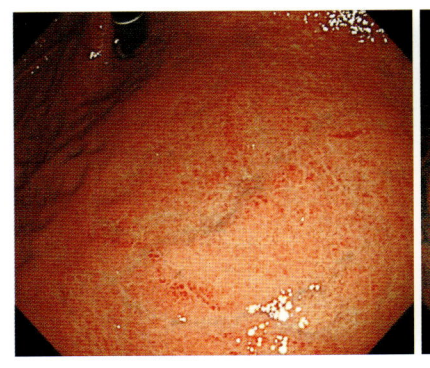
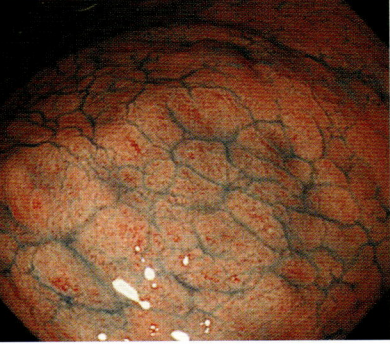

Fig. 26 Spotty redness

Spotty redness frequently occurs in the fornix and upper body. When observed up close, the redness has a smooth surface and the sizes and shapes vary. There is diffuse redness in the background.

4) Diffuse redness (Figs. 27 & 28)

In *H. pylori* currently infected cases, non-atrophic mucosa in the body exhibits uniform redness. This is called diffuse redness. Unlike spotty redness, it is designated as planar redness with continuity. Diffuse redness correlates with the degree of neutrophil infiltration[20]. When the infection is eradicated, neutrophil infiltration is reduced and reddened mucosa will change to faded or flesh-colored mucosa in a few months[20, 21].

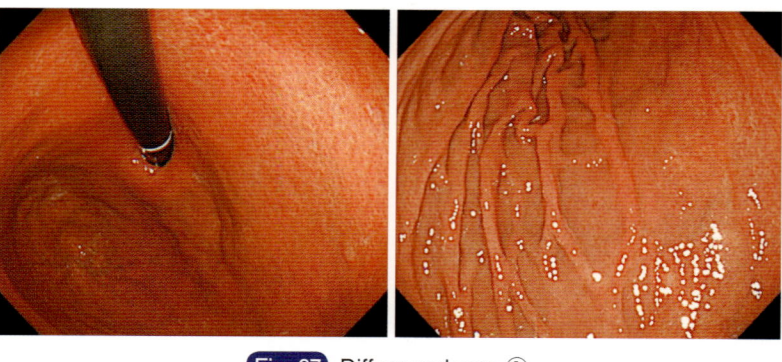

Fig. 27 Diffuse redness ①

Diffuse redness is uniform with no gradations. The degree of redness differs depending on the case. It also varies according to the setting of the endoscope and monitor.

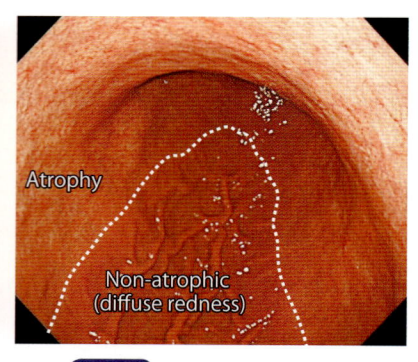

Fig. 28 Diffuse redness ②

In cases where the atrophic border is clear, the contrast between the diffuse redness of non-atrophic mucosa and the faded color of atrophic mucosa is also clear. Diffuse redness occurs on non-atrophic mucosa.

5) Enlarged and tortuous folds (Fig. 29)

Hyperplastic foveolar epithelium due to chronic gastritis and edematous changes in stroma causes the folds in the greater curvature of the body to become enlarged and tortuous. As the mucosa shows edematous changes, it is soft when it is pushed with forceps.

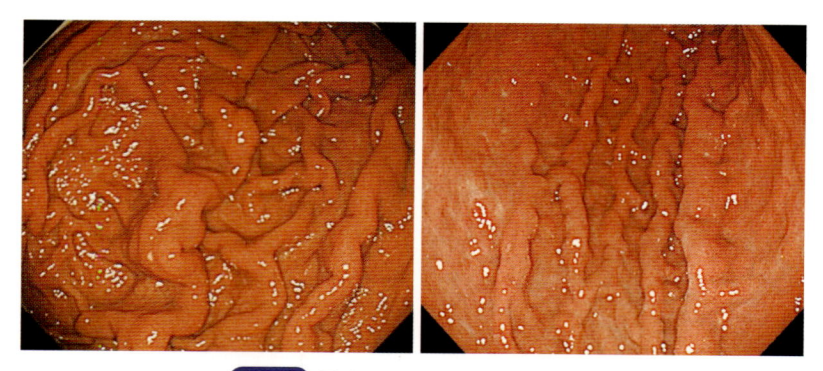

Fig. 29 Enlarged and tortuous folds

Even when the lumen of the stomach is stretched, the folds are still thick. The degree of enlargement and tortuosity differs depending on the case.

6) Sticky mucus (Fig. 30)

Sticky mucus is dirty-looking, whitish and opaque mucus often observed in *H. pylori* currently infected cases. It is highly viscous and sticks firmly to the mucosa, making it difficult to wash off. Eradication of the *H. pylori* infection will quickly ameliorate sticky mucus.

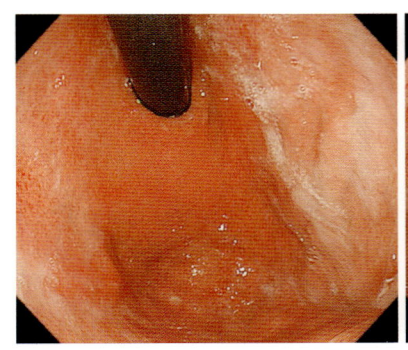
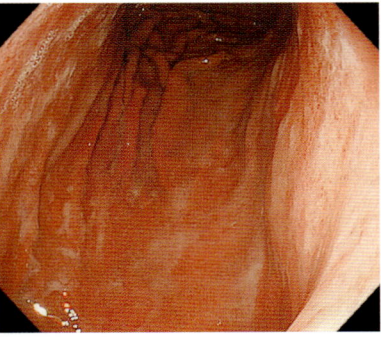

Fig. 30 Sticky mucus

Sticky mucus is stubbornly resistant to removal, making it a hindrance to observation. In a case like this where there is a lot of sticky mucus, it is quite likely that a small gastric cancer would be missed, making it necessary to perform endoscopy again after *H. pylori* eradication.

7) Mucosal swelling (Fig. 31)

H. pylori infection causes inflammatory cell infiltration and edematous changes in the lamina propria mucosae. In endoscopic observation, the mucosa looks soft and thick. It sometimes exhibits unevenness as seen in enlarged areae gastricae[11]. Mucosal swelling can be ameliorated by *H. pylori* eradication..

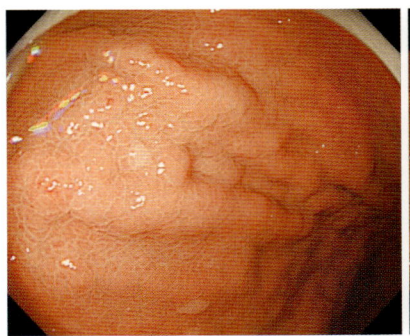
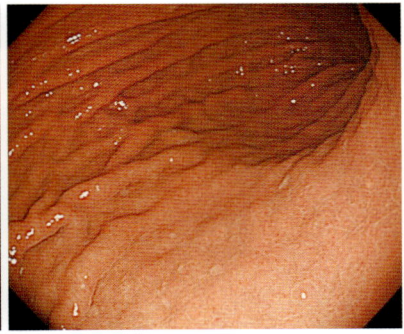

Fig. 31 Mucosal swelling

The mucosa is soft and appears thick. The areae gastricae have become enlarged and exhibit a variety of sizes. Taut yet soft hill-shaped elevations can be seen.

8) Hyperplastic polyps (Figs. 32–35)

Hyperplastic polyps are extremely erythematous polyps caused by hyperplasia of the foveolar epithelium. When observed at a close distance, they exhibit coarse mucosal patterns that are described as long tube-like, gyrus-like, and squamous. Dilated openings can also be seen. Their morphology might also feature a white coating known as "rotten strawberry." About 80% of hyperplastic polyps diminish after *H. pylori* eradication[22]. Small polyps can be safely left alone and observed in follow-up examinations, but larger ones must be treated with caution because, although rare, they may become cancerous.

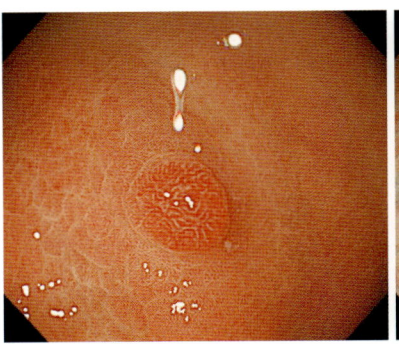
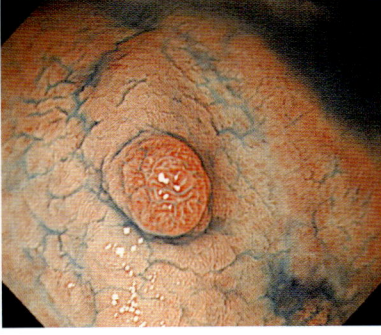

Fig. 32 Hyperplastic polyp ①

This is a 3-mm hyperplastic polyp, exhibiting a coarse mucosal pattern that resembles cerebral gyri.

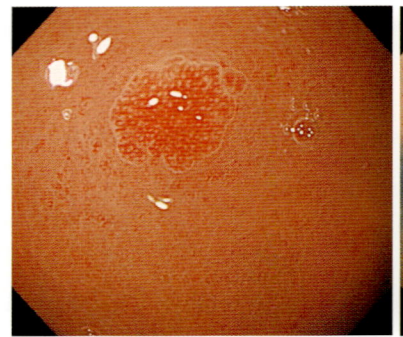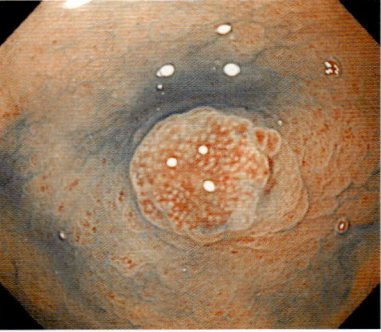

Fig. 33 Hyperplastic polyp ②

This is a 3-mm hyperplastic polyp with an erythematous flat elevation. Dilated crypt openings with shapes varying from round to oval can be seen.

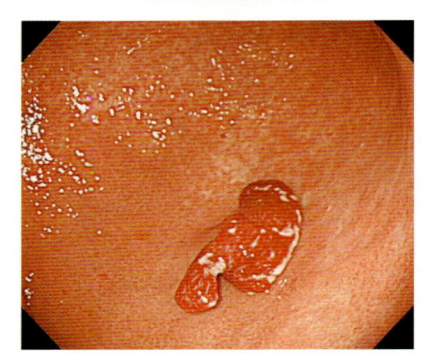

Fig. 34 Hyperplastic polyp ③

Exhibiting strong erythema, this 10-mm hyperplastic polyp has a white coating. Polyps showing such remarkable redness — described as a "rotten strawberry" — have abundant blood flow. Hence, bleeding sometimes causes iron-deficiency anemia.

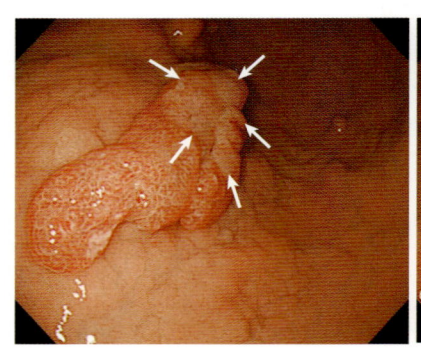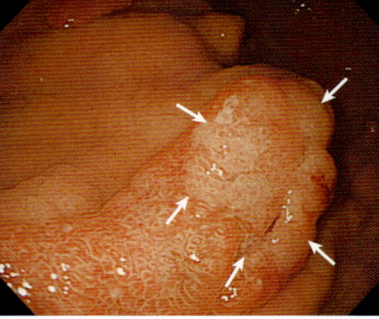

Fig. 35 Hyperplastic polyp ④ : Accompanied by carcinoma

This is a 20-mm protruded type polyp. Hyperplastic polyp and carcinoma coexist in this case. Carcinoma (tub1) is observed in locations indicated by the arrows. Other areas show hyperplastic changes.

9) Nodular gastritis (Fig. 36)

Nodular gastritis frequently occurs in the antrum of young females. It is distinguished by multiple small granular elevations that resemble goosebumps. Nodular gastritis is an early-stage immune response to *H. pylori* infection. Histopathologically, nodular gastritis is hyperplasia of the lymphoid follicles[23]. Reports suggest that it indicates a high risk of undifferentiated-type gastric cancer[24]. Once the *H. pylori* infection has been eradicated, nodular gastritis gradually disappears over a period of a few years.

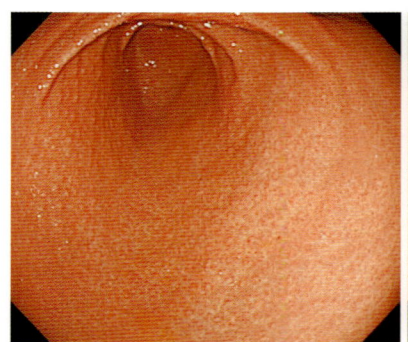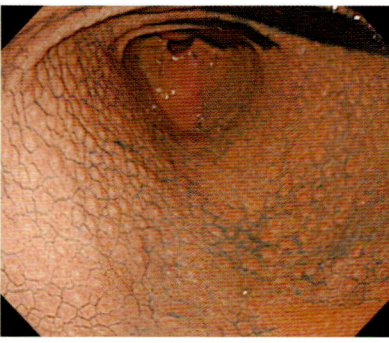

Fig. 36 Nodular gastritis

Small uniform granular elevations about 2 mm in size are found in multiple locations in the antrum. Indigo carmine spraying makes them look clearer. Their crests are slightly whitish.

10) Xanthoma (Fig. 37)

A xanthoma is a yellowish lesion that ranges in size from a few mm to about 1 cm with clear margins. Most are elevated, but some are depressed. When viewed up close, fine granular changes can be seen. These changes are believed to be caused by the accumulation of macrophages with phagocytosed lipids. Xanthomas do not change and remain even after the *H. pylori* infection has been eradicated.

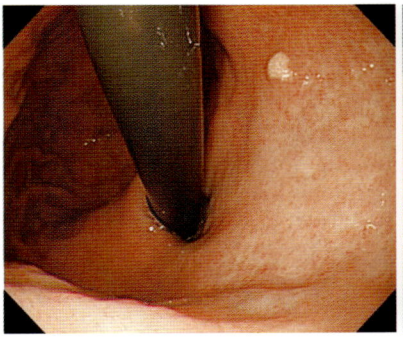 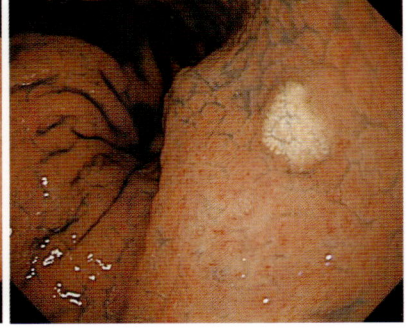

Fig. 37 Xanthoma

A slightly elevated yellowish lesion about 3 mm in size can be seen in the lesser curvature of the body. The margins are clear, when viewed up close, a fine granular pattern is observed. It can be diagnosed from the characteristic color tone and granular structure.

② Findings often seen in *H. pylori* past infection

H. pylori past infection includes spontaneous disappearance of *H. pylori* as a result either of eradication or advanced atrophy. Histopathologically, neutrophil infiltration quickly begins to disappear, while lymphocyte infiltration takes some time to recede.

As for endoscopic findings, diffuse redness begins to improve immediately after eradication and turns into flesh-colored mucosa. Spotty redness, mucosal swelling, enlarged/tortuous folds, and sticky mucus also decrease and disappear in a relatively short period of time. However, atrophy and intestinal metaplasia show virtually no improvement or only slight improvement in some parts over a long period. Typical findings after eradication include noticeable map-like redness in the antrum and body[10]. Hematin attachment and erosion in the body and antrum may also emerge accompanied by improvement in acid secretion capacity.

<Map-like redness (Fig. 38)>

After *H. pylori* eradication, erythematous depression with clear margins emerges in the region from the antrum to the body. This is called map-like redness. The degree of erythema can range from strong to weak. Morphologies also vary in size and shape, with shapes that include oval, mottled, patchy, linear, and extensive map-like shapes.

When map-like redness is biopsied, intestinal metaplasia is more prominent than in the surrounding area[25]. This happens because the intestinal metaplasia — which was slightly reddish in the first place — becomes more noticeable as a fairly erythematous depressed surface following *H. pylori* eradication, which reduces redness and edema, causing the surface of the non-atrophic mucosa to change from diffuse redness to flesh-colored mucosa[26]. This is called the "color reversal phenomenon"[27].

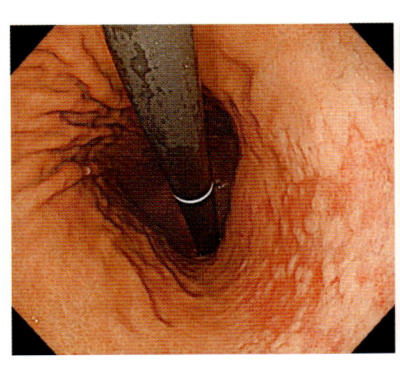 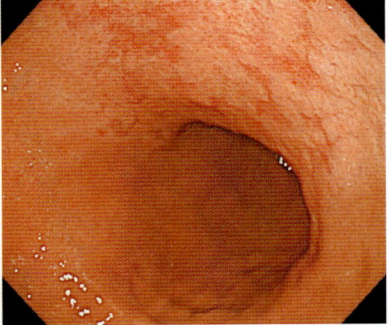

Fig. 38 Map-like redness

Map-like redness extends through the lesser curvature of the body. It has clear margins and is slightly depressed.

The relationships between *H. pylori* infection and the endoscopic findings we have discussed so far are shown in Table 1.

Table 1 Endoscopic findings of gastritis and *H. pylori* infection

Region	Endoscopic findings	*H. pylori* uninfection	*H. pylori* current infection	*H. pylori* past infection
Entire gastric mucosa	Atrophy	×	○	○ - ×
	Diffuse redness	×	○	×
	Hyperplastic polyp	×	○	○ - ×
	Map-like redness	×	×	○
	Xanthoma	×	○	○
	Hematin attachment	○	△	○
	Red streak	○	△	○
	Intestinal metaplasia	×	○	○ - △
	Mucosal swelling	×	○	×
	Patchy redness	○	○	○
	Depressive erosion	○	○	○
Body	Enlarged folds, tortuous folds	×	○	×
	Sticky mucus	×	○	×
Body to fornix	Fundic gland polyp	○	×	△
	Spotty redness	×	○	△ - ×
	Multiple white and flat elevated lesions	○	△	○ - △
Lesser curvature of lower body to lesser curvature of angulus	RAC	○	×	× - △
Antrum	Nodular gastritis	×	○	△ - ×
	Raised erosion	○	△	○

○ : Frequently observed ×: Not observed △ : Sometimes observed

[Excerpted with partial modification from Kyoto Classification of Gastritis[10].]

Side Note 🖍 How frequently is gastric cancer missed?

What is the miss rate for gastric cancer when an endoscope is used? In other words, what is endoscopy's false-negative rate (the proportion of gastric cancer cases that cannot be detected using endoscopes)? Hosokawa et al. defined cases registered as gastric cancer within 3 years of an endoscopy in which cancer was not diagnosed as false-negative cases. They reported a false-negative rate of 22.2%[a]. According to Tsuchiya et al., cases in which advanced cancer is found within 2 years from the first endoscopy and cases in which submucosal invasive cancer or 2-cm-or-larger mucosal cancer is found within 1 year of the first endoscopy can be defined as false-negative. They found a false-negative rate of 7.7%[b]. Although the frequency differs depending on the definition of false-negative, the reality is that a not insignificant number of gastric cancers are missed in endoscopy, emphasizing just how difficult it can be diagnosed gastric cancer against the background of gastritis..

a) Hosokawa O, Hattori M, Takeda T, et al. [Accuracy of endoscopy in detecting gastric cancer.] J Gastroenterol Mass Survey. 2004; 42: 33–39. (In Japanese)
b) Tsuchiya H, Harada K, Yamazaki T, et al. [Long term survey of gastric cancer in endoscopically negative group: a study of reliability of panendoscopy.] Gastroenterol Endosc. 1990; 32: 2199–2211. (In Japanese.)

The difference is clear when the pictures of the mucosa before and after eradication are placed side by side.

Before eradicatio ➡ 1 year after eradication

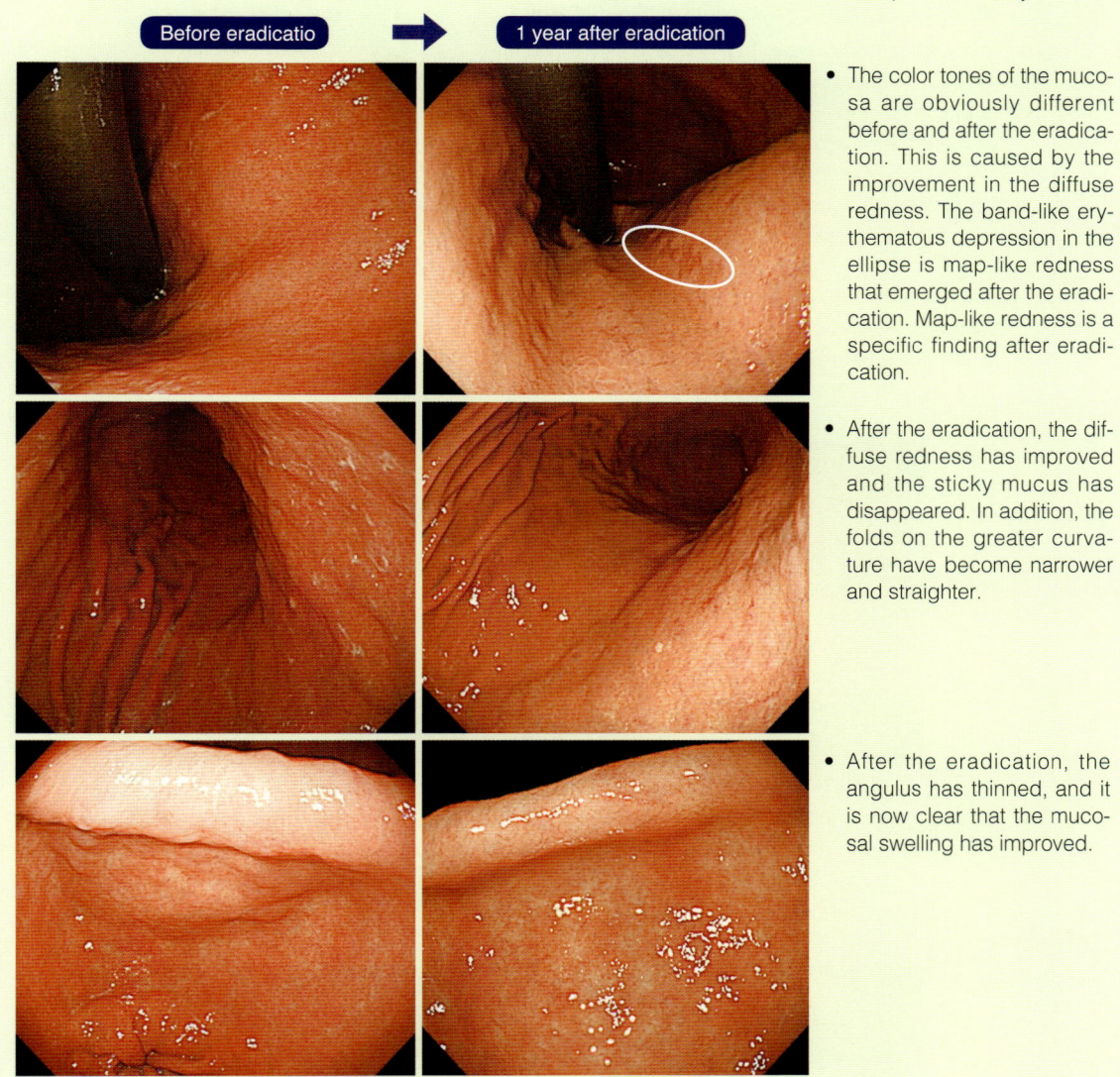

- The color tones of the mucosa are obviously different before and after the eradication. This is caused by the improvement in the diffuse redness. The band-like erythematous depression in the ellipse is map-like redness that emerged after the eradication. Map-like redness is a specific finding after eradication.

- After the eradication, the diffuse redness has improved and the sticky mucus has disappeared. In addition, the folds on the greater curvature have become narrower and straighter.

- After the eradication, the angulus has thinned, and it is now clear that the mucosal swelling has improved.

Areae gastricae

The surface of gastric mucosa is divided into small sections roughly 3 to 5-mm in width called areae gastricae. These are separated by shallow grooves that form a reticular network. The morphology of the areae gastricae in the pyloric gland is different from that in the fundic gland. There are also differences in the areae gastricae found in normal uninfected mucosa and atrophic mucosa. Areae gastricae are difficult to see under standard observation, but when sprayed with indigo carmine, their visibility improves.

Because the grooves between areae gastricae in normal uninfected mucosa are shallow and narrow, they may be indistinct and difficult to see. When atrophy occurs, the grooves between areae gastricae become deeper and wider, bringing the boundaries between areae gastricae into clearer relief. As the atrophy progresses, the grooves between areae gastricae expand and fuse, resulting in areae gastricae of different sizes and shapes. As the atrophy becomes more prominent, the areae gastricae begin to shrink, assuming a more granular texture. At the same time, the spaces between areae gastricae continue to expand. The morphology of areae gastricae corresponds with the degree of mucosal atrophy[a].

Since the morphology of areae gastricae differs from one case to the next, in order to detect gastric cancer it is important to first verify the original shapes of background areae gastricae and track any changes.

[*H. pylori*-uninfected normal gastric mucosa]

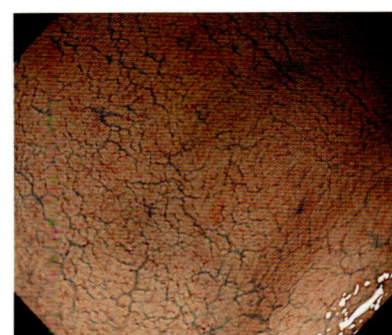 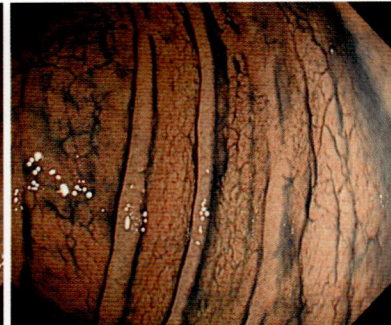

Lesser curvature of the antrum   Lesser curvature of the lower body

In normal *H. pylori*-uninfected mucosa, the grooves separating the areae gastricae are shallow and extremely narrow so the areae gastricae appear indistinct. In the antrum (pyloric gland region), areae gastricae exhibit regular, fine crepe-like patterns. In the body (fundic gland region), on the other hand, areae gastricae exhibit fine, cracked patterns and are harder to see than in the antrum.

[Atrophic gastritis]

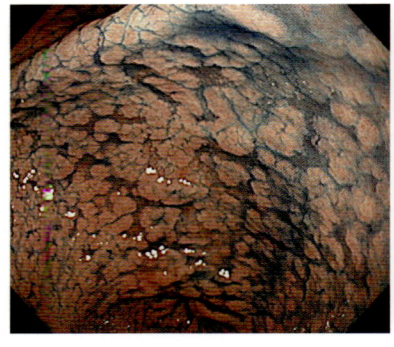 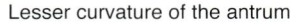 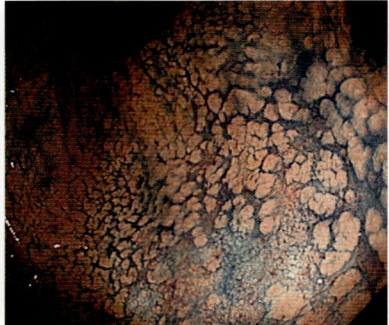

Lesser curvature of the antrum   Lesser curvature of the lower body

As atrophic gastritis progresses, the grooves between the areae gastricae grow deeper and wider both in the antrum and body, highlighting a variety of clear patterns. As the atrophy progresses and the grooves continue to expand, the areae gastricae shrink and the patterns gradually lose coherence and disappear.

a) Takechi K, Miyagawa H, Ozaki M, et al. [Endoscopic study on areae gastricae of the fundic mucosa.] Gastroenterol Endosc. 1984; 26: 194–200. (In Japanese.)

Basic Knowledge in Gastric Cancer Detection

Practice Exercise

> ▸ Male in his 50s.
> ▸ Endoscopy was performed as part of a medical checkup. He did not have a history of *H. pylori* eradication.

Diagnose the condition of the gastritis by examining the pictures below.

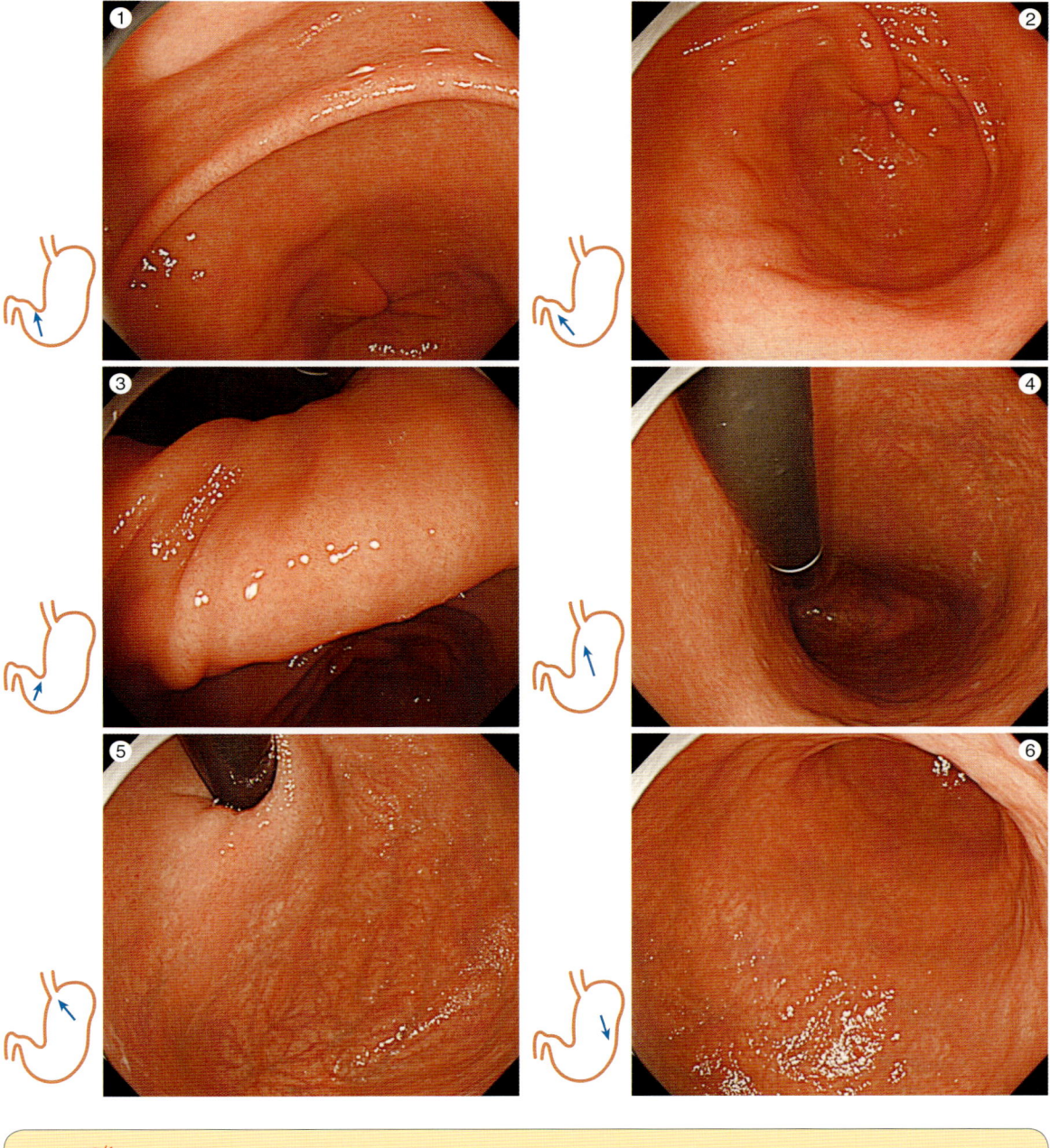

Hint 💡   Where is the atrophy?

The body has severe atrophy.   The antrum has no atrophy.

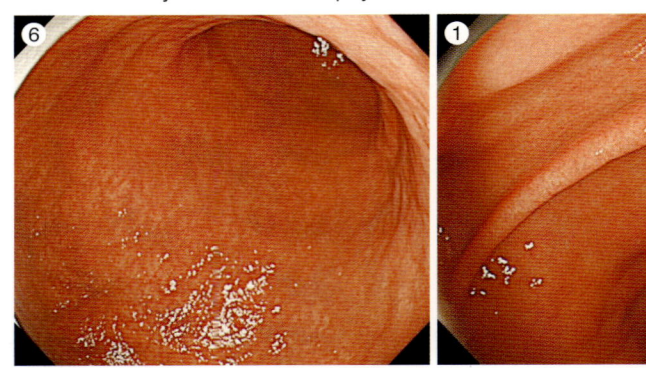

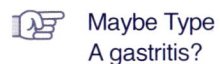 Maybe Type A gastritis?

- Severe atrophy can be seen from the body to the fornix. However, the mucosa in the antrum has no irregularities and is glossy, showing no atrophy. Note that the antrum is part of the pyloric gland region and absence of RAC does not equal to atrophy.
- When you see a pattern opposite to ordinary atrophy like in this case, the first thing that should come to mind is Type A gastritis.

 Let's check the gastrin.

- Serum gastrin level: ················· 5,500 pg/mℓ
- Anti-parietal cell antibodies: ··········· Positive
- Anti-intrinsic factor antibodies: ········ Positive
- Serum anti-*H. pylori* antibodies ····· Negative
- Urea breath test: ························· Negative

It's Type A gastritis!

Type A gastritis (autoimmune gastritis) and gastric carcinoid tumor

Chronic gastritis is classified into two types: Type B gastritis, which is caused by *H. pylori* infection and is the most common; and Type A gastritis, which is caused by an autoimmune response. The pathology of Type A gastritis is the destruction of the fundic glands caused by autoantibodies (including anti-parietal cell antibodies and anti-intrinsic factor antibodies) attacking and destroying parietal cells in the fundic glands. This leads to severe atrophy in the fundic gland region. Gastric acid secretion also decreases, triggering a feedback mechanism that causes excessive secretion of gastrin by the G cells in the pyloric gland region.

The gastrin stimulates the gastric endocrine cells (enterochromaffin-like [ECL] cells) in the fundic gland region to produce histamine. This causes carcinogenesis, generating multiple carcinoid tumors in the stomach. A carcinoid tumor that develops in Type A gastritis is classified as Rindi's Type I (**Figs. 39 & 40**; see page 165 for Rindi's Classification). Meanwhile, Rindi's Type II carcinoid occurs in the context of a gastrin-secreting tumor, and Rindi's Type III carcinoid tumor occurs sporadically, regardless of whether gastrin is present or not.

In addition to carcinoid tumors, Type A gastritis is often complicated by gastric cancer.

In some cases, vitamin B_{12} absorption deficiency is caused by intrinsic factor deficiency and accompanied by macrocytic anemia.

<Watch for the "reverse atrophy" exhibited by Type A gastritis>

Type A gastritis is relatively rare and likely to be diagnosed as Type B by physicians not familiar with it. In Type B gastritis, atrophy starts at the antrum and extends towards the proximal side. In Type A, on the other hand, there is no atrophy in the antrum because the pyloric glands do not affect an autoimmune mechanism; instead, severe atrophy is exhibited only in the body. This condition is known as "reverse atrophy." The key to successful discovery of Type A gastritis is to pay attention to the difference between atrophy in the antrum and in the body

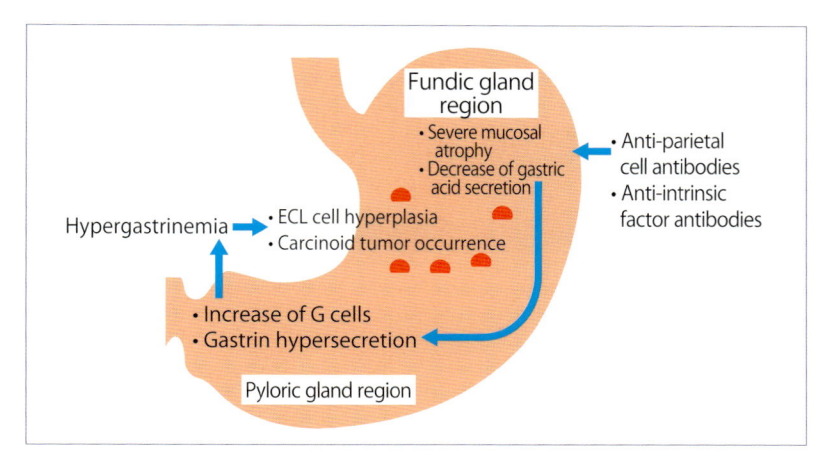

Fig. 39 Pathogenetic mechanism of carcinoid tumors (Rindi's Type I)

Carcinoid tumors arise from Type A gastritis through the mechanism shown in this figure. In *H. pylori*-infected Type B gastritis, on the other hand, a decrease in gastric acid secretion becomes evident as atrophy of the body progresses. Atrophy of the pyloric glands also occurs, thus the increase in gastrin secreted by the pyloric glands is relatively low.

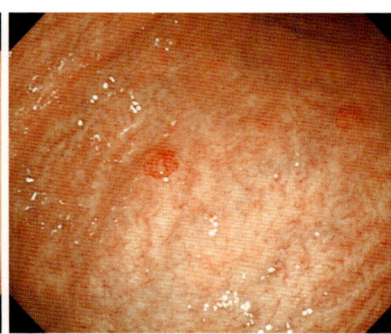
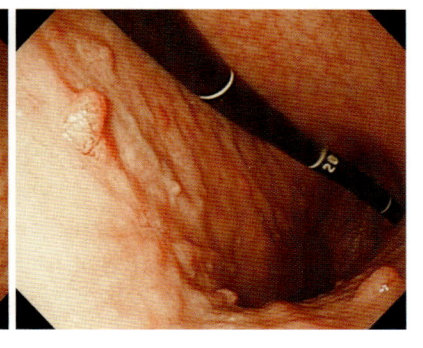

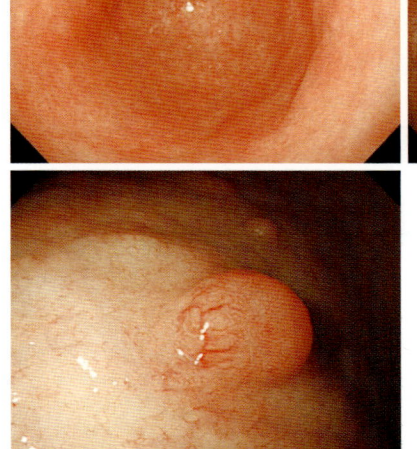

Fig. 40 Carcinoid tumor accompanied by Type A gastritis (Rindi's Type I)

Fine branched vascular patterns are visible on the mucosa of the body, and there is severe atrophy. However, since the antrum is shiny, this case should be diagnosed as being without atrophy and therefore Type A gastritis. Polyps that occur in multiple locations in Type A gastritis should be considered as potential carcinoid tumors. Carcinoid tumors arising from Type A gastritis are flat and protruded polyp patterns, while color tones vary and can include red, yellow, and normal. What most distinguishes this type of tumor is the prominent visibility of dilated capillaries.

[Excerpted from: Hirasawa T. [Gastric carcinoid (application part 19)]. Watanabe M, Fujishiro M, ed. [Gastrointestinal diseases found with images, vol. 1, upper gastrointestinal tract.] Tokyo: Igaku Shuppan. 2013: 144–147. (In Japanese.)[28]]

Side Note 🖍 **Carcinoid tumor and NET**

The term "carcinoid" was coined In 1907 by Siegfried Oberndorfer, who pointed out that this type of lesion featured the low cellular atypia and cellular architecture characteristic of a tumor, but its slow growth and lack of metastasis indicated it was benign. He dubbed the tumor "carcinoid" by combining "carcinoma" with "-oid," a suffix meaning like or resembling.

Subsequently, when it became evident that carcinoids shared characteristics with neuro endocrine cells, they came also to be called neuroendocrine tumors. As reports began coming in of cases in which malignant processes such as metastasis and invasion occurred, many argued that the term "carcinoid" was no longer inappropriate appropriate. Consequently, the 2000 WHO classification did not use the term. The 2010 WHO classification introduced the general term "neuroendocrine neoplasms" (NENs) for pancreatic and gastrointestinal tumors with the properties and phenotypes of the endocrine system. NENs are classified into well-differentiated neuroendocrine tumors (NETs) and poorly differentiated neuroendocrine carcinomas (NECs). NETs are further subclassified into Grades 1 and 2 (NET G1 and NET G2) based on the cell proliferation capability derived according to mitotic and Ki67 indices.

The Japanese Classification of Gastric Carcinoma (14th edition) edited by the Japanese Gastric Cancer Association classifies neuroendocrine tumors into two types: carcinoid tumors and endocrine cell carcinomas, continuing usage of the term carcinoid.

2 Classification of gastric cancer and clinical characteristics

I Classification of gastric cancer

Gastric cancer is a malignant tumor arising from the gastric epithelium. It shows a wide variety of tumor histologies. We will first discuss the classification.

① Classification of histological types of gastric cancer[29]

According to the Japanese Classification of Gastric Carcinoma (3rd. English edition)[29], gastric cancer is classified as shown in **Fig. 1**. Papillary adenocarcinoma (pap) and tubular adenocarcinoma (tub) are subclassified as differentiated-type gastric cancer while poorly differentiated adenocarcinoma (por) and signet ring cell carcinoma (sig) are subclassified as undifferentiated-type gastric cancer. Mucinous carcinoma (muc) is subclassified as differentiated-type gastric cancer and undifferentiated-type gastric cancer depending on the histological morphology of component cancer cells (Nakamura-Sugano Classification)

Differentiation refers to changes in cells as they grow into mature tissues. While differentiated-type gastric cancer (Fig. 2) has a glandular structure similar to a normal glandular structure, undifferentiated-type gastric cancer (**Fig. 3**) is deficient in glandular formation. When differentiated-type gastric cancer and undifferentiated-type gastric cancer coexist, the histological images of the cancer that is quantitatively superior should be used. Differentiated-type gastric cancer and undifferentiated-type gastric cancer are also different from each other in terms of clinical characteristics and endoscopic images, naturally making the method of how to find them different as well.

Malignant epithelial tumors (common types)

a. Papillary adenocarcinoma (pap)
b. Tubular adenocarcinoma (tub)
　(1) Well differentiated (tub1)
　(2) Moderately differentiated (tub2)
　　　　　　　　　　　　　　　Differentiated type*

c. Poorly differentiated adenocarcinoma (por)
　(1) Solid type (por1)
　(2) Non-solid type (por2)
　　　　　　　　　　　　　　　Undifferentiated type*
d. Signet-ring cell carcinoma (sig)

e. Mucinous adenocarcinoma (muc)

Fig. 1 Histological classification of malignant epithelial gastric tumors
[Excerpted from Japanese Classification of Gastric Carcinoma (3rd. English edition)[29]]
*Nakamura and Sugano classification

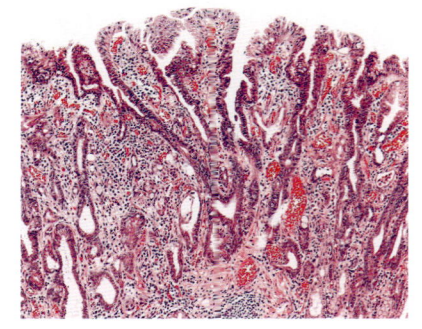

Fig. 2 Differentiated-type gastric cancer (cancer showing glandular formation)

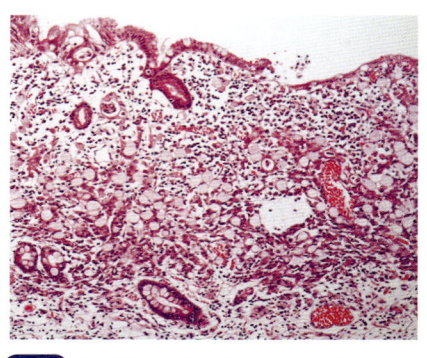

Fig. 3 Undifferentiated-type gastric cancer (cancer deficient in glandular formation)

② Macroscopic type classification (Fig. 4)[29]

The macroscopic morphology often seen in cases where the depth of tumor invasion is confined within the submucosa (**Fig. 5**) is classified as superficial type (Type 0). In cases where the invasion has penetrated the muscularis propria or deeper, the macroscopic morphology often manifested is classified as an advanced type (Types 1–4). The superficial type is subclassified as 0–I, 0–IIa, 0–IIb, 0–IIc, or 0–III (**Figs. 6–14**). With mixed superficial types, the subclassification names are combined with "+" in descending order of the extent of lesions.

Carcinomas limited to the mucosa or submucosa are called early cancer, regardless of the presence or absence of lymph node metastasis. Carcinomas that have invaded the muscularis propria or beyond are called advanced cancer.

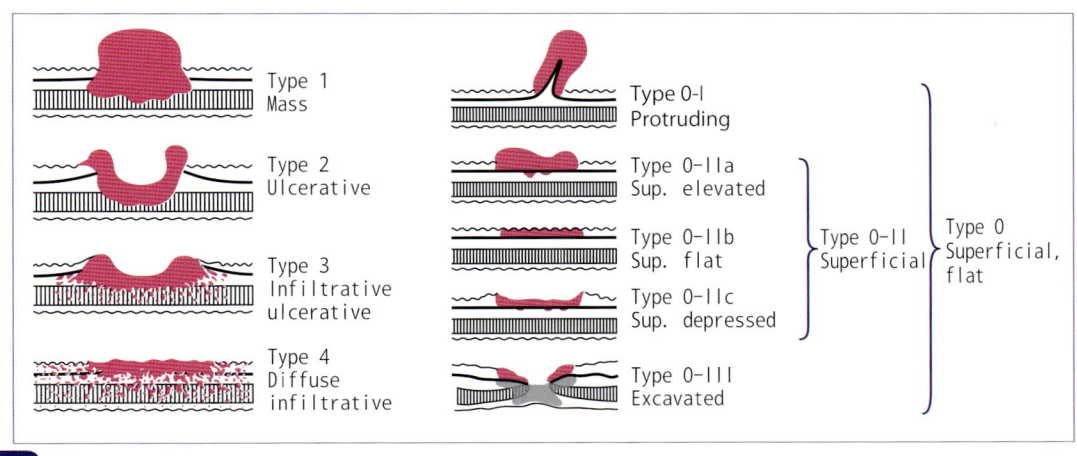

Fig. 4 Macroscopic types

[Excerpted from Japanese Classification of Gastric Carcinoma (3rd. English edition)[29]]

③ Depth of tumor invasion (T) (Table 1)[29]

Table 1 Depth of tumor invasion (T)

- TX : Depth of tumor unknown.
- T0 : No evidence of primary tumor.
- T1 : Tumor confined to the mucosa (M) or submucosa (SM).
- T1a : Tumor confined to the mucosa (M).
- T1b : Tumor confined to the submucosa (SM[1]).
- T2 : Tumor invades the muscularis propria (MP).
- T3 : Tumor invades the subserosa (SS).
- T4 : Tumor invasion is contiguous to or exposed beyond the serosa (SE) or tumor invades adjacent structures (SI).

    T4a : Tumor invasion is contiguous to the serosa or penetrates the serosa and is exposed to the peritoneal cavity (SE[2]).

    T4b : Tumor invades adjacent structures (SI[3]).

[1] SM may be subclassified as SM1 or T1b1 (tumor invasion is within 0.5 mm of the muscularis mucosae) or SM2 or T1b2 (tumor invasion is 0.5 mm or more deep into the muscularis mucosae).

[2] Tumor extending into the greater or lesser omentum without visceral peritoneal perforation is classified as T3.

[3] Invaded adjacent structures should be recorded. The adjacent structures of the stomach are the liver, pancreas, transverse colon, spleen, diaphragm, abdominal wall, adrenal gland, kidney, small intestine, and retroperitoneum. Serosal invasion with involvement of the greater and lesser omentum is classified as T4a, not T4b. Invasion of the transverse mesocolon is not T4b unless it extends to the colic vessels or penetrates the posterior surface of the mesocolon.

[Excerpted from Japanese Classification of Gastric Carcinoma (3rd. English edition)[29]]

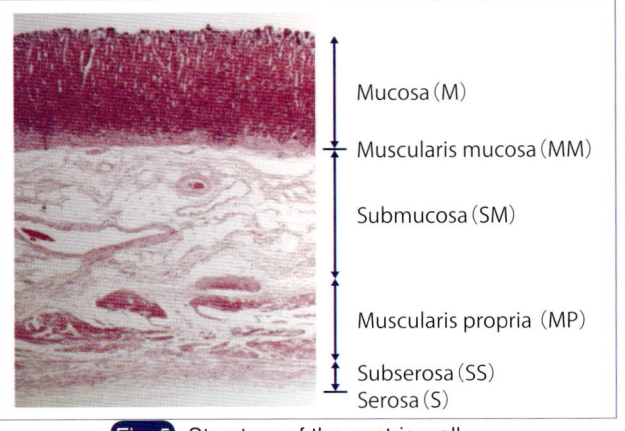

Mucosa (M)

Muscularis mucosa (MM)

Submucosa (SM)

Muscularis propria (MP)

Subserosa (SS)
Serosa (S)

Fig. 5 Structure of the gastric wall

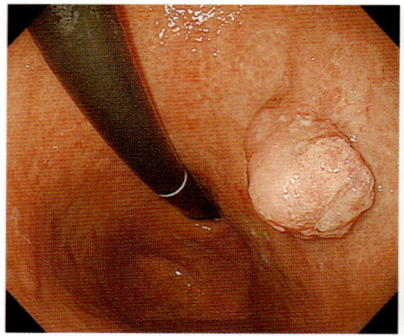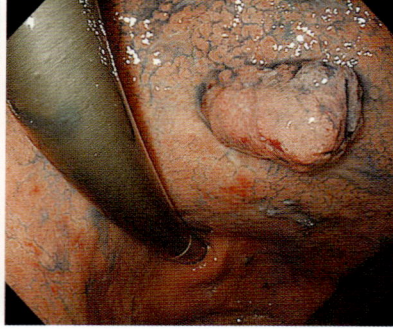

Fig. 6 Superficial type 0-I

0-I is a polypoid tumor of which height is over 3 mm.
▶ Anterior wall of the middle body, 0-I, 20 mm, tub1, T1b(SM), UL (−)

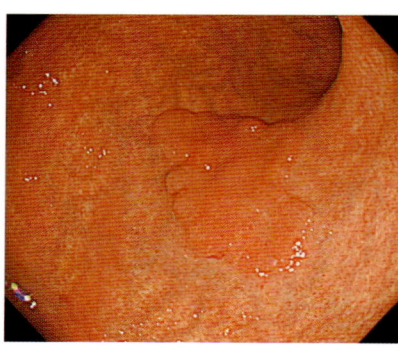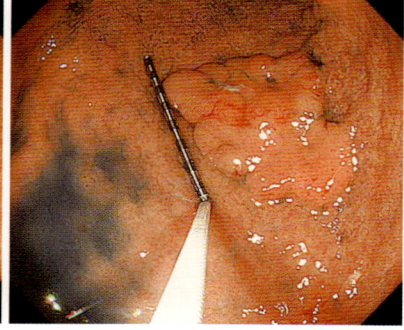

Fig. 7 Superficial type 0-IIa

0-IIa is slightly elevated tumor. The height of the tumor is between 2 and 3 mm.
▶ Posterior wall of the lower body, 0-IIa, 35 mm, tub1>2, T1a (M), UL (−)

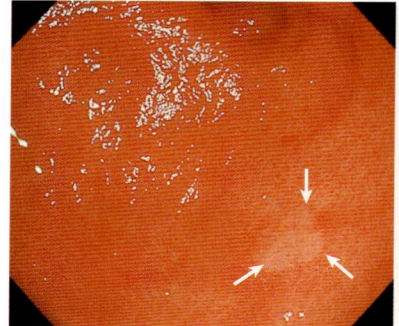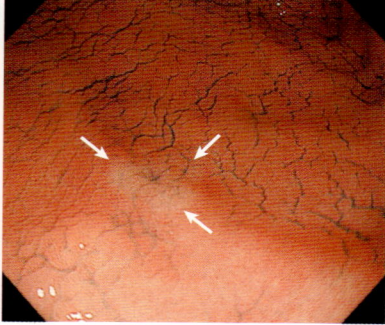

Fig. 8 Superficial type 0-IIb

0-IIb is tumor without elevation or depression. In terms of elevation or depression, it shows no marked differences from the irregularities seen on normal mucosa.
▶ Greater curvature of the angulus, 0-IIb, 4 mm, sig, T1a (M), UL (−)

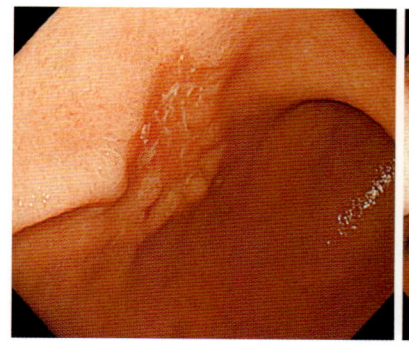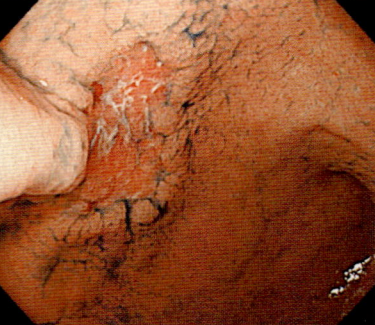

Fig. 9 Superficial type 0-IIc

0-IIc is a slightly depressed tumor.
▶ Anterior wall of the lower body, 0-IIc, 25 mm, tub2>por, T1b (SM), UL (+)

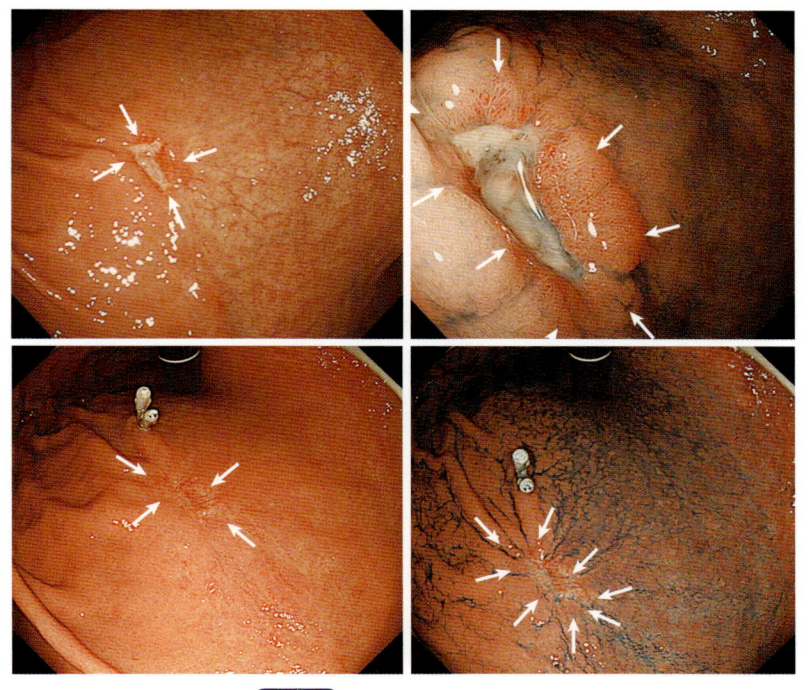

Fig. 10 Superficial type 0–III

Top row : 0–III is a tumor with deep depression. In general, this applies to tumors in which a peptic ulcer forms inside a cancerous lesion. Cancer is not found on the ulcer base, but is present to some degree on the inner edge of the ulcer. Unadulterated 0–III is rare, and many 0–III tumors show signs of 0–IIc in the peripheral areas. In the case shown in the pictures in the top row, the ulcerous area is 0–III and the surrounding erythematous area is 0–II.

▶ Anterior wall of middle body, 0–III+IIc, 18 mm, tub2, T1a (M), UL (+)

Bottom row : These are pictures of the same case one month after PPI medication. The ulcer has disappeared and turned into a 0–IIc lesion. As in this case, the peptic ulcer formed within the cancer lesion sometimes goes through repeated phases of healing and relapsing. This phenomenon is called a "malignant cycle."

• A cancerous ulcer is one in which an ulcer base seen in Type 2 and Type 3 advanced cancers has a cancerous mass underneath. PPI medication does not improve it.

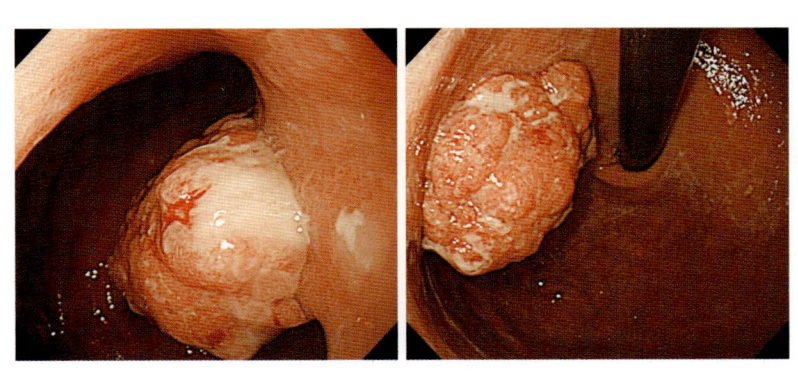

Fig. 11 Advanced type 1 (Type 1)

Type 1 is a polypoid tumor, which sharply demarcated from the surrounding mucosa.

▶ Posterior wall of the upper body, Type 1, 38 mm, tub1>pap, T2 (MP)

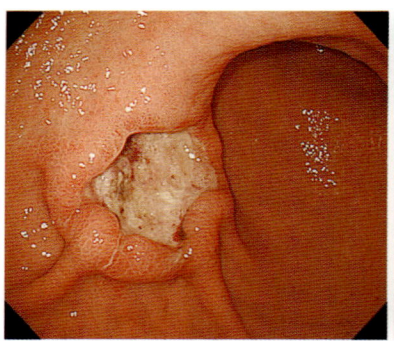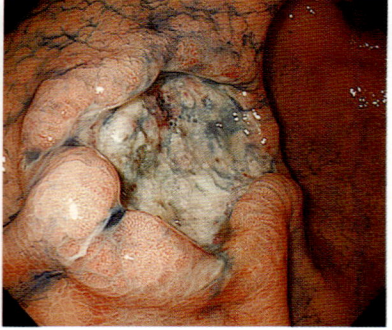

Fig. 12 Advanced type 2 (Type 2)

Type 2 is an advanced type — among ulcerous lesions accompanied by raised rims — where the boundary between the raised rim of the ulcer and the surroundings is clear. The raised rim has a steep inclination.
- ▶ Greater curvature of the lower body, Type 2, 36 mm, por>sig, T4a (SE)

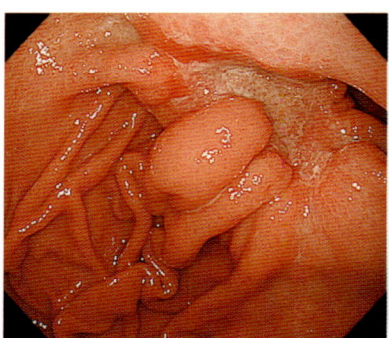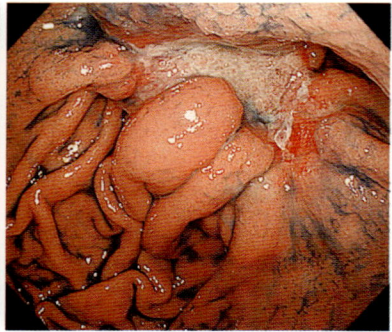

Fig. 13 Advanced type 3 (Type 3)

Type 3 is an advanced type — among ulcerous lesions accompanied by raised rims — where the boundary between the raised rim of the ulcer and the surroundings is unclear.
- ▶ Anterior wall of the greater curvature of the middle body, Type 3, 55 mm, por>sig, T4a (SE)

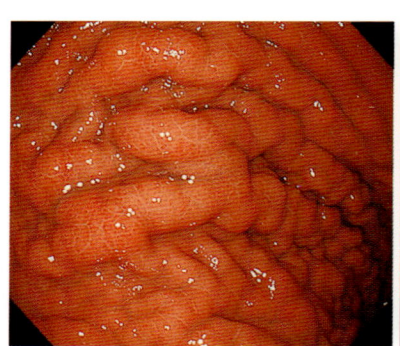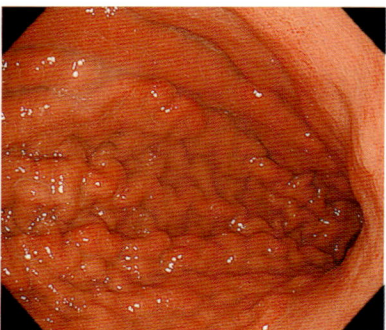

Fig. 14 Advanced type 4 (Type 4)

Type 4 is an advanced type — with neither prominent ulcer formation nor raised rims and showing thickening and hardening of the gastric wall — where the boundary with non-cancerous mucosa is unclear.
- ▶ Fornix to antrum, Type 4, 180 mm, sig>por, T4a (SE)

Pitfall to be avoided

Advanced superficial type cancers

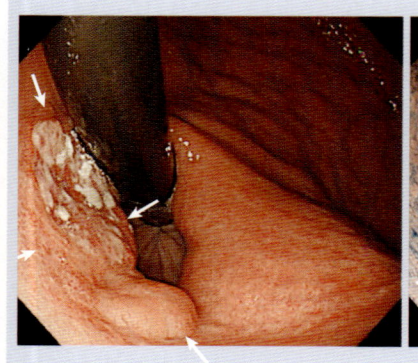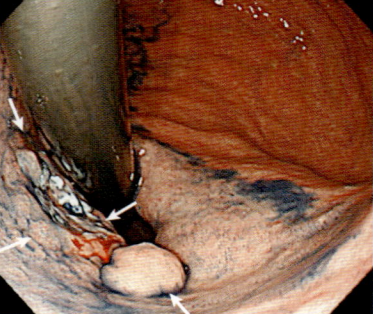

- The classification of the macroscopic type should be determined regardless of invasion depth, and the invasion depth should always be recorded. So, for example, if the invasion depth is muscularis propria (MP) even if the macroscopic type is 0–IIc superficial type, enter "0–IIc, T2 (MP)".
- In the picture on the left, a flat elevation lesion can be seen in the lesser curvature of the cardia while a depressed surface has formed on the anterior wall. When an undifferentiated-type gastric cancer exhibits elevation, the invasion depth is often deep.
- ▶ Lesser curvature of the cardia, 0–IIa+IIc, 22 mm, por, T2 (MP)

II Histogenesis and growth patterns of gastric cancer and clinical characteristics

1 Undifferentiated-type gastric cancer (Figs. 15–17)

Proper gastric mucosa without intestinal metaplasia can provide a base for the genesis of undifferentiated-type gastric cancer. In many cases, undifferentiated-type gastric cancer arises from the glandular neck region (cell proliferation zone) in the fundic gland region. While destroying the basement membrane of the glandular neck region and not forming glandular ducts, undifferentiated-type gastric cancer invades and extends into the lamina propria mucosae scatteringly. In the initial stage of carcinogenesis, undifferentiated-type gastric cancer invades horizontally only in the middle layer of the mucosa, exhibiting the characteristics of Type 0–IIb covered by non-cancerous epithelium. As the cell volume and density gradually increases, proliferative zone and proper gastric glands are destroyed. As a result, the foveolar epithelium on the surface falls off and a depressed surface with steep cliff-like edges is formed. The background mucosa shows no signs of atrophy and is fairly thick so the lesion's depression is deeper[30), 31)]. Once the glands have been destroyed, the mucosal patterns on the depressed surface disappear and become struc-

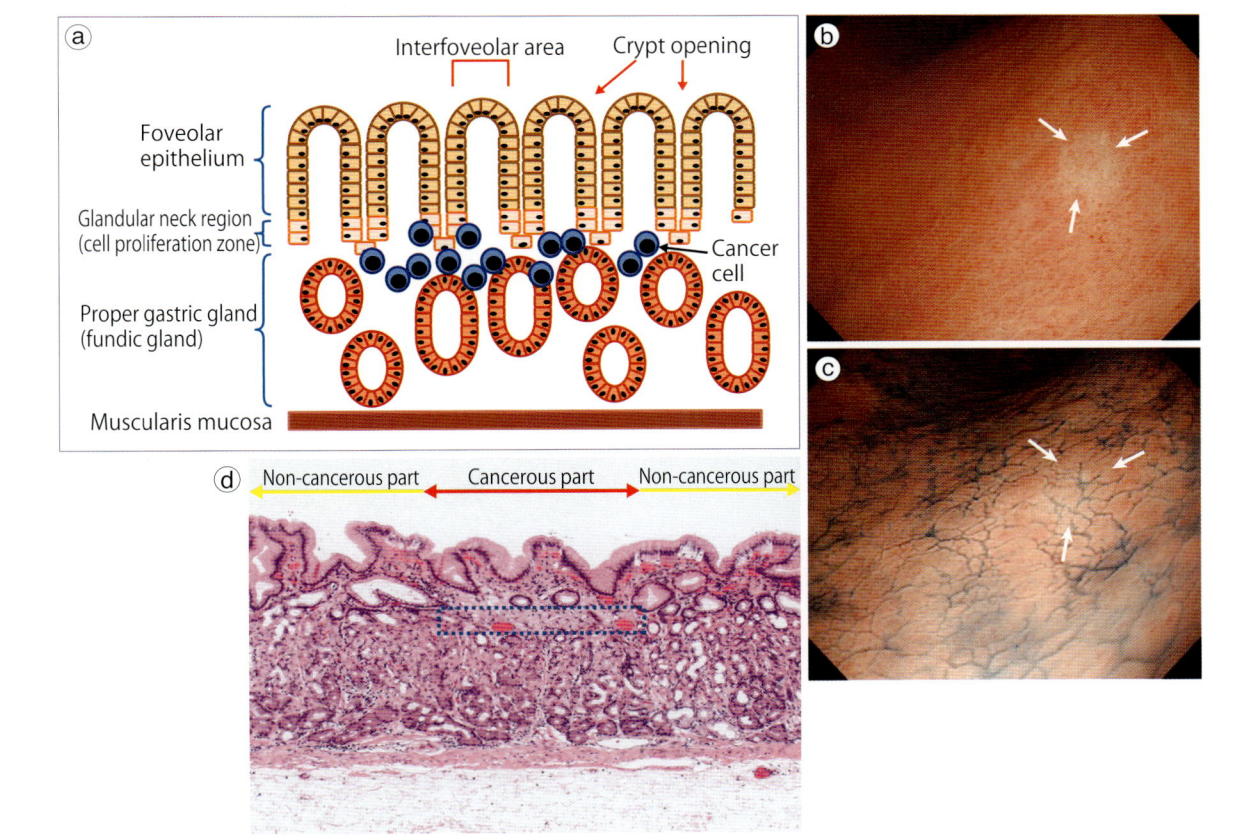

Fig. 15 Growth and development patterns of undifferentiated-type gastric cancer ①

a : Schematic diagram. Undifferentiated-type gastric cancer arises from the fundic gland region without atrophy. Cancer cells are generated from the glandular neck region, which is a cell proliferation zone. They break through the basement membrane and invade the middle layer of the mucosa in the horizontal direction.

b, c : Endoscopic images. The lesion can be seen as faded mucosa without irregularities. Mucosal patterns show no changes from the surrounding area. Greater curvature of the angulus, 0–IIb, 3 mm, sig, T1a (M), UL (–)

d : Histopathological image. Signet ring cell carcinoma is present only in the middle layer of the mucosa (glandular neck region) in ⌐ ¬, and glands are not affected.

tureless.

Since formation of glands and basement membrane is weak in undifferentiated-type gastric cancer, the defense mechanism against gastric acid deteriorates, making it more likely that erosions, ulcers, and regenerative changes will occur[32]. Any areas of foveolar epithelium that have not been destroyed by cancer cells along with any regenerative epithelium produced by erosion or ulcers may stand out on the surface like islands. In Japan, this phenomenon is called "*insel*," derived from the German word for "island".

The initial stage of undifferentiated-type gastric cancer is classified as 0–IIb. As the cancer invades in the vertical direction, it forms a depression. It rarely forms an elevation. The color is basically faded, but the regenerative epithelium of ulcer and erosion exhibits redness. The background mucosa shows few signs of atrophy, and the difference between the color tones of the background and lesion is so clear that even a small lesion can easily be found.

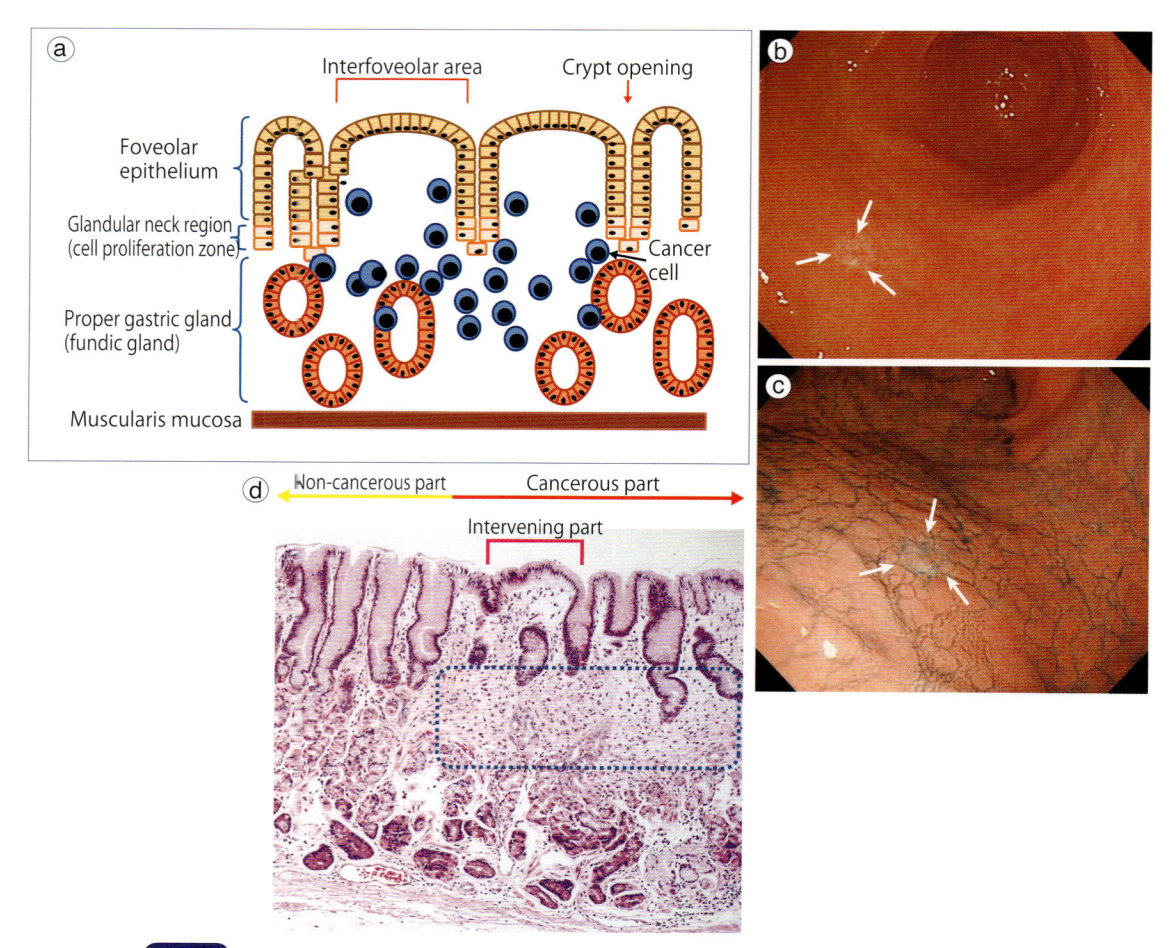

Fig. 16 Growth and development patterns of undifferentiated-type gastric cancer ②
- a : Schematic diagram. As the cancer cells gradually invade in the vertical direction, crypts and fundic glands are destroyed. Intervening part are dilated.
- b, c : Endoscopic images. The lesion appears as faded mucosa with an extremely shallow depression. The areae gastricae are not as clear as the surrounding mucosa. Greater curvature of the antrum, 0–IIc, 5 mm, sig, T1a (M), UL (–)
- d : Histopathological image. Signet ring cell carcinoma is invading in the middle layer of the mucosa, destroying the glands and reducing their number. This expands the intervening part.

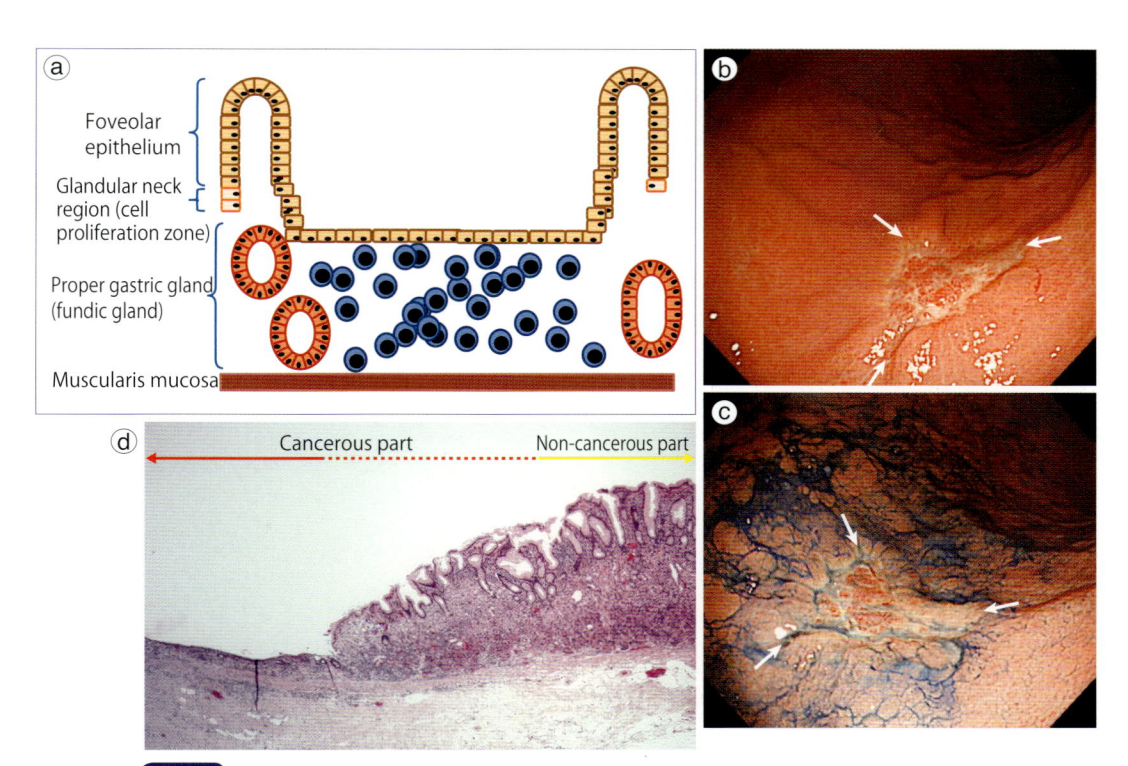

Fig. 17 Histogenesis and growth patterns of undifferentiated-type gastric cancer ③

a：Schematic diagram. Continued destruction of the fundic glands and crypts eventually leads to complete disappearance of the ducts. The margin of the depressed surface forms clear edges (cliff-like).

b, c：Endoscopic images. This is a depressed lesion with faded color accompanied by regenerative epithelium generated during the ulcer healing process. The margin is cliff-like. No glandular structure is visible except in the region of the regenerative epithelium. Anterior wall of the greater curvature of the middle body, 0–IIc, 23 mm, sig>por, T1a (M), UL (+)

d：Histopathological image. The mucosa of the inner side of cancer is thinning, and the glands have disappeared(left). The non-cancerous mucosa, on the other hand, shows no signs of atrophy and is relatively thick(right). As a result, the margin between the cancerous and non-cancerous mucosa is cliff-like. In the section marked by the red dotted line(peripheral side of cancer), the cancer is not exposed on the surface and is present only in the middle layer of the mucosa. As can be seen here, cancer sometimes invades in the middle layer of the mucosa on the marginal side of undifferentiated-type gastric cancer, so caution needs to be exercised in the extent diagnosis.

Side Note 🖊 Can the detection rate of gastric cancer be improved by training?

At the Cancer Institute Hospital of JFCR, the gastric cancer detection rates among young doctors are announced at the year-end party as part of the training. The detection rates for gastric cancer and gastric adenoma are between 1.9% and 6.5%, excluding known lesions. These detection rates can vary quite significantly depending on the endoscopist. However, the detection rates are steadily improving thanks to the training. Six months after they start their training, the trainees gradually become able to detect even small gastric cancers. According to one report, two-year training programs can improve gastric cancer detection rates from 0.4% to 1.9%[a].

Ideally, doctors should be trained at facilities with an established system of endoscopy training. In practice, however, there are not many opportunities for specialized instruction. In this book, we have tried to document the details of the training received daily by our residents and to incorporate as many clinical cases as possible. We hope this book will prove useful in practical endoscopic diagnosis and treatment.

a) Yamazato, T., Oyama, T., Yoshida, T., et al. Two years' intensive training in endoscopic diagnosis facilitates detection of early gastric cancer. Intern. Med. 2012 ; 51: 1461–1465

We have reported that the progress of undifferentiated-type gastric cancer in the vertical direction in the mucosa can be estimated with magnifying NBI images[33), 34)]. It used to be considered difficult to make an extent diagnosis when the cancer was present only in the middle layer of the mucosa and was not exposed on the surface. Today, however, NBI magnifying observation enables you to make an extent diagnosis by observing the dilatation of the interfoveolar areas[35)].

[Vertical progression of undifferentiated-type gastric cancer and magnifying NBI images]

- When the cancer is present only in the middle layer of the mucosa, the glands are relatively unaffected although there may be some decrease. In such a case, the intervening part will exhibit dilatation under NBI magnifying observation. When the cancer extends close to the superficial layer, disappearance of the glands will accelerate. Under NBI magnifying observation, so-called "wavy microvessels" will be seen. These are dilated and tortuous vessels on the superficial microstructure. When the cancer extends through all layers, the glandular structures will be completely destroyed. Under NBI magnifying observation, the superficial microstructure becomes unclear and so-called "corkscrew-pattern vessels" are observed[35)].

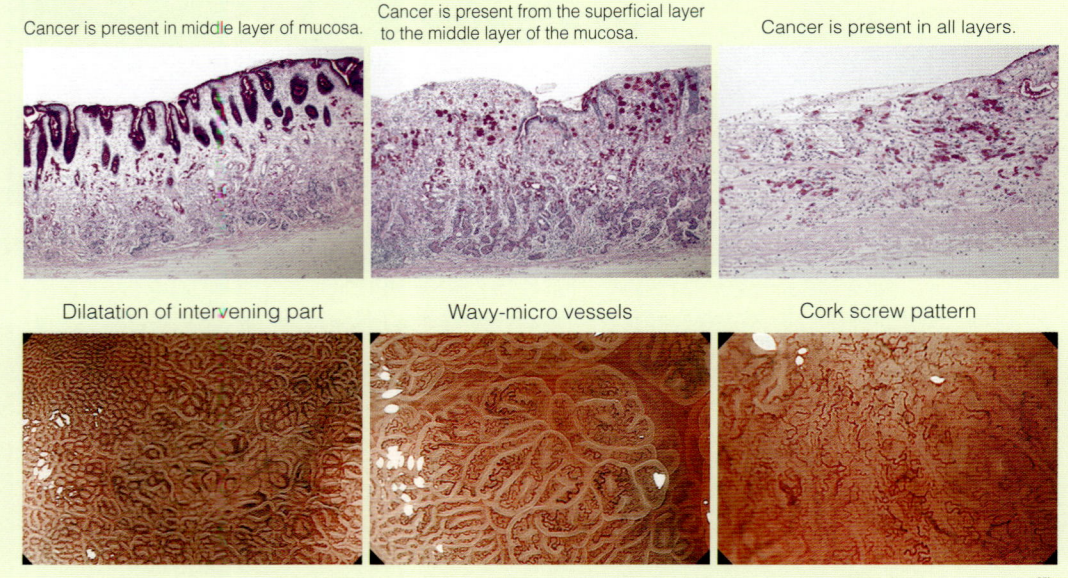

Cancer is present in middle layer of mucosa.　　Cancer is present from the superficial layer to the middle layer of the mucosa.　　Cancer is present in all layers.

Dilatation of intervening part　　Wavy-micro vessels　　Cork screw pattern

[Excerpted from Horiuchi Y, et al. Gast Cancer. 2016 ;19 : 515–523[35)]]

[Dilatation of interfoveolar areas and extent diagnosis]

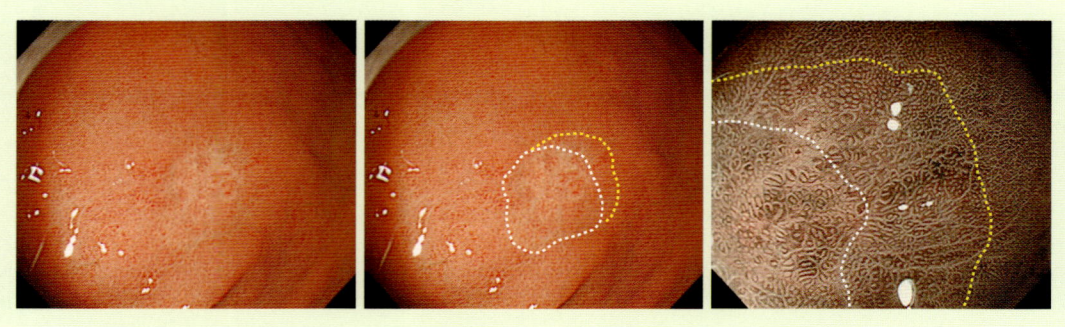

- Under WLI observation, the extent of a lesion is estimated from the faded depression and the margin of the lesion is as shown by the white dotted line.
- When the dilatation of the intervening part on the distal side is analyzed with NBI magnifying observation, dilatation of the intervening part extends as far as the yellow broken line.
▶ Greater curvature of the lower body, 0–IIc+IIb, 15 mm, sig, T1a (M), UL (–)

② Differentiated-type gastric cancer (Figs. 18–20)

Differentiated-type gastric cancer mainly arises from the mucosa with intestinal metaplasia. The cell proliferation zone of intestinal metaplasia is located in the glandular base. As differentiated-type gastric cancer generated in that region progresses, cancer cells replace non-cancerous glands[30]. Consequently, mucosal patterns produced by glandular structures — such as granular and villous — are likely to be seen. When the cancerous glands proliferate towards the superficial layer, they do so while collapsing slightly towards the deeper layer, thereby exhibiting a depressive type.

With the depressive type, cancer invades along the grooves of the areae gastricae. Thus, the edges take form thorn-like projections. Because the background mucosa has been thinned by the atrophy, the depression is not as deep as with undifferentiated-type cancer, resulting in a gently sloping margin. In the area around the depression, hyperplastic changes are produced, creating what is called a reactive elevation. The color tones range from reddish to homochromatic. In the flat elevation type, occasionally, whitish tones are shown. There are also lesions that are difficult to detect because of background atrophy and intestinal metaplasia.

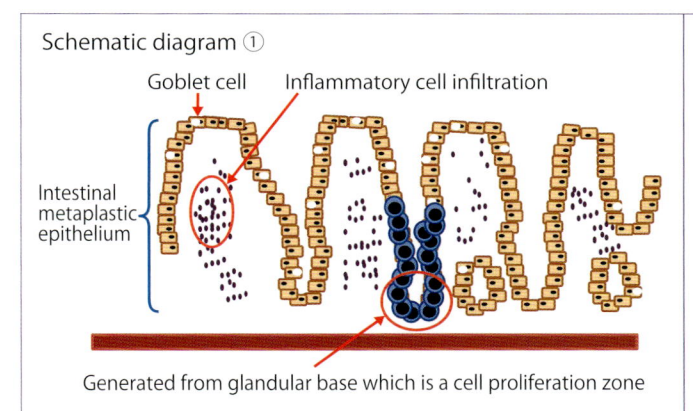
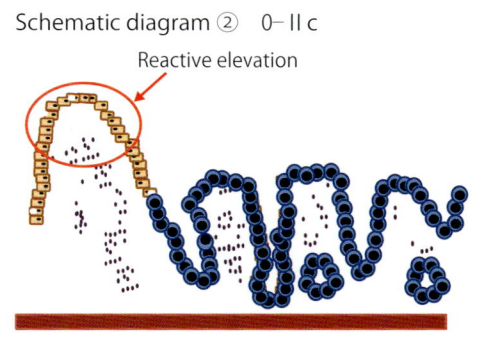

Fig. 18 Growth and development patterns of differentiated-type gastric cancer

① : Differente-type gastric cancer arises from the intestinal metaplastic epithelium. In intestinal metaplastic epithelium, the cell proliferation zone is located in the glandular base. The cancer cells generated from the glandular base invade continuously, replacing the existing glandular structures without destroying the basement membrane.

② : There are two types of cancer cell growth: growing towards the surface and assuming the shape of 0–IIa or gradually depressing and taking the shape of 0–IIc. The morphology can differ depending on the degree of cell atypism, cell density, and surface directivity. At any rate, as the cells grow, they form glands. With the depressive type, the margin of the depression slopes gently, sometimes forming a reactive elevation in non-cancerous areas around the periphery.

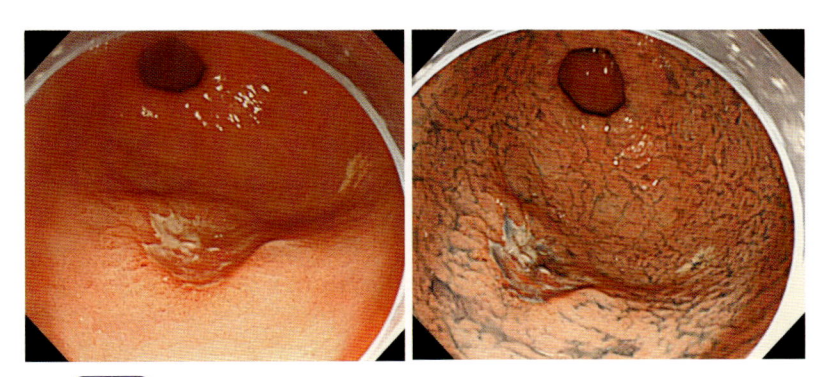

Fig. 19 Differentiated-type gastric cancer: Endoscopic images

A reddish depressive lesion can be seen in the greater curvature of the antrum. Some mucus is attached. The margin of the depression slopes gently, and the periphery is slightly elevated.

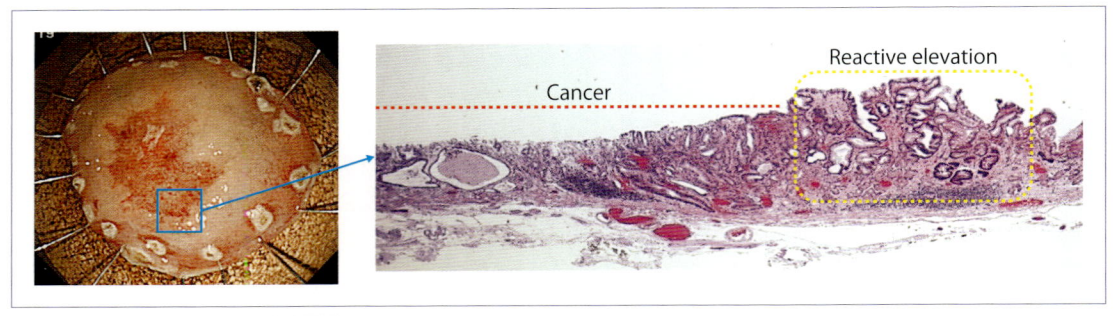

Fig. 20 Differentiated-type cancer: Histopathological image

Shown above is a histopathological image of the edge of a lesion. The extent of the cancer corresponds to the depressed surface marked by the red dotted line. The marginal elevation is a reactive elevation caused by hyperplasia.

▶ Greater curvature of antrum, 0–IIc, 12 mm, tub1>tub2, T1a (M), UL (–)

The clinical characteristics of differentiated-type and undifferentiated-type early gastric cancers are shown in **Table 2**.

Table 2 Clinical characteristics of differentiated-type and undifferentiated-type early gastric cancers

	Differentiated type (pap, tub1, tub2)	Undifferentiated type (por, sig)
Age	Mainly elderly	Relatively young
Sex	2:1 gender ratio	1:1 gender ratio
Background mucosa	Intestinal metaplasia	Fundic gland region without atrophy
Color tone	Reddish, whitish	Faded
Macroscopic classification	Mainly IIa and IIc	IIb in early stage; IIc when advanced; rarely IIa
Encroachment of depressed type	Thorn-like, asteroid	Cliff-like
Mucosal surface of depressed type	Areae gastricae pattern, fine granular	Dilatation of intervening part in early stage; structureless or island-like (insel) when advanced
Ulcer formation	Sometimes	Frequently

Side Note Is it really "undifferentiated carcinoma"?

The term "undifferentiated carcinoma" (without "type") is sometimes used erroneously at conferences and presentation. According to the Japanese Classification of Gastric Carcinoma, "undifferentiated carcinoma" is classified as a special type of malignant epithelial tumor. This classification defines it as a cancer that does not differentiate into adenocarcinoma or squamous cell carcinoma in any part of the lesion and considers it an exceptional histological type. The present author has seen thousands of gastric cancer cases at the Cancer Institute Hospital of JFCR but experienced only one case of "undifferentiated carcinoma" in the stomach. On the other hand, "undifferentiated type" (with "type," which we refer to it as "undifferentiated-type gastric cancer" in this book) is a classification method that combines poorly differentiated adenocarcinoma and signet ring cell carcinoma (Nakamura-Sugano Classification). In spite of the similarity of the terms, they present completely different histopathological images.

Just as "type" is frequently dropped when it should be used, it is also added when it is unnecessary.

Well-differentiated-type adenocarcinoma (inadequate) → Well-differentiated tubular adenocarcinoma (adequate)

Moderately differentiated-type adenocarcinoma (inadequate) → Moderately differentiated tubular adenocarcinoma (adequate)

Poorly differentiated-type adenocarcinoma (inadequate) → Poorly differentiated adenocarcinoma (adequate)

The use of "type" as a designation of differentiation has been practiced traditionally and is not erroneous per se. However, to avoid confusion with the Nakamura-Sugano Classification ("type" is not used either in the Japanese Classification of Gastric Carcinoma), its use should be avoided. The terms should not be used indiscriminately (see page 36).

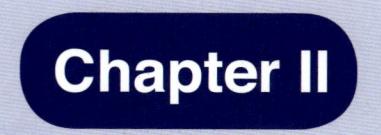

How to Detect Gastric Cancer

1 Findings you need to consider in order to detect gastric cancer

- If you perform a cursory endoscopy, you won't detect gastric cancer. Generally, depending on the lesion, you will be looking for a finding that is barely detectable. To make it easier, we've put together a collection of tips on how to detect gastric cancer — such as points you need to bear in mind and findings you need to pay attention to.

2 Factors and findings which make gastric cancer easy to miss

- To help minimize the possibility of missing a cancerous lesion, we will point out those locations that are likely to be blind spots in endoscopy and discuss types of lesions that are hard to find.

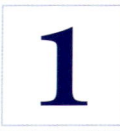

1 Findings you need to consider in order to detect gastric cancer

What findings should be considered in order to detect gastric cancer?

- **Relationship with the background**
  - State of gastritis in the background mucosa
  - Is there a similar lesion in the surrounding area?
- **Findings on the surface (cancerous area)**
  - Irregular morphology
  - Changes in the surface structure
  - Changes in color tone
  - Disappearance of vascular patterns
  - Spontaneous bleeding
- **Findings on the margins**
  - Clear margin
  - Encroachment (thorn-like, asteroid, cliff-like)
  - Margin elevation

I Relationship with the background mucosa

1 State of gastritis in the background mucosa (Figs. 1–10)

Depending on the state of the gastritis in the background mucosa, there are specific characteristics of gastric cancer which are likely to be exhibited in the histological type, macroscopic type, and color tone. In the fundic gland region and atrophic border, look for faded mucosa and a depression where fading and redness coexist. In areas where atrophy or intestinal metaplasia is present, look for a reddish depression or a flat elevation with a color tone that ranges from whitish to a one that is similar to that of the surrounding mucosa. Differentiated-type gastric cancer can arise in these kinds of conditions.

Points to observe

- Fundic gland region without atrophy, atrophic border
  - Undifferentiated-type gastric cancer frequently arises here.
  - ⇒ Look for faded mucosa !

- Atrophy, intestinal metaplasia
  - Differentiated-type gastric cancer frequently arises here.
  - ⇒ Look for a reddish depression or a whitish flat elevation !

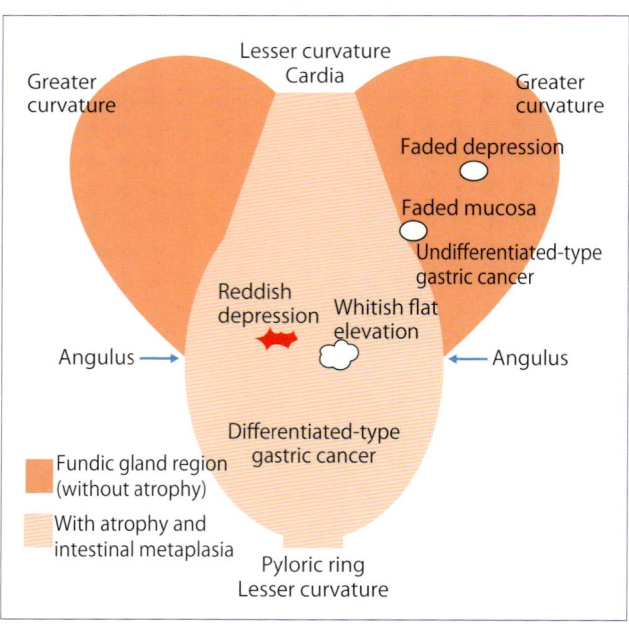

Fig. 1 Background mucosa and gastric cancer

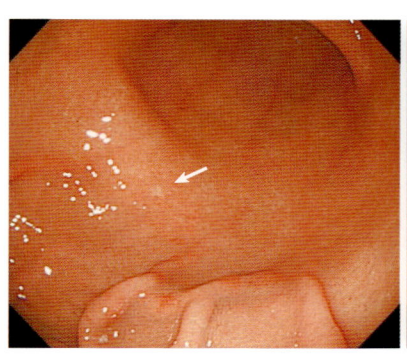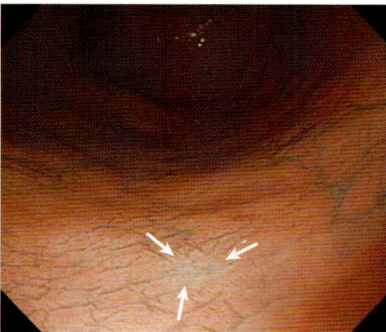

Fig. 2 Background mucosa : Non-atrophic ①

The background mucosa has no atrophy and is glossy and reddish-orange in color. Even though the lesion is small, fading is easily visible against the reddish-orange background and is noticeable from a distance. In closed-up view with indigo carmine spraying, it was found that the lesion was distinguished only by a change in color tone and exhibited virtually no surface irregularities.

▶ Greater curvature of the lower body, 0–IIb, 2 mm, sig, T1a (M), UL (–)

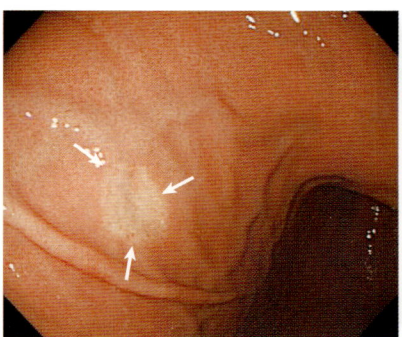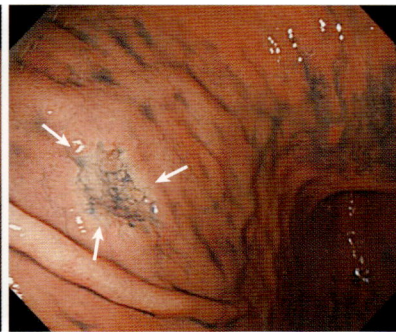

Fig. 3 Background mucosa : Non-atrophic ②

RAC can be seen in the background mucosa. This is fundic gland mucosa without atrophy. A depressed lesion with faded color and clear margins can be seen on the anterior wall of the middle body.

▶ Anterior wall of the middle body, 0–IIc, 20 mm, sig>por, T1a (M), UL (–)

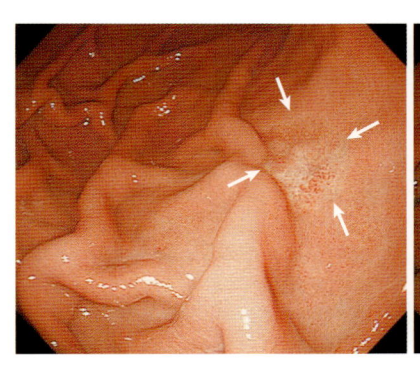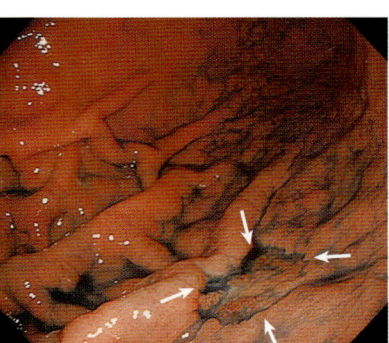

Fig. 4 Background mucosa : Non-atrophic ③

This case exhibits diffuse redness as well as enlarged and tortuous folds in the background mucosa, suggesting a current *H. pylori* infection. Despite these findings, however, there is no atrophy. Regenerative epithelium and redness caused by insel can be seen in the faded depression. When indigo carmine is sprayed, the depression appears to have a cliff-like structure.

▶ Posterior wall of the greater curvature of the middle body, 0–IIc, 20 mm, sig, T1a (M), UL (–)

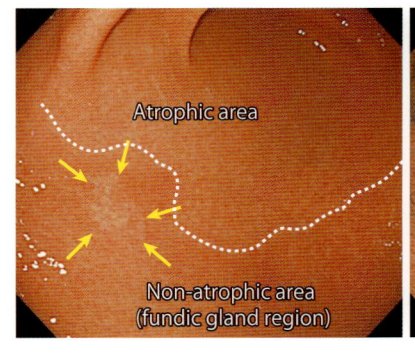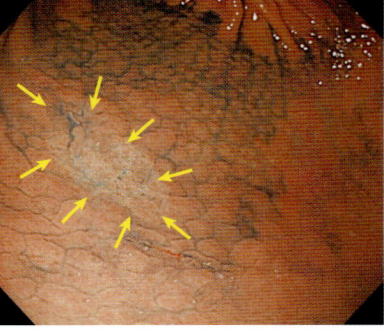

Atrophic area

Non-atrophic area (fundic gland region)

Fig. 5 Background mucosa : Proximal side of the atrophic border

Faded mucosa can be seen in the fundic gland region on the proximal side of the atrophic border (dotted line). When indigo carmine is sprayed, a shallow depression becomes visible. The atrophic area looks like nodular gastritis.

▶ Greater curvature of the lower body, 0–IIc, 16 mm, sig, T1a (M), UL (–)

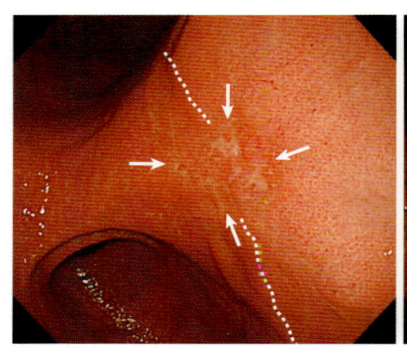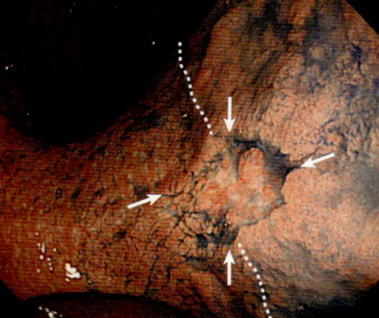

Fig. 6 Background mucosa : Atrophic border

The background mucosa exhibits diffuse redness. A depressed lesion with fading and redness along the atrophic border (dotted line) can be seen on the posterior wall of the angulus. When undifferentiated-type gastric cancer consists of only signet ring cell carcinoma, it often exhibits fading. However, once poorly differentiated adenocarcinoma is intermingled, both fading and redness are often exhibited.

▶ Posterior wall of angulus, 0–IIc, 20 mm, por>sig, T1a (M), UL (–)

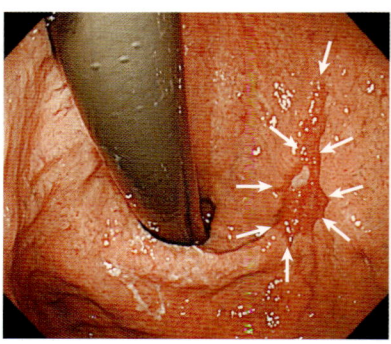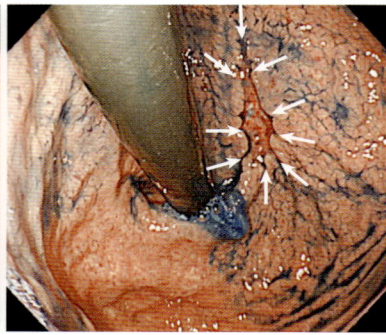

Fig. 7 Background mucosa: Atrophy and intestinal metaplasia ①

The background mucosa features conspicuous intestinal metaplasia. An extremely red depressed lesion can be seen on the anterior wall of the upper body. The margins exhibit thorn-like projections.

▶ Anterior wall of the upper body, 0–IIc, 28 mm, tub1>tub2, T1b (SM), UL (–)

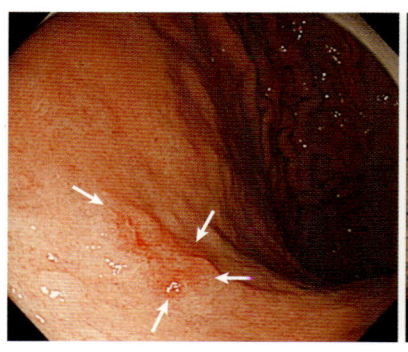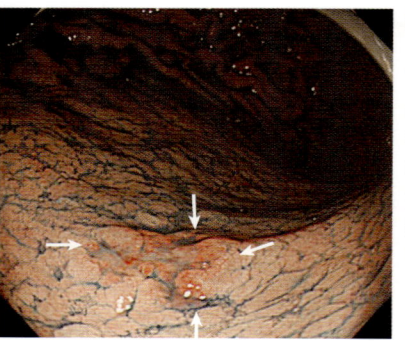

Fig. 8 Background mucosa: Atrophy and intestinal metaplasia ②

The background mucosa exhibits atrophy and intestinal metaplasia. A reddish depressed lesion with an irregular shape can be seen on the posterior wall of the upper body. The margins are clear.

▶ Posterior wall of the upper body, 0–IIc, 12 mm, tub1>tub2, T1a (M), UL (–)

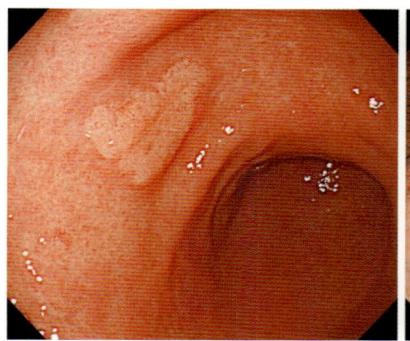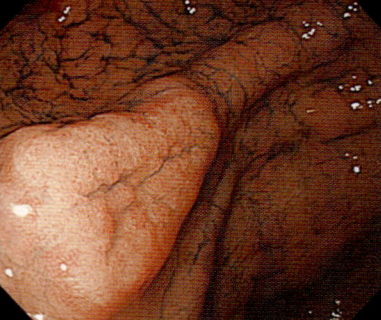

Fig. 9 Background mucosa: Atrophy and intestinal metaplasia ③

The background mucosa has minor atrophy. A whitish flat elevated lesion with clear margins can be seen on the anterior wall of the lesser curvature of the antrum. The center is slightly depressed.

▶ Anterior wall of the lesser curvature of the antrum, 0–IIa+IIc, 15 mm, tub1, T1a (M), UL (–)

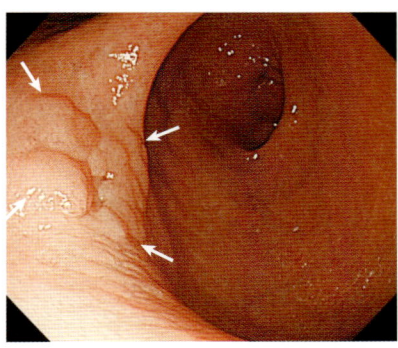
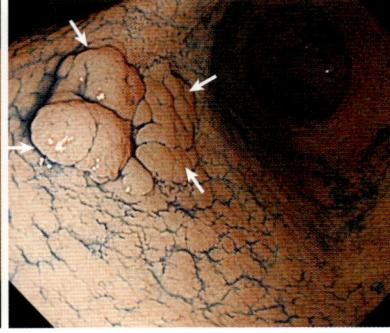

Fig. 10 Background mucosa :
Atrophy and intestinal
metaplasia ④

The background mucosa exhibits atrophy. A lobulated flat elevation with a clear margin can be seen. The color tone is similar to the area around the lesion.
▶ Anterior wall of the angulus, 0–IIa, 15 mm, tub1, T1a (M), UL (−)

---

② Are there multiple similar lesions in the surrounding area? (Figs. 11 & 12)

When the legion occurs at only one site, cancer should be suspected. When there are multiple lesions, gastri- tis or lymphoma should be considered.

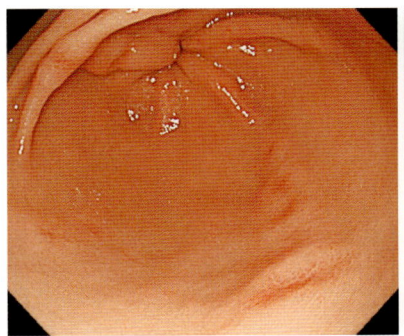
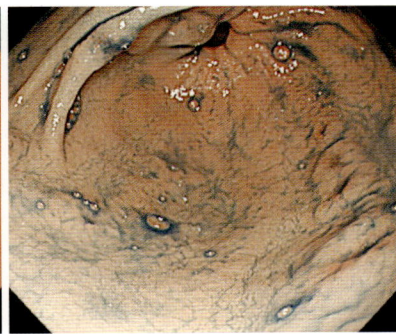

Fig. 11 Multiple lesions :
Benign erosion

There are multiple reddish depressed lesions in the antrum. These are benign elevated erosions. When multiple lesions are present as in this case, the likelihood of cancer is low.

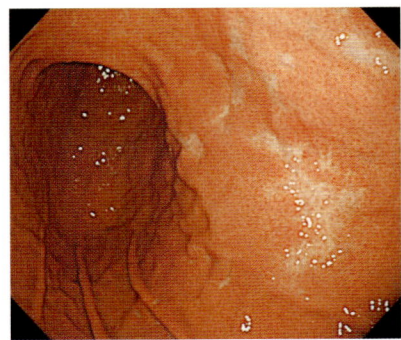
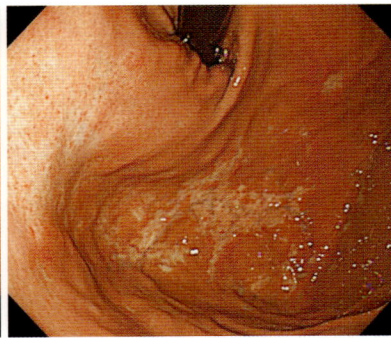

Fig. 12 Multiple lesions : MALT lymphoma

There are multiple faded depressed lesions with map-like patterns. When faded depressed lesions occur in multiple locations, MALT lymphoma is likely.

Ⅱ Findings on the surface (cancerous area)

Findings on the lesion's surface — such as a depressed or elevated surface, as well as a finely patterned surface structure — should be observed in detail. When the lesion has a large surface area, cancer should be suspected.

① Irregular morphologies (Figs. 13 & 14)

Although "regular" and "irregular" are frequently used in endoscopy terminology, their meaning has not been clearly defined. In most cases those words are used empirically, and what is meant by the term can vary depending on the individual who uses it. Generally speaking, "irregular" refers to morphologies where the lesion is round, almost round, or oval, while "irregular" is used to refer to lesions that are asymmetrical and exhibit uneven surface conditions.

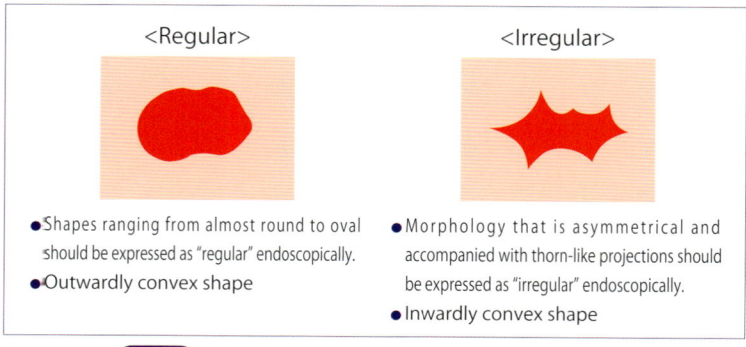

Fig. 13 Definitions of "regular" and "irregular"

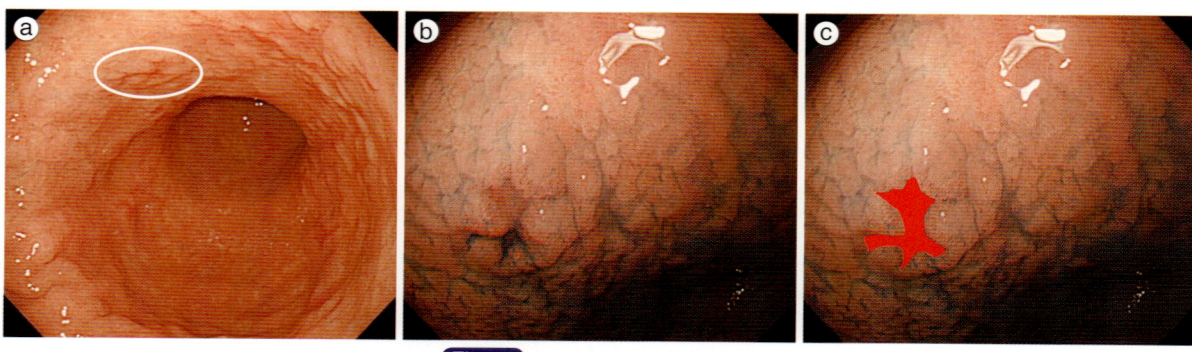

Fig. 14 Irregular morphologies

a : Map-like redness can be seen in the background mucosa, which is in a post-*H. pylori* eradication condition. It is difficult to detect gastric cancer when the mucosa exhibits map-like redness. The circled reddish depression has an irregular shape, which makes it stand out. However, because there are similar reddish depressions at multiple locations in the surrounding area, it cannot be diagnosed as cancer in conventional endoscopy.

b, c : When indigo carmine is sprayed on the site and it is examined carefully, thorn-like projections can be seen on the irregularly shaped reddish depression. This increases the likelihood of cancer. The slight elevation around the perimeter further reinforces the likelihood of cancer.

▶ Anterior wall of the lesser curvature of the middle body, 0–Ⅱc, 5 mm, tub1, T1a (M), UL (−)

② Changes in the surface structure (Figs. 15 & 16)

The first thing you have to do is thoroughly acquaint yourself with the current condition (e.g., areae gastricae disrupted by gastritis) of the background mucosa of the case under examination. Using that condition as a reference, look for a region where there is a change in the surface structure of the mucosa. With cancer, the areae gastricae are likely to have become indistinct, often causing mucosa to lose its shine. With differentiated-type gastric cancer, fine granular changes may be exhibited.

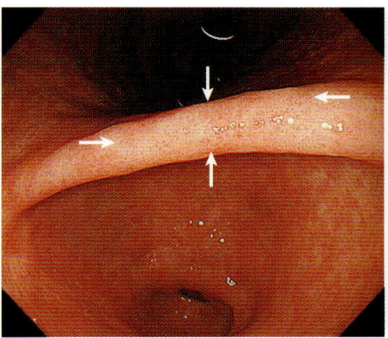 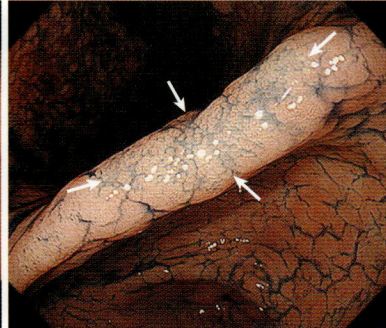

Fig. 15 Changes in the surface structure ①

The background mucosa shows signs of atrophic gastritis. It is difficult to see the lesion with conventional endoscopy. When indigo carmine is sprayed, a depressed lesion with a fine-grained surface structure and indistinct areae gastricae can be seen on the lesser curvature of the angulus. This can be diagnosed as cancer.
▶ Lesser curvature of the angulus, 0–IIc, 16 mm, tub1>tub2, T1a (M), UL (–)

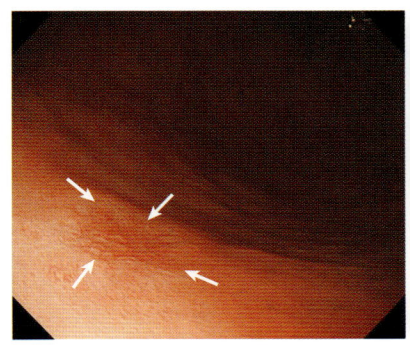 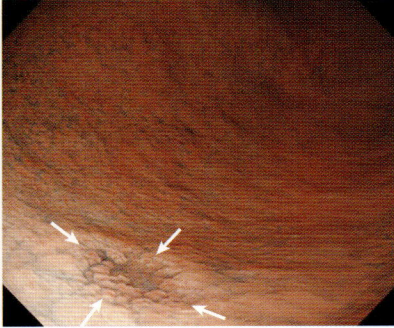

Fig. 16 Changes in the surface structure ②

Even in conventional endoscopy, finely detailed irregularities can be seen that stand out from the surrounding mucosa. Spraying indigo carmine helps clarify a minute granular mucosal structure. When a mucosal structure like this is seen, differentiated-type cancer should be suspected. Unless close-up observation is performed, such a small cancer will normally be missed.
▶ Greater curvature of the lower body, 0–IIc, 5 mm, tub1, T1a (M), UL (–)

③ Changes in color tones (Figs. 17–21)

Evaluate any subtle differences in color tone between the region of interest and the background mucosa. The color tones can vary — such as faded with undifferentiated-type gastric cancer and reddish, normal, and whitish with differentiated-type gastric cancer. Since there is no mucosal atrophy in cases of undifferentiated-type cancer, the color tone of the background mucosa is a uniform reddish-orange — which makes it easy to detect any fading even if the lesion is very small. In differentiated-type gastric cancer, on the other hand, the color tones of the background mucosa are not consistent due to the presence of atrophy and/or intestinal metaplasia. This can make it more difficult to detect cancer when relying solely upon changes in coloration.

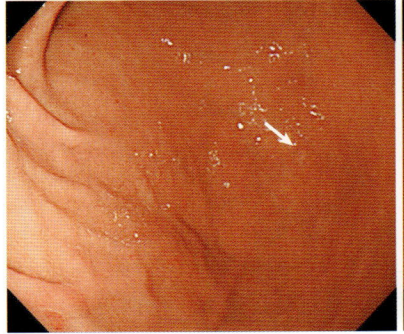 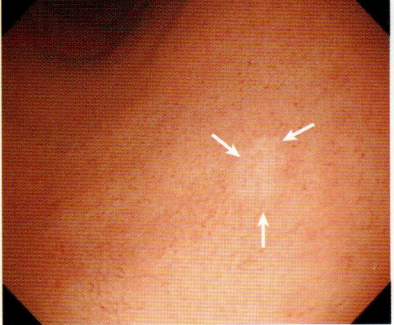 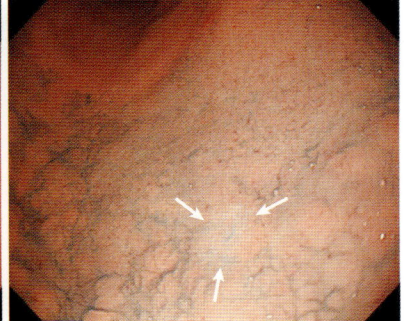

Fig. 17 Changes in color tone ①
There is no atrophy on the background mucosa. Experienced endoscopists will be able to detect the faded mucosa even from a distance. In closed-up view, the faded mucosa shows no signs of unevenness or of any other change to the mucosal surface structure, aside from the color tone.
▶ Greater curvature of the angulus, 0–IIb, 3 mm, sig, T1a (M), UL (–)

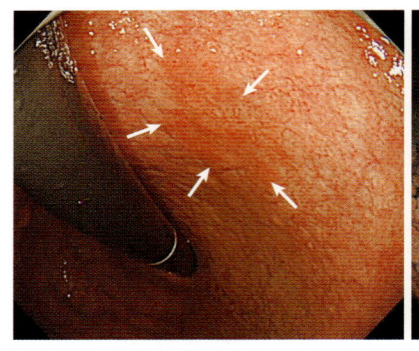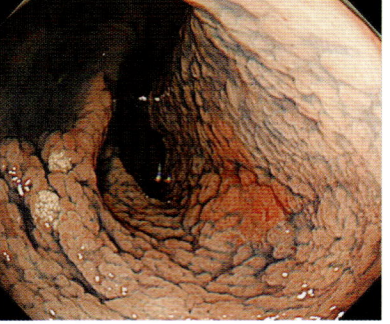

Retroflexed view | Antegrade view

Fig. 18 Changes in color tone ②

In conventional endoscopy, a large area that is redder than the area around it can be seen in the atrophic mucosa. Vascular patterns have disappeared — which is another reason to suspect cancer. In indigo carmine chromoendoscopy, the dye collects in the grooves between the areae gastricae around the lesion, making the mucosa look bluish. However, as very little dye attaches to the lesion because the areae gastricae inside the lesion has shallow grooves, there is no effect on the degree of redness so the contrast between the color tone of the lesion and its surroundings is emphasized.

▶ Lesser curvature of the upper body, 0–IIb, 18 mm, tub2, T1a (M), UL (–)

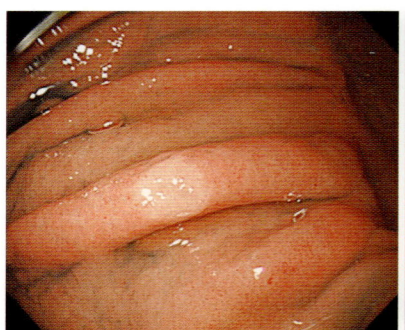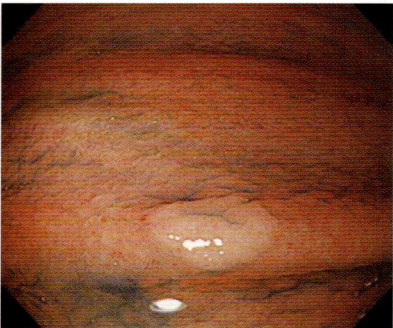

Fig. 19 Changes in color tone ③

This is the part of the remnant stomach after distal gastrectomy. The background is reddened due to residual stomach gastritis; however, whitish mucosa with clear margins can be seen on the greater curvature of the body. Spraying indigo carmine reveals that the whitish mucosa is slightly elevated. This leads to the suspicion that the whitish flat elevation is an adenoma or a very well-differentiated adenocarcinoma.

▶ Greater curvature of the remnant stomach, 0–IIa, 6 mm, tub (very well-diff.), T1a (M), UL (–)

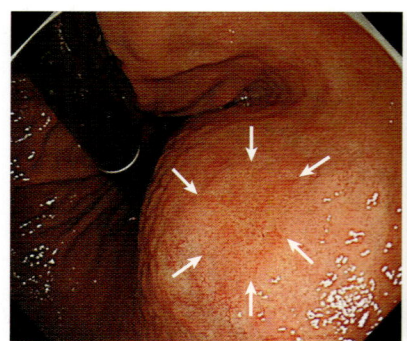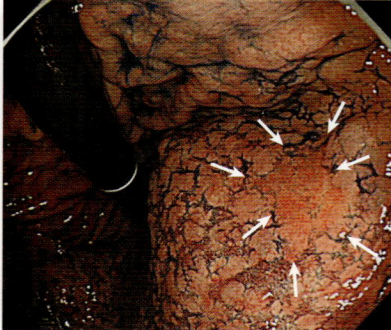

Fig. 20 Changes in color tone ④

Atrophy and intestinal metaplasia are seen in the background mucosa. On the posterior wall of the middle body, the mucosa is slightly yellower than the surrounding mucosa. When the site is sprayed with indigo carmine, it becomes obvious that the area gastrica patterns have disappeared. The indigo carmine also makes the margin of the affected area more distinct. Differentiated-type gastric cancer can often be detected by changes in mucosal coloration and will appear slightly yellower than the surrounding mucosa.

▶ Posterior wall of the middle body, 0–IIc, 12 mm, tub1, T1a (M), UL (–)

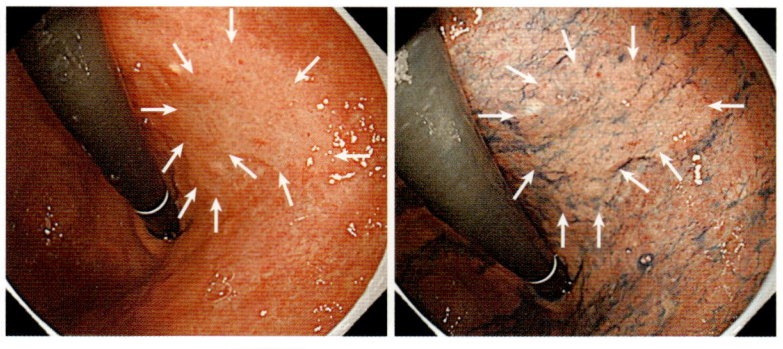

Fig. 21 Changes in color tone ⑤

The background mucosa exhibits diffuse redness. Mucosa that is slightly more yellow-ish-white than the surroundings can be seen in the lesser curvature of the upper body. Although changes in the lesion's coloration cannot be confirmed from edge to edge in conventional endoscopy, a clearly visible margin has formed in some areas, making cancer a definite possibility. When indigo carmine is sprayed, the margin becomes clear around the entire circumference. The color tone of the background mucosa varies widely depending on the individual. To find cancer, you have to be able to detect slight changes in the mucosa by comparing it with the background mucosa.

▶ Lesser curvature of the upper body, 0–IIa, 25 mm, tub1>tub2, T1a (M), UL (–)

④ Disappearance of vascular patterns (Figs. 22 & 23)

When atrophy is present, submucosal vascular patterns will be visible. However, if a tumor develops, the vascular patterns will disappear because of the thickness of the tumor and the increase in cell density. In a clinical case where vascular patterns are prominent in the background, look for regions where the vascular patterns have disappeared.

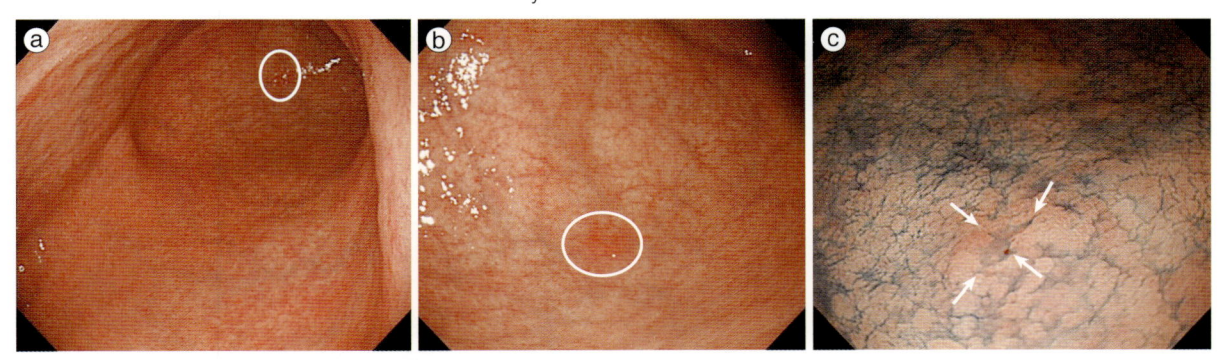

Fig. 22 Disappearance of vascular patterns ①

a, b : The background mucosa has O–3 atrophy, and vascular patterns are visible. Reddened areas (circled in the pictures) where vascular patterns have disappeared can be seen in the greater curvature of the angulus.

c : When indigo carmine is sprayed, it can be seen that the area indicated by the arrows is a depressed lesion. As there is no similar lesion in the surrounding area and the indigo carmine spraying stimulated some bleeding, this finding suggests cancer.

▶ Greater curvature of the angulus, 0–IIc, 3 mm, tub1, T1a (M), UL (–)

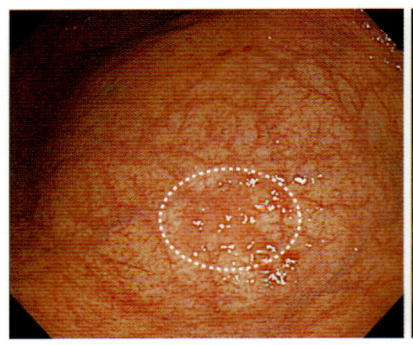
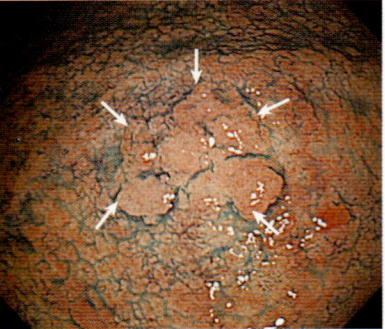

Fig. 23 Disappearance of vascular patterns ②

The background mucosa is severely atrophied and vascular patterns are visible. There is a spot on the anterior wall of the middle body where the blood vessels cannot be seen clearly. It is too early at this point to diagnose this spot as cancer, but it is clearly different from its surroundings. When indigo carmine is sprayed, we can see that it is a flat elevated lesion and diagnose it as cancer.

▶ Anterior wall of the middle body, 0–IIa, 12 mm, tub1, T1a (M), UL (–)

⑤ Spontaneous bleeding (Figs. 24 & 25)

Cancerous tissue is more sensitive and hemorrhagic than normal tissue. In some cases, it may already be bleeding when the endoscope is inserted; in other cases, it may start bleeding when irritated by insufflation or irrigation. This bleeding does, however, make it possible to detect cancer more easily.

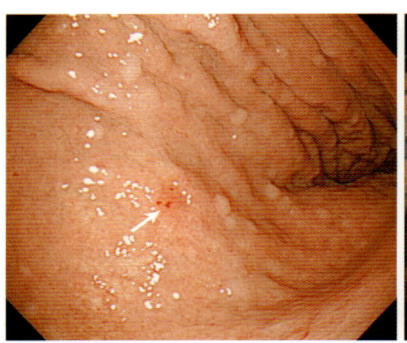
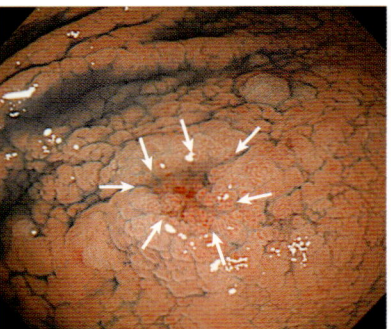

Fig. 24 Spontaneous bleeding ①

A whitish elevation produced by intestinal metaplasia is clearly visible on the background mucosa. A reddish depressed lesion with fresh blood attached can be seen on the greater curvature of the upper body. Since fresh blood stands out even from a distance, it can frequently lead to the discovery of small gastric cancers.

▶ Greater curvature of the upper body, 0–IIc, 6 mm, tub1, T1a (M), UL (–)

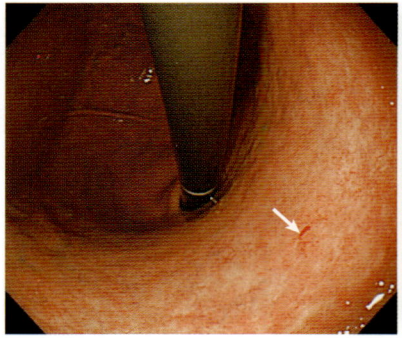
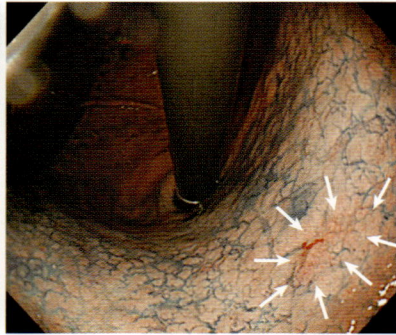

Fig. 25 Spontaneous bleeding ②

In conventional endoscopy, a tiny amount of fresh blood can be seen in the atrophic region. On its own, this is insufficient for a cancer diagnosis, but it is possible that the spontaneous bleeding could be caused by cancer. Consequently, the site was observed more closely. Extent diagnosis was difficult even after indigo carmine had been sprayed. A lesion was found in the region where the areae gastricae had disappeared (indicated by the arrows in the picture on the right). A lesion like this would be difficult to detect if there were no spontaneous bleeding.

▶ Lesser curvature of the middle body, 0–IIb, 5 mm, tub1, T1a (M), UL (–)

Ⅲ Findings on the margins

Gastric cancer is a malignant tumor that develops on the epithelium of the mucosal surface. This means that the cancer is exposed on the mucosal surface and forms clear boundaries with non-cancerous areas. With signet ring cell carcinoma — where the cancer is present only in the middle layer of the mucosa without being exposed to the surface — and with the "hand-shaking" type cancer of moderately differentiat-ed-type tubular adenocarcinoma, these boundaries or margins are relatively indistinct. These are exceptions, however. With all other types of cancer, it is safe to say that margins are formed. While some cancers may not have fully circumferential margins, parts of those margins usually are quite distinct. In other words, if the margin is indistinct throughout the full circumference, there is high likelihood that it is not a cancer.

Compare ! Margins of benign lesions

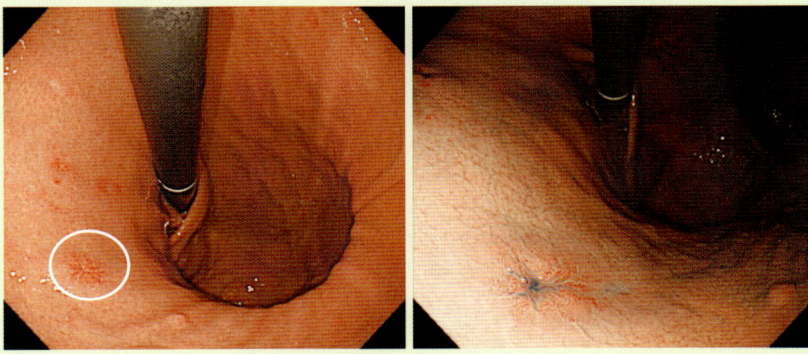

- A reddish depressed lesion (circled in the above left picture) can be seen on the posterior wall of the lesser curvature of the upper body. Redness and dilated crypt openings are prominent in the center of the lesion but gradually disappear into the background mucosa at the edges. The margins of the lesion are unclear, so it is diagnosed as a benign erosion. The fact that there are similar lesions in multiple locations in the surrounding area also supports the diagnosis that it is benign.

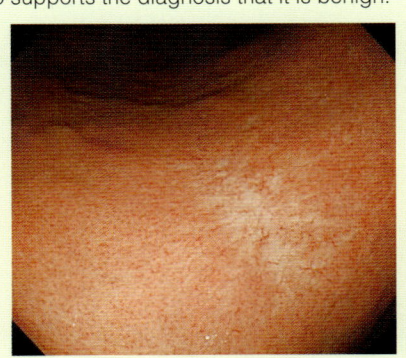

- Faded mucosa can be seen near the anterior wall of the lesser curvature of the lower body. The fading gradually loses intensity towards the edges, making it difficult to accurately track the margin. It is diagnosed as a benign ulcer scar (S2).
- An ulcer scar on the lesser curvature of the body often exhibits fading that gradually increases from the periphery to the center without folds convergence.

① Encroachment (Fig. 26)

Margins play a critical role in the search for cancer. The margins between depressed gastric cancer and non-cancerous mucosa are irregular like the edges of a mulberry leaf eaten by a silkworm. This irregularity is described as "encroachment." It indicates a condition where one intrudes into the other as if the silkworm ate the mulberry leaves. It is one of the most important findings for the diagnosis of gastric cancer.

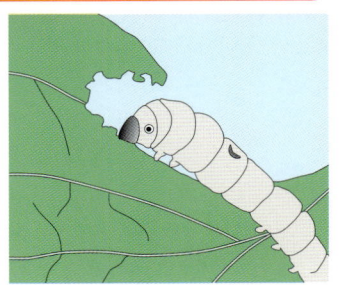

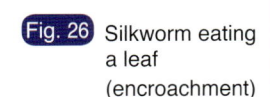 Silkworm eating a leaf (encroachment)

1) Undifferentiated-type gastric cancer (Figs. 27 & 28)

Undifferentiated-type gastric cancer exhibits clear, cliff-like margins around depression. Because the background mucosa where undifferentiated-type cancer arises is not atrophied and is relatively thick, the depression formed by the lesion is able to penetrate deeper.

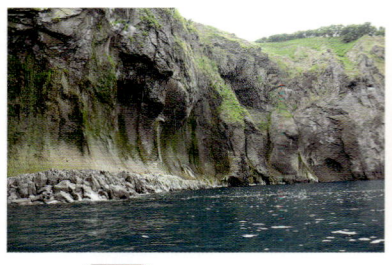

Fig. 27 "Cliff" margin

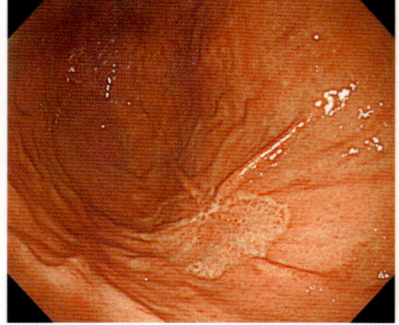 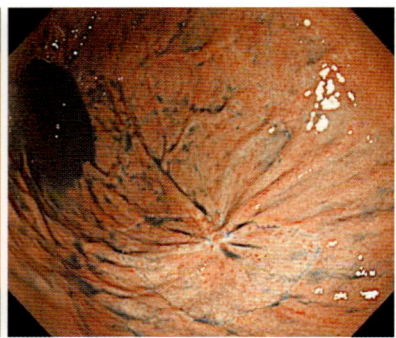

Fig. 28 Encroachment of undifferentiated-type gastric cancer: Cliff-like margin
Diffuse redness can be seen in the background mucosa, indicating a current *H. pylori* infection. However, there is no atrophy in the background mucosa. The lesion is a depression with faded color tones and partially accompanied by redness. The margin of the depression is straight with a clear and consistent height as if cut with a knife. The appearance of the margin is described as "cliff-like." It is a typical finding of encroachment of undifferentiated-type gastric cancer.
▶ Anterior wall of the greater curvature of the upper body, 0–IIc, 35 mm, por>sig, T1b (SM), UL (+)

2) Differentiated-type gastric cancer (Figs. 29–31)

Differentiated-type gastric cancer forms margins that look like the thorns of a rose or beams of starlight. Those edges are described as "thorn-like" or "asteroid." Because the background mucosa has been thinned by atrophy, the difference between the level of a depression and the surrounding mucosa is not as obvious as it is with undifferentiated-type gastric cancer. The relatively gentle slopes of the depression make the margins unclear. A hyperplastic change called reactive elevation is sometimes seen on the periphery of the depression.

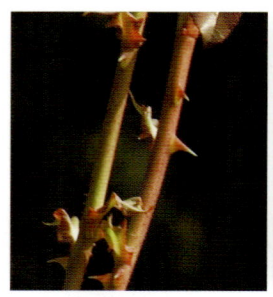 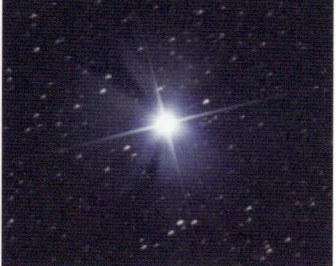

Fig. 29 "Thorn-like" (left) and "asteroid" margins (right)

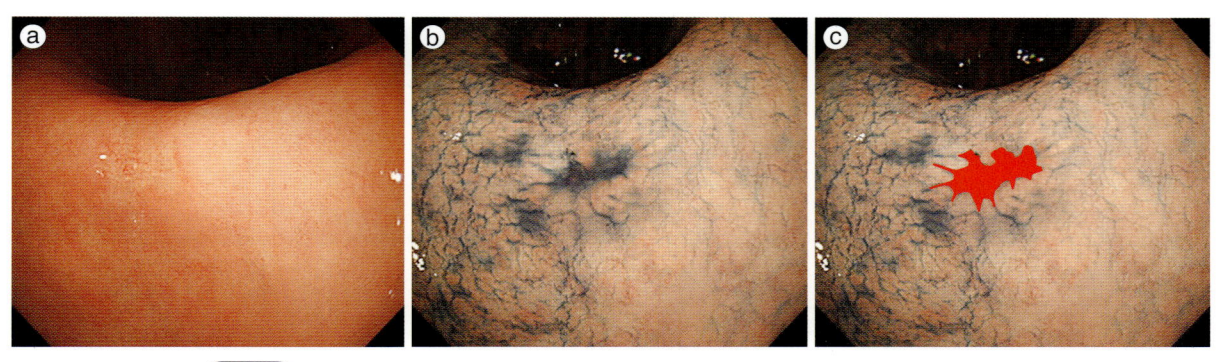

Fig. 30 Encroachment of differentiated-type gastric cancer: Thorn-like and asteroid

a : Atrophy and intestinal metaplasia are present on the background mucosa. In conventional endoscopy, a depressed surface that is slightly more whitish than its surroundings can be seen, but the encroachment is not clear.

b, c : When indigo carmine is sprayed, the margin of the depression can be seen to protrude outward like needles. This shape is described as "thorn-like" or "asteroid." This is a typical image of encroachment of differentiated-type gastric cancer. Because the cancer progresses along the grooves of the areae gastricae, the margin forms a thorn-like shape. The overall surface of the depression is uneven. The non-cancerous areas on the edges have a slight reactive elevation. Unlike undifferentiated-type gastric cancer, clear visualization of encroachment is often impossible with differentiated-type gastric cancer unless indigo carmine is sprayed.

▶ Lesser curvature of the antrum, 0–IIc, 12 mm, tub1, T1a (M), UL (–)

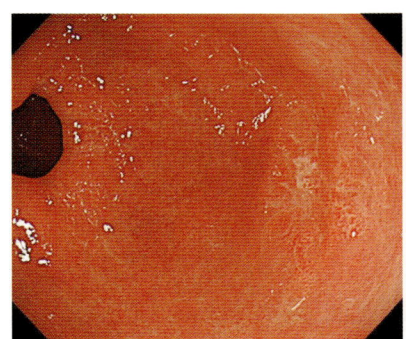 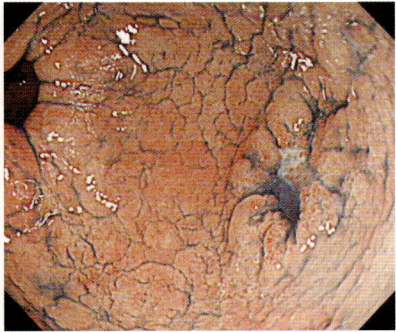

Fig. 31 Encroachment of differentiated-ed-type gastric cancer: A case with conspicuous reactive elevation

In this case, in addition to the thorn-like encroachment, the elevation around the depression stands out. This is not a result of cancer; rather, it is a hyperplastic change created reactively. A reactive elevation is one of the findings that suggests cancer.

▶ Posterior wall of the antrum, 0–IIc, 10 mm, tub1, T1a (M), UL (–)

Side Note 　Anisakiasis

One morning, I was woken up by sudden epigastric pain. It was a kind of pain I had never experienced before. It didn't get better even after I took a PPI and loxoprofen that I happened to have on hand. My mind was going through differential diagnosis like, "Could it be an initial symptom of appendicitis? Or myocardial infarction of the inferior wall?" Then I suddenly remembered that I had sushi with a friend last night. So I self-diagnosed anisakiasis.

I had eaten some slightly broiled mackerel marinated in salt and vinegar the night before. Enduring the pain, I went to my hospital and asked one of my colleagues to perform endoscopy on me. As I suspected, there was an Anisakis biting at the gastric wall. As soon as it was removed with forceps, the pain went away immediately. The Anisakis does not die even when marinated in vinegar; it is rendered harmless only when it is heated or frozen (at –20°C for over 24 hours). I knew all this, but it never occurred to me that I would get it one day. But as the proverb goes, "the danger past and God forgotten," I still enjoy eating delicious mackerel.

According to the revision of Japan's Food Sanitation Law in 1999, any doctor who has diagnosed a patient suspected to have food poisoning from Anisakis is required to report it to the nearest public health center within 24 hours. Yet in fiscal 2015, there were only 127 reports. It would appear that many cases are going unreported.

2 Factors and findngs which make gastric cancer easy to miss

Two main reasons why gastric cancer is often hard to detect

One reason is that the cancerous site can be difficult to observe with an endoscope; the other is that the morphology of the lesion itself can make it difficult to distinguish the cancer from the background gastritis.

I Sites that are easy to overlook
- Lesser curvature of the cardia: Hidden by the endoscope shaft
- Anterior wall of the body, posterior wall of the angulus : Likely to be aligned in the tangential direction
- Greater curvature of the body: Hidden between the folds due to insufficient stretching
- Antrum: Concealed by peristalsis or hidden behind the constriction ring

II Lesions that are difficult to be found
- Minute gastric cancer
- 0–IIb lesion
- Gastritis resembling carcinoma

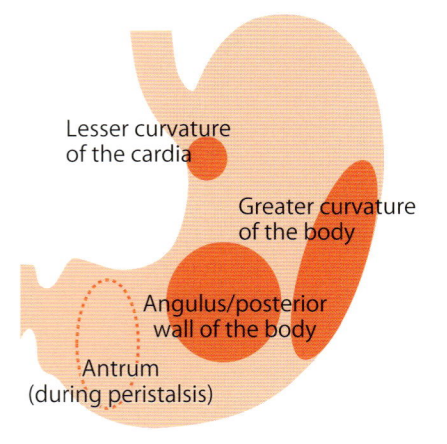

Lesser curvature of the cardia

Greater curvature of the body

Angulus/posterior wall of the body

Antrum (during peristalsis)

【Sites that are easy to overlook】

I Sites that are easy to overlook

① Lesser curvature of the cardia (Figs. 32 & 33)

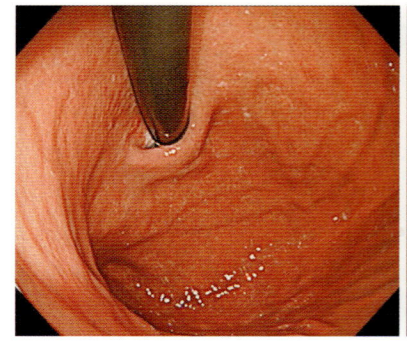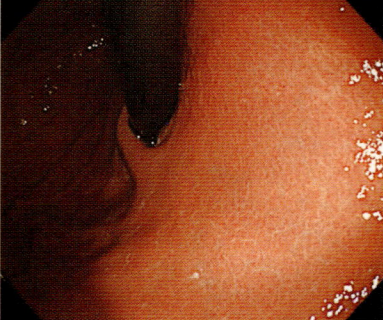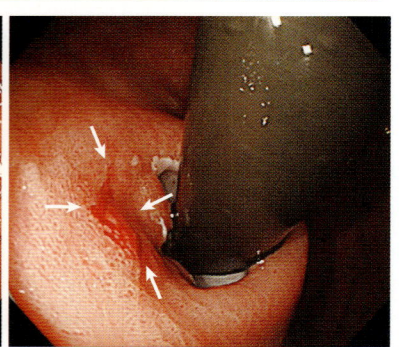

Fig. 32 Lesser curvature of the cardia ①

In endoscopic observation from the anterior and posterior walls, the lesion sitting directly on the lesser curvature of the cardia is hidden behind the endoscope shaft and cannot be seen. However, when the endoscope shaft is turned in a J-turn and observation is performed as the endoscope tip is moved to the lesser curvature side, the depressed lesion (indicated by the arrows) comes into view. Sites on the lesser curvature of the cardia are especially difficult to observe in cases where there is no esophageal hiatal hernia. Extra care should be taken in such a case.
▶ Lesser curvature of the cardia, 0–IIc, 6 mm, tub1, T1a (M), UL (−)

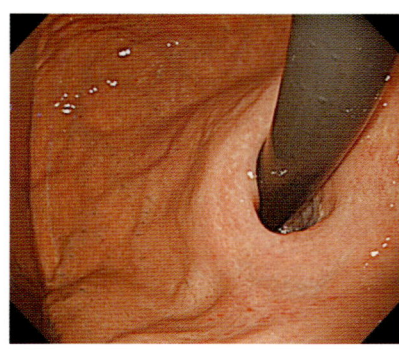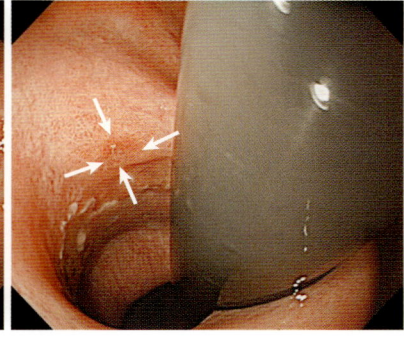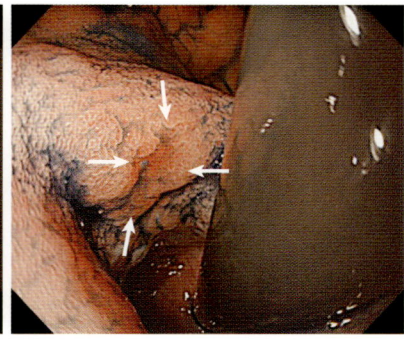

Fig. 33 Lesser curvature of the cardia ②

At first glance, there didn't appear to be anything in the lesser curvature of the cardia. However, when the endoscope was moved in closer so that a better view could be obtained of the anterior wall of the lesser curvature of the cardia, a small reddish depression was observed. Whenever you are observing the cardiac region, you will need to come as close as this.
▶ Near the anterior wall of the lesser curvature of the cardia, 0–IIc, 4 mm, tub1, T1a (M), UL (–)

② Posterior wall of the body, posterior wall of the angulus (Figs. 35 & 33)

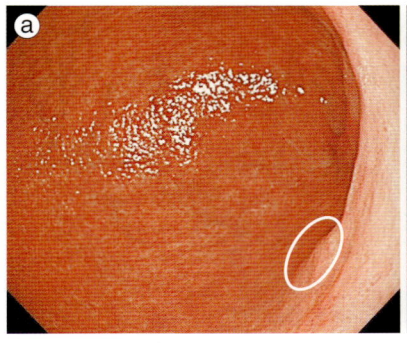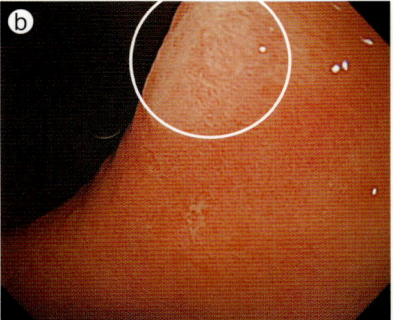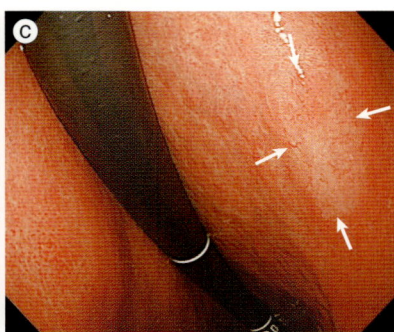

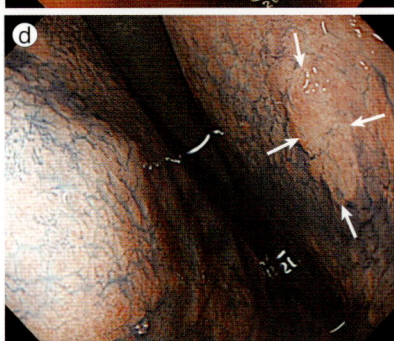

Fig. 34 Posterior wall of the lower body

a : The circled site on the posterior wall of the lower body comes in the tangential direction when viewed towards the distal side, which makes the lesion difficult to observe.

b : When the endoscope is retroflexed, it cannot be moved back far enough to view the entire site.

c, d : When the endoscope is pushed in further using additional force and then retroflexed, the entire lesion — which is slightly whiter than its surroundings — can be seen (indicated by the arrows). After twisting the endoscope counterclockwise, the tip is angulated to the left and the area is slightly deaerated. Now the lesion can be viewed from right front. Unless you keep in mind the need to deliberately push in the endoscope and retroflex it like this, there will be a blind spot in the posterior wall of the lower body.

▶ Posterior wall of the lower body, 0–IIa, 12 mm, tub1, T1a (M), UL (–)

 Side Note What is the detection rate of gastric cancer ?

The detection rate of gastric cancer differs depending on the characteristics of the population. While the detection rate of gastric cancer is high in populations that include many older males who are more likely to be infected with *H. pylori* — which presents a high risk of gastric cancer, the detection rate is lower in younger populations where *H. pylori* is less prevalent. In Japan, the detection rate for gastric cancer in endoscopy check-ups performed primarily on symptom-free patients was 0.22% of all gastrointestinal cancer screenings performed nationwide in fiscal 2013. At hospitals specializing in cancer treatment, the detection rate is higher than in ordinary hospitals because they are better equipped to find synchronous and asynchronous multiple lesions.

At the Cancer Institute Hospital of JFCR, 2,459 upper GI endoscopies were performed during the period from March to May of 2015. 73 cases (3.0%) of gastric cancer and adenoma excluding known lesions were detected.

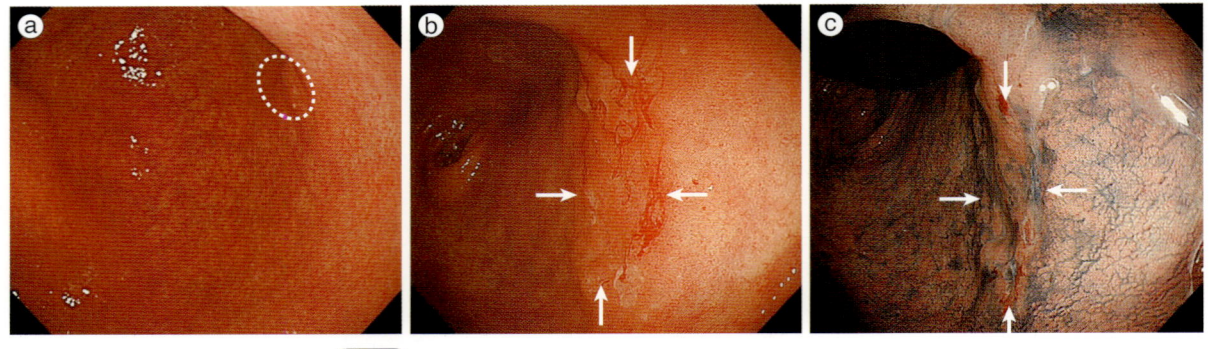

Fig. 35 Posterior wall of the angulus (undetected lesion)

a : Although irregularities were slightly conspicuous (shown in the dotted circle), the lesion was in the tangential direction and could not be discerned.

b, c : Under observation a year later, a depressed reddish lesion (indicated by the arrows) that was friable and slightly thick was detected.
  ▶ Posterior wall of the angulus, 0–IIc, 22 mm, tub2, T1b (SM), UL (−)

③ Greater curvature of the body (Fig. 36)

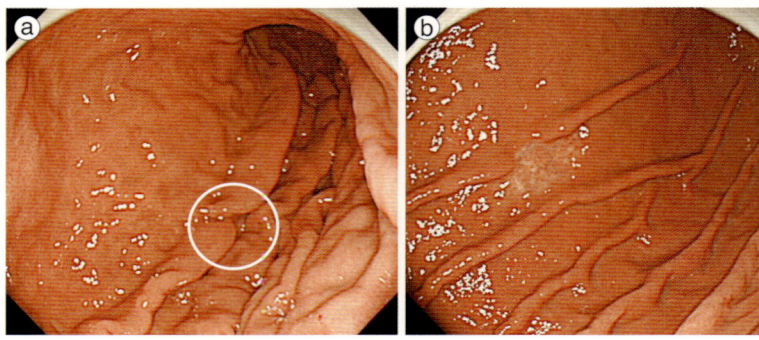

Insufficiently stretched   Sufficiently stretched

Fig. 36 Greater curvature of the body

In the greater curvature of the body, lesions tend to be hidden behind the fold and are likely to be missed. When the greater curvature is not stretched sufficiently as in a, the lesion (shown in the circle) cannot be seen. When the greater curvature is stretched sufficiently as in b, the lesion will not be missed. It is necessary to stretch the stomach until the folds in the greater curvature run in parallel to each other.
  ▶ Greater curvature of the middle body, 0–IIc, 30 mm, sig, T1a (M), UL (+)

④ Antrum (peristalsis) (Fig. 37)

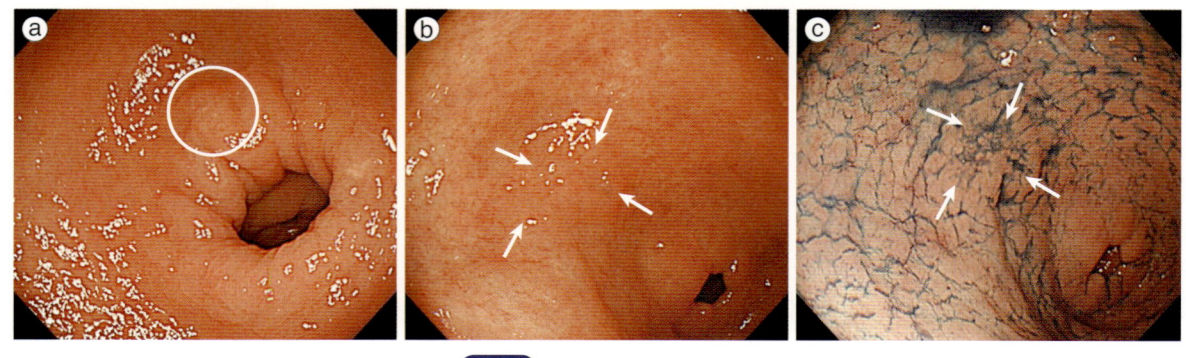

Fig. 37 Antrum (peristalsis)

a : Rapid peristalsis often occurs in the antrum. The circled lesion cannot be seen due to the peristalsis.

b, c : Once the peristalsis has stopped, a 0–IIc lesion can be seen on the lesser curvature of the antrum.
  ▶ Lesser curvature of the antrum, 0–IIc, 8 mm, tub1, T1a (M), UL (−)

II Lesions that are difficult to be found

① Minute gastric cancer (Figs. 38 & 39)

A tumor with a diameter of 5 mm or less is defined as minute gastric cancer. It exhibits few of the characteristic findings of cancer, making it difficult to discover.

However, with more detailed observation, cancer findings can be detected.

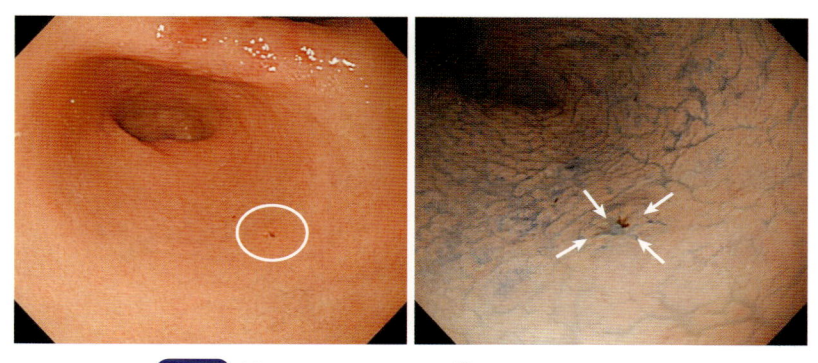

Fig. 38 Minute gastric cancer ① : Differentiated type

An erosion with hematin attached (shown in the circle) can be seen on the posterior wall of the greater curvature of the antrum. When indigo carmine is sprayed, numerous depressions in the surrounding area become visible. Their color tone is somewhat yellowish-white and they exhibit thorn-like encroachment (indicated by the arrows), leading to a suspicion of cancer.

▶ Posterior wall of the greater curvature of the antrum, 0–IIc, 3 mm, tub1, T1a (M), UL (–)

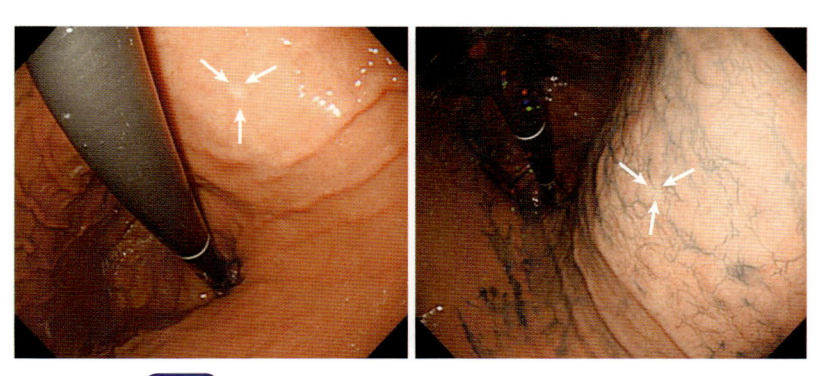

Fig. 39 Minute gastric cancer ② : Undifferentiated type

Because the background mucosa is not atrophied in undifferentiated-type gastric cancer, it is possible to find even a small lesion (indicated by the arrows) as you familiarize yourself with the technique. This case is an *H. pylori*-uninfected case without inflammation, so it is easy to find the lesion under conventional endoscopy — even from a distance. However, a lesion like this — which only has changes in color tone and has no surface irregularities — may be difficult to see with indigo carmine spraying.

▶ Posterior wall of the middle body, 0–IIb, 2 mm, sig, T1a (M), UL (–)

A lesion composed only of 0-IIb is a macroscopic type and is very rare, accounting for just 1% of all gastric cancers. Due to its lack of surface irregularities, it is difficult to detect[36), 37)]. To detect this type of lesion, look for color alterations that extend over a relative- ly wide area, disappearance of vascular patterns in atrophic mucosa, bleeding that is spontaneous or is induced by irrigation, and changes in area gastrica patterns.

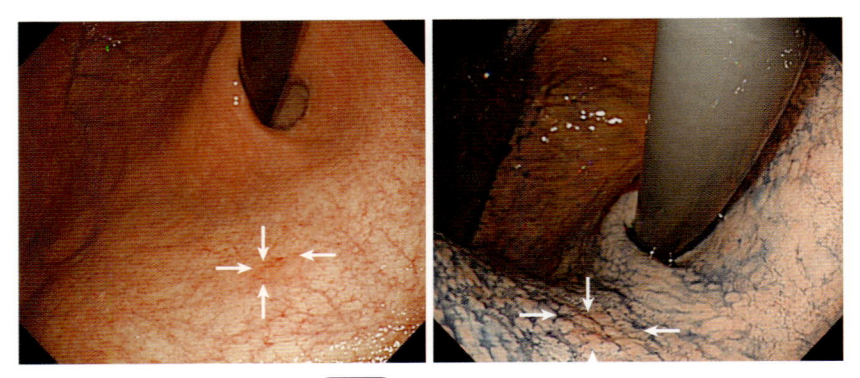

Fig. 40 0-IIb lesion ①

Severe atrophy is present in the background mucosa, and vascular patterns can be discerned. Faint redness where vascular patterns have disappeared (indicated by the arrows) can be seen on the anterior wall of the upper body. Moreover, fresh blood is present, further reinforcing the suspicion of cancer. Spraying indigo carmine makes the red area more clearly visible as the dye does not attach to the surface.

▶ Anterior wall of the upper body, 0-IIb, 3 mm, tub1, T1a (M), UL (−)

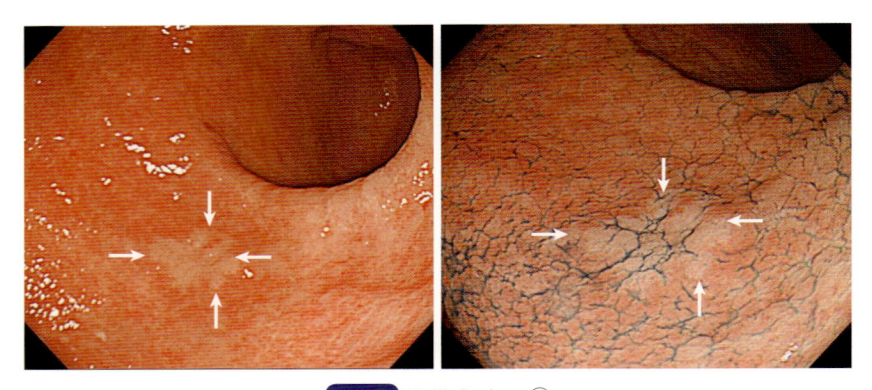

Fig. 41 0-IIb lesion ②

The background mucosa has whitish patches due to intestinal metaplasia. A relatively large area of whitish mucosa (indicated by the arrows) can be seen. Because it is slightly whiter than the surrounding intestinal metaplasia and because the area is fairly large, cancer is suspected. Spraying indigo carmine clarifies that the lesion has no surface irregularities.

▶ Greater curvature of the angulus, 0-IIb, 8 mm, tub1, T1a (M), UL (−)

③ Carcinoma resembling gastritis (Figs. 42 & 43)

Occasionally, a type of gastric cancer may be encountered which can be described as "gastritis resembling carcinoma"[38]. In this case, it is difficult to differentiate between gastritis and gastric cancer. Generally, this type of cancer is a differentiated-type gastric cancer arising from severe gastritis. It is necessary to spray indigo carmine to observe in detail the changes in the mucosal surface structure.

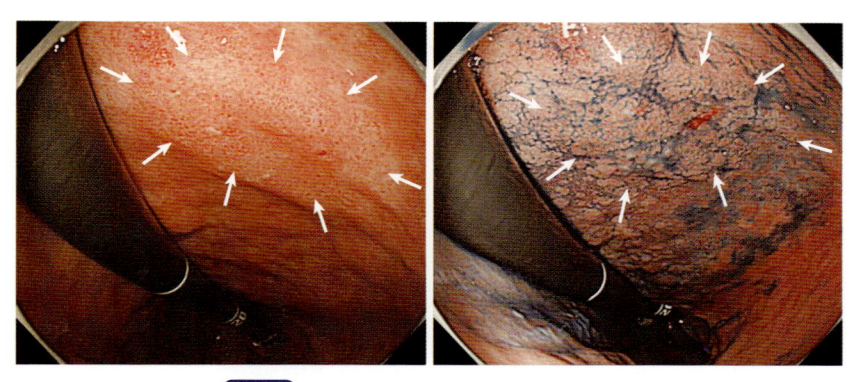

Fig. 42 Gastritis resembling carcinoma ①

Diffuse redness and atrophy are observed in the background mucosa. In addition, mucosa that is slightly more yellowish-white than the surrounding mucosa can also be seen. The margins between the yellowish-white mucosa and the surrounding mucosa are not clear. When indigo carmine is sprayed, a rough, finely granular mucosal structure is exhibited, while the margins become a little easier to distinguish. The fact that the indigo carmine spraying has induced bleeding adds to the likelihood of cancer.

▶ Posterior wall of the lower body, 0–IIb, 20 mm, tub1, T1a (M), UL (−)

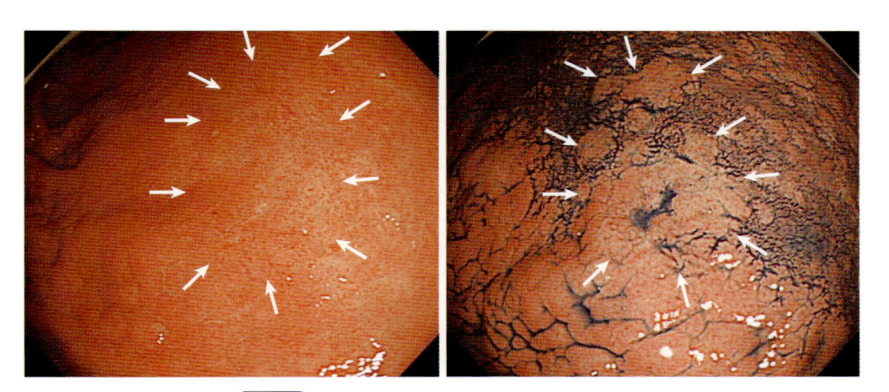

Fig. 43 Gastritis resembling carcinoma ②

Atrophy is recognized in the background mucosa. In conventional endoscopy, it is difficult to see the lesion; however, reddish spots that are slightly more conspicuous than the surrounding mucosal surface can be seen on the atrophic side of the atrophic border. When indigo carmine is sprayed, the lesion can be identified as the area where the fine mucosal patterns produced by atrophy have disappeared.

▶ Anterior wall of the middle body, 0–IIb, 18 mm, tub1, T1a (M), UL (−)

III Indigo carmine — a magic potion that unveils hidden cancers

A surprisingly large number of lesions can be found by spraying indigo carmine. The time from spraying to observation only takes 30 seconds to a minute. It is recommended that you spray indigo carmine when observing any area where atrophy or intestinal metaplasia is present.

Lesions that can be detected by spraying indigo carmine

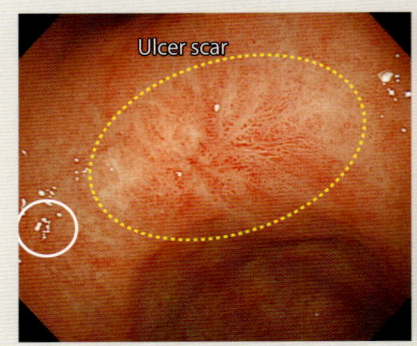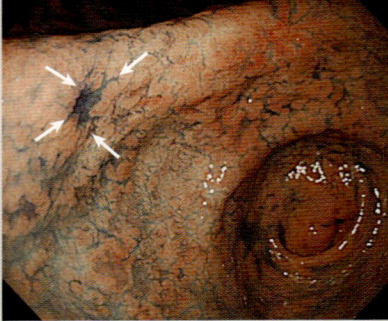

Fig. 44
The background is atrophic mucosa, and an ulcer scar (inside the yellow dotted-line circle) can be seen in the lesser curvature of the angulus. In conventional endoscopy, the cancer (inside the white solid-line circle) cannot be detected. When indigo carmine is sprayed, a depressive lesion accompanied by thorn-like encroachment (indicated by the arrows) becomes visible, making possible diagnosis of differentiated-type cancer.
▶ Anterior wall of the angulus, 0–IIc, 5 mm, tub1, T1a (M), UL (–)

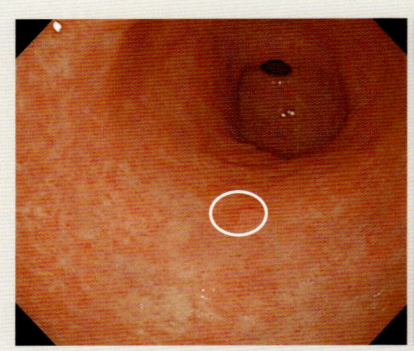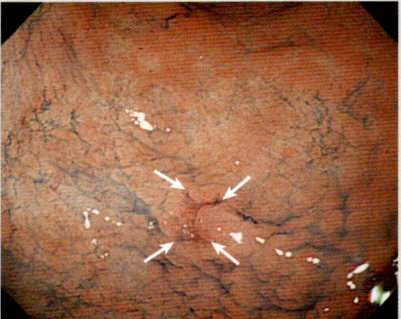

Fig. 45
The background mucosa is atrophic with conspicuous irregularities on the surface. Although the irregularities shown in the circle were visible in conventional endoscopy, the lesion was not noticeable because of irregularities in the surrounding area. Spraying indigo carmine made it possible to recognize the depressed lesion (indicated by the arrows) accompanied by thorn-like encroachment within the irregularities, making it possible to diagnose the lesion as differentiated-type cancer.
▶ Greater curvature of the antrum, 0–IIc, 4 mm, tub1, T1a (M), UL (–)

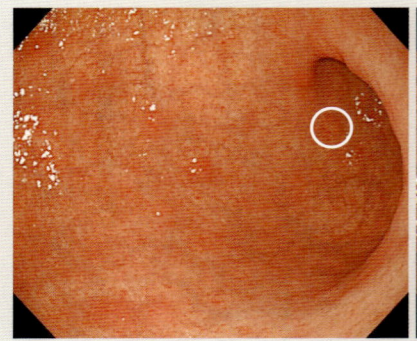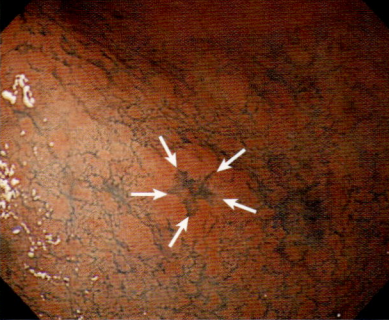

Fig. 46
The background is atrophic mucosa, and multiple erythematous patches are present. In conventional endoscopy, the cancer shown in the circle could not be seen. However, when indigo carmine was sprayed, a thorn-like encroachment (indicated by the arrows) could be seen in an erythematous patch on the anterior wall of the greater curvature of the angulus, allowing diagnosis of differentiated-type cancer.
▶ Anterior wall of the greater curvature of the angulus, 0–IIc, 4 mm, tub1, T1a (M), UL (–)

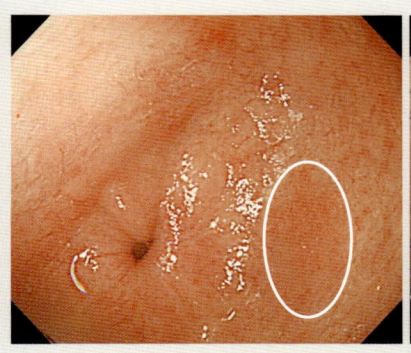
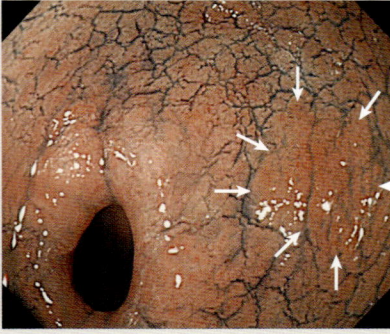

Fig. 47

Although erythematous mucosa (in the circle) can be seen on the posterior wall of the antrum in conventional endoscopy, no signs of cancer are visible. Spraying indigo carmine obscures the areae gastricae at the site of the lesion, while highlighting the finely granular mucosal structure (indicated by the arrows). Consequently, it can be diagnosed as cancer.

▶ Posterior wall of the prepyloric region, 0–IIb, 6 mm, tub1, T1a (M), UL (–)

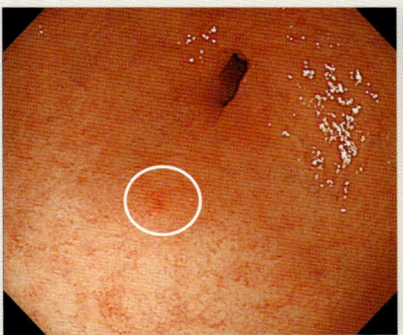
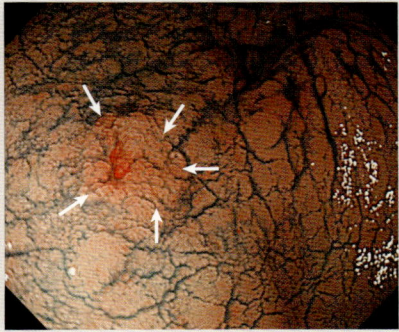

Fig. 48

There was atrophic mucosa in the background, and the lesion in the circle could not be recognized. Despite inducing bleeding, spraying indigo carmine made it possible to observe the minute changes (indicated by the arrows) on the surface of the mucosa, clarifying that the lesion exhibited a more finely granular morphology than the surrounding area. As for the color tone, the redness became more prominent.

▶ Greater curvature of the angulus, 0–IIb, 3 mm, tub1, T1a (M), UL (–)

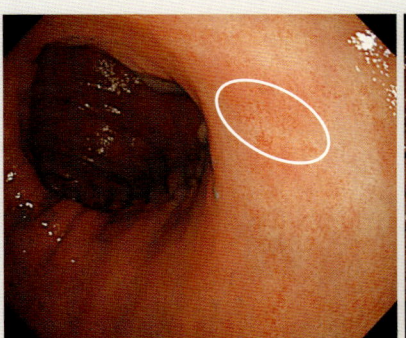
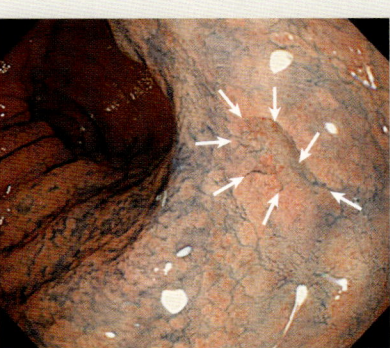

Fig. 49

After distal gastrectomy and Roux-en-Y reconstruction for gastric cancer, the background mucosa exhibits atrophy and intestinal metaplasia. Slightly whitish mucosa (in the circle) can be seen on the posterior wall of the body in conventional endoscopy; however, it cannot be distinguished from intestinal metaplasia. Spraying indigo carmine makes it possible to see the depressed surface (indicated by the arrows) and clarifies the margins.

▶ Posterior wall of the body of remnant stomach, 0–IIb, 6 mm, tub1>tub2, T1a (M), UL (–)

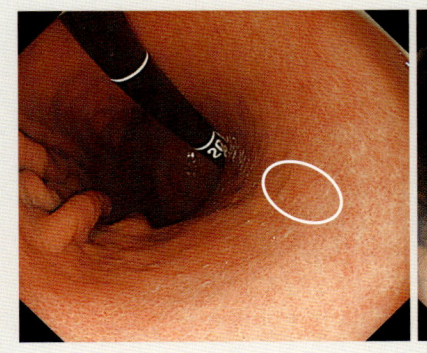
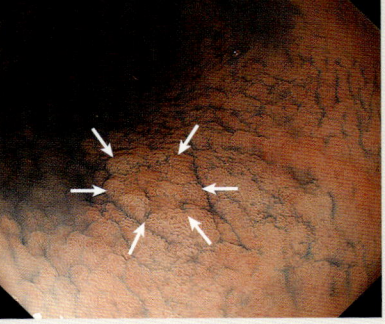

Fig. 50

The background mucosa exhibits atrophy and intestinal metaplasia. Even though minor surface irregularities (in the circle) exist near the anterior wall of the lesser curvature of the lower body, it is difficult to confirm that this site is a lesion. Spraying indigo carmine makes it possible to recognize it as a flat elevated lesion with its center slightly depressed (indicated by the arrows).

▶ Lesser curvature of the lower body, 0–IIa, 7 mm, tub1>tub2, T1a (M), UL (–)

Washing away gastric mucus

Mucus on the surface of gastric mucosa is one of the reasons why gastric cancer may go undetected. If the mucus and bubbles attached to the stomach lining are not carefully washed off, not only are minute lesions likely to be missed but so are larger lesions. Moreover, indigo carmine sticks to the mucus, making it impossible to observe the mucosal surface structure. Therefore, it is important to wash away mucus thoroughly before indigo carmine is sprayed.

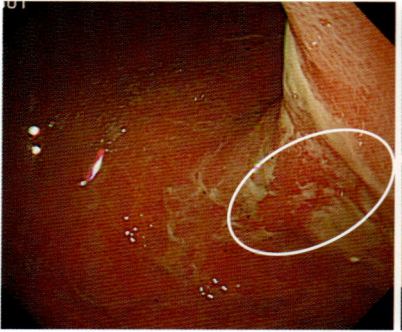 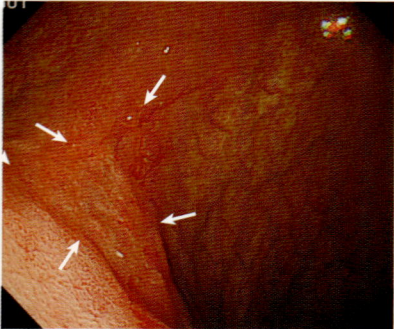

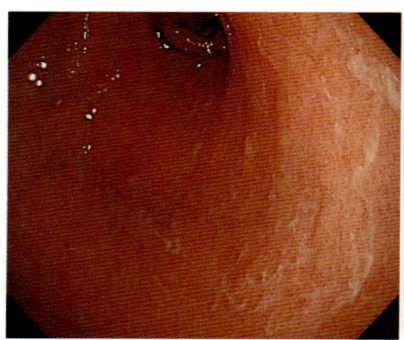 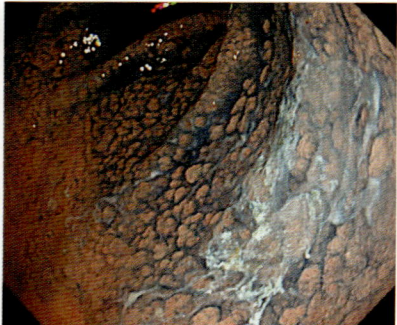

[Gastric cancer made visible after mucus has been removed]

· This case has a current *H. pylori* infection with substantial attachment of mucus. It is difficult to see the gastric cancer until the mucus is washed away as shown in the photo on the left. Once the mucus has been thoroughly washed off, the lesion becomes visible as shown in the picture on the right.

▶ Posterior wall of the upper body, 0–IIc, 30 mm, tub1>tub2, T1b (SM), UL (+)

· If indigo carmine is sprayed when mucus is attached to the surface, mucus sticks to the indigo carmine, making it impossible to clearly image the area gastrica patterns.

Generally, the stomach lining is washed with tap water mixed with a small amount of Gascon® in a 20-ml syringe. The cleaning fluid is injected from the instrument port of an endoscope. However, this method can be problematic when there is a large amount of mucus. At the Cancer Institute Hospital of JFCR, we use the Water Please® endoscopic irrigation system to wash the interior of the stomach. At the press of a foot pedal, irrigation at 700 ml/minute is possible. The interior of the stomach can be washed efficiently, and once you have used this, you won't want to perform a procedure without it.

The secret to effective washing is to wash the interior of the stomach thoroughly. Advance the endoscope as far as the antrum and wash thoroughly. Then while retroflexing the endoscope and pulling it to the proximal side, wash the body and fornix. Keeping the scope retroflexed, suction the irrigation fluid that has collected in the greater curvature of the upper body while being careful not to damage the mucosal surface. Once the stomach has been thoroughly cleaned, you can begin observation inside the stomach.

Washing a friable lesion like a cancerous lesion with strong water pressure may cause bleeding, making extent diagnosis and magnifying observation more difficult. Keep in mind that a friable lesion must be washed gently or its peripheries washed first before washing the lesion.

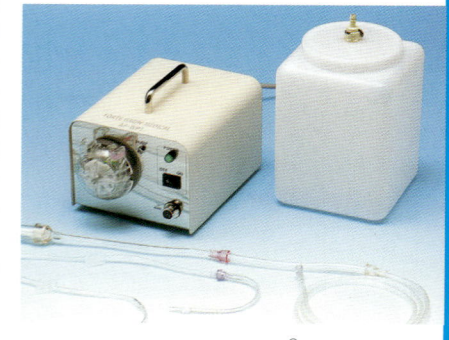

Water Please®
(mfd. by Forte Grow Medical)

Chapter III

Where's the Gastric Cancer?
— Detection and diagnosis —

- To treat gastric cancer endoscopically, you first have to find a lesion that's still at an early stage.
- Finding a lesion can be quite difficult, however, as they are sometimes hidden in the background gastritis.
- Skill and experience also play a role. Different doctors can view the exact same image and some will spot the cancer and some won't.
- Can you find the hidden cancerous lesion? Please also try to predict the size and histological type of the cancer.
- All the pictures show the cancer at the time of discovery. Nothing has been affected by biopsy. (Note, however, that some simultaneous multiple lesions were previously biopsied.)
- Also think about the presence/absence of *H. pylori* infection.

1

Screening endoscopy at the cancer screening center ①

▶ Male in his 60s.
▶ A screening endoscopy was performed at the Cancer Screening Center of the Cancer Institute Hospital.

Can you specify the location of the gastric cancer?

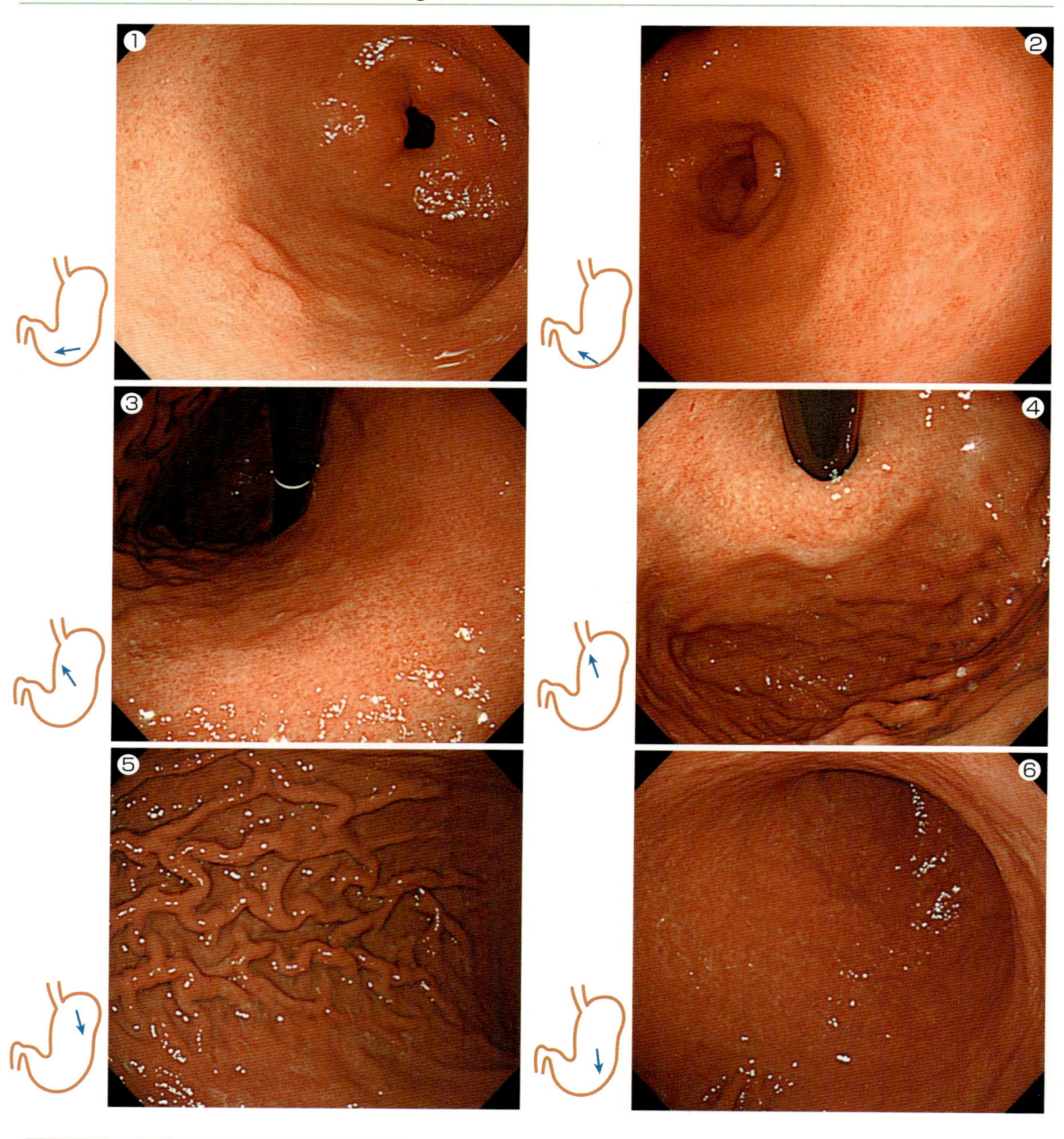

> **Hint** 💡 Pay attention to surface irregularities in the mucosa.

The answer and diagnosis are on page 124.

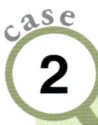
Screening endoscopy at the cancer screening center ②

▶ Male in his 60s.

▶ A screening endoscopy was performed at the Cancer Screening Center of the Cancer Institute Hospital.

Can you specify the location of the gastric cancer?

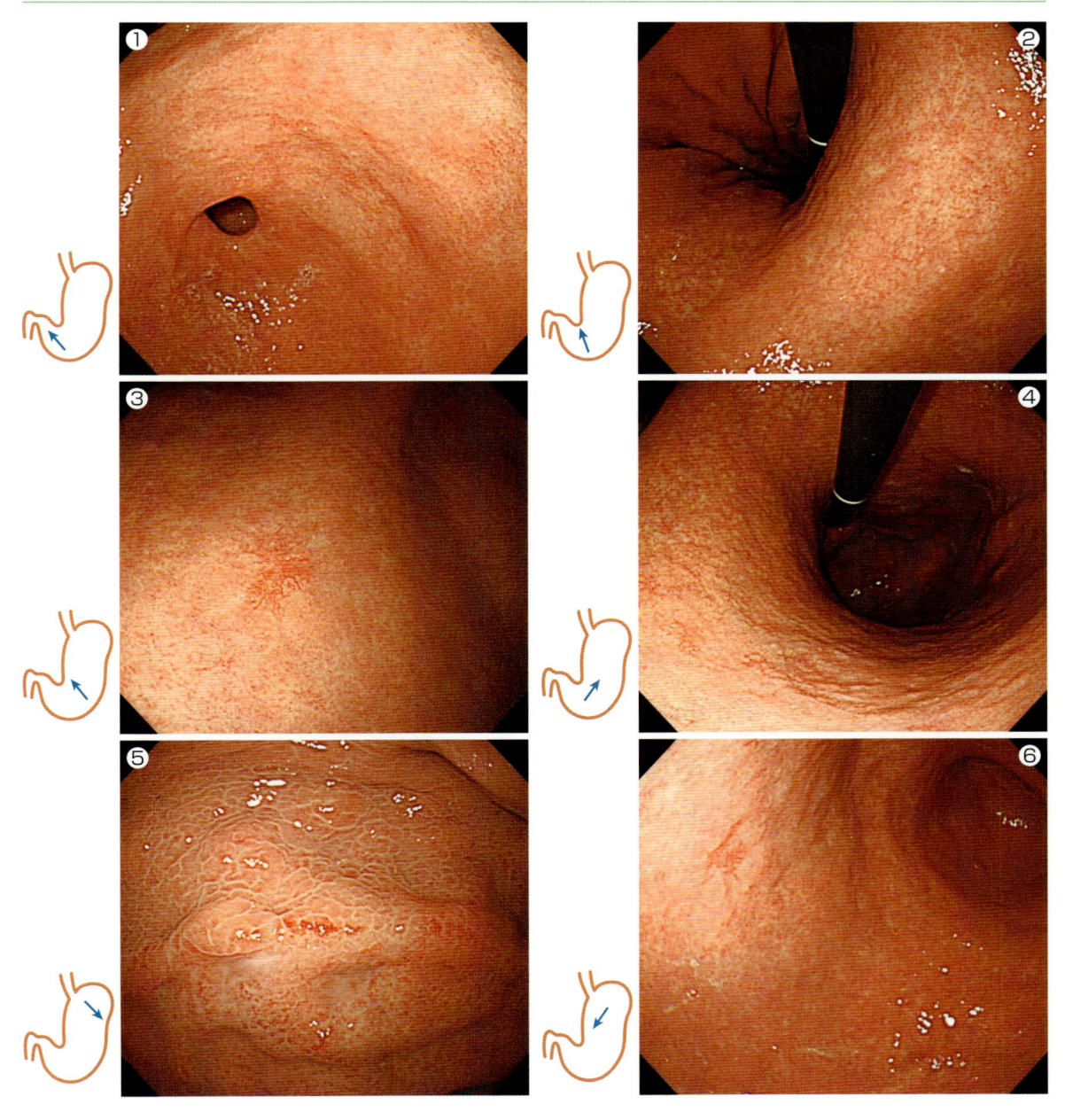

Hint Look for an erythematous depression that looks conspicuous to you.

The answer and diagnosis are on page 126.

Screening endoscopy at the cancer screening center ③

▶ Male in his 40s.
▶ A screening endoscopy was performed at the Cancer Screening Center of the Cancer Institute Hospital.
▶ No history of *H. pylori* eradication, serum anti-*H. pylori* antibodies negative, urea breath test negative, serum pepsinogen test method negative.

Can you specify the location of the gastric cancer?

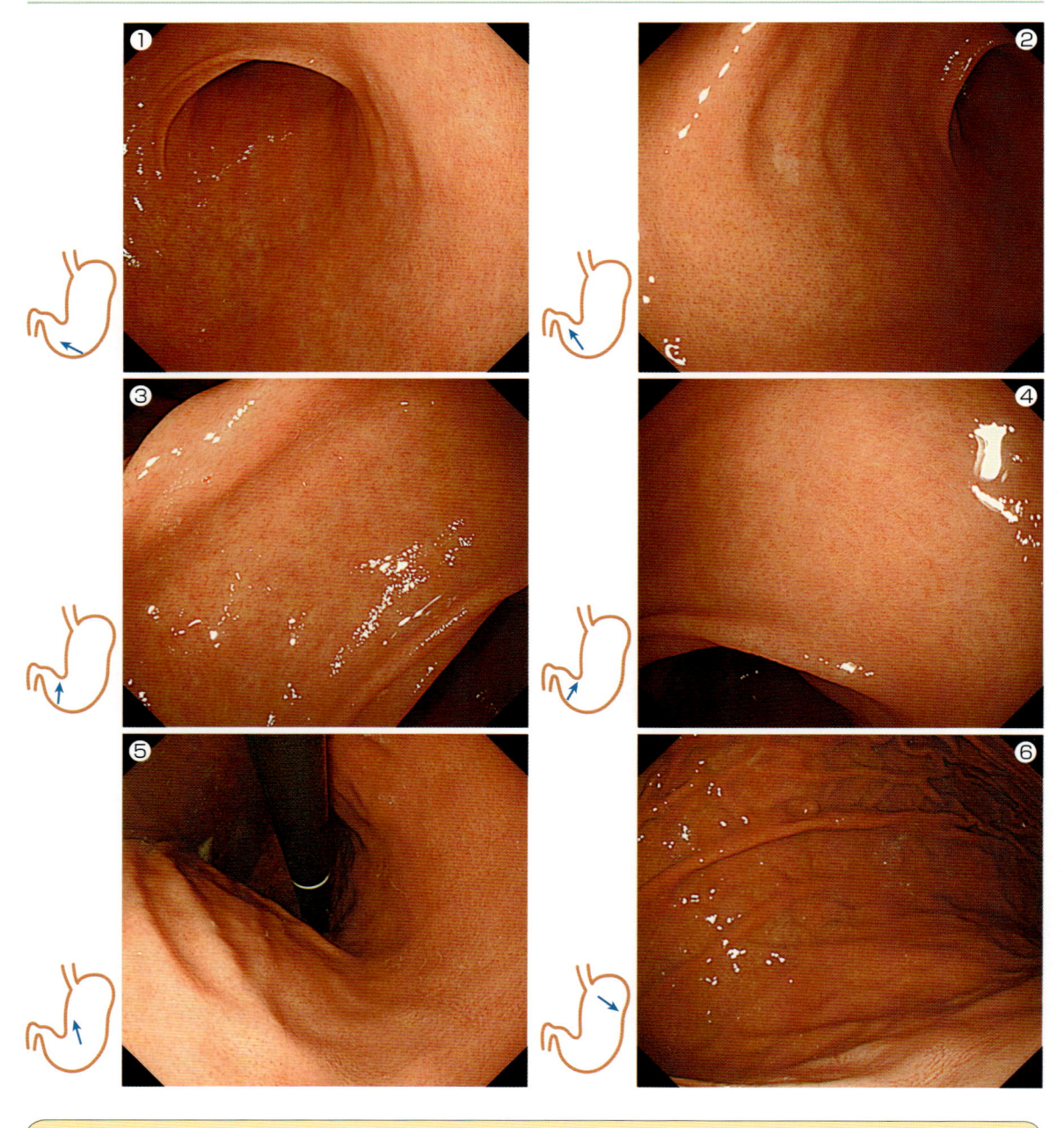

> **Hint** 💡   Look for fading.

The answer and diagnosis are on page 127.

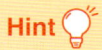

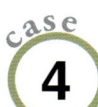

case 4

Screening endoscopy at the cancer screening center ④

- ▶ Male in his 70s.
- ▶ A screening endoscopy was performed at the Cancer Screening Center of the Cancer Institute Hospital. The patient was under PPI medication for long periods due to GERD.
- ▶ No history of *H. pylori* eradication, serum anti-*H. pylori* antibodies negative, urea breath test negative, serum pepsinogen test method negative.

Can you specify the location of the gastric cancer?

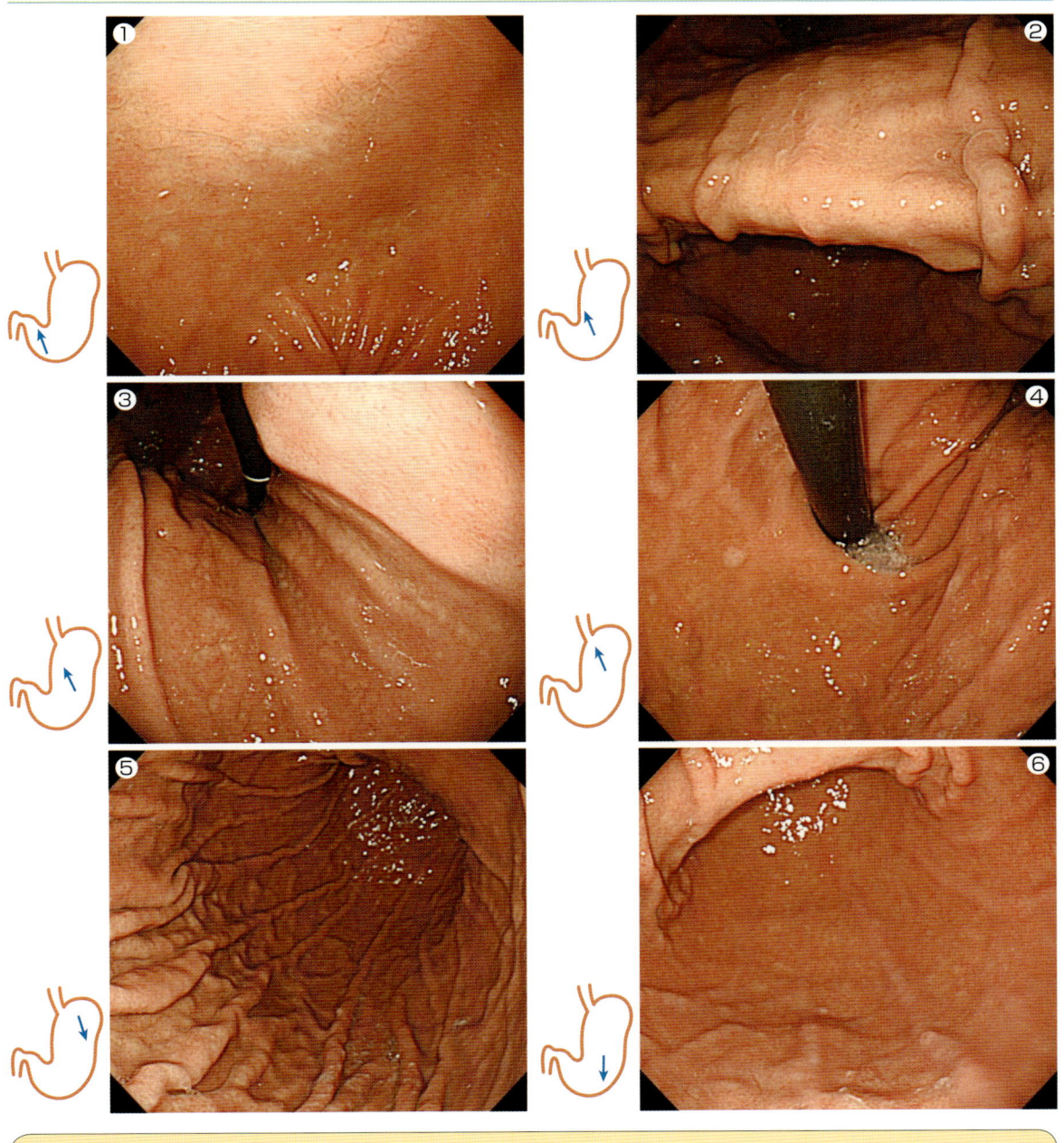

| Hint 💡 | Look for fading. |

The answer and diagnosis are on page 129.

73

Screening endoscopy at the cancer screening center ⑤

- ▶ Male in his 40s.
- ▶ A screening endoscopy was performed at the Cancer Screening Center of the Cancer Institute Hospital.
- ▶ No history of *H. pylori* eradication, serum anti-*H. pylori* antibodies negative, urea breath test negative, serum pepsinogen test method negative.

Can you specify the location of the gastric cancer?

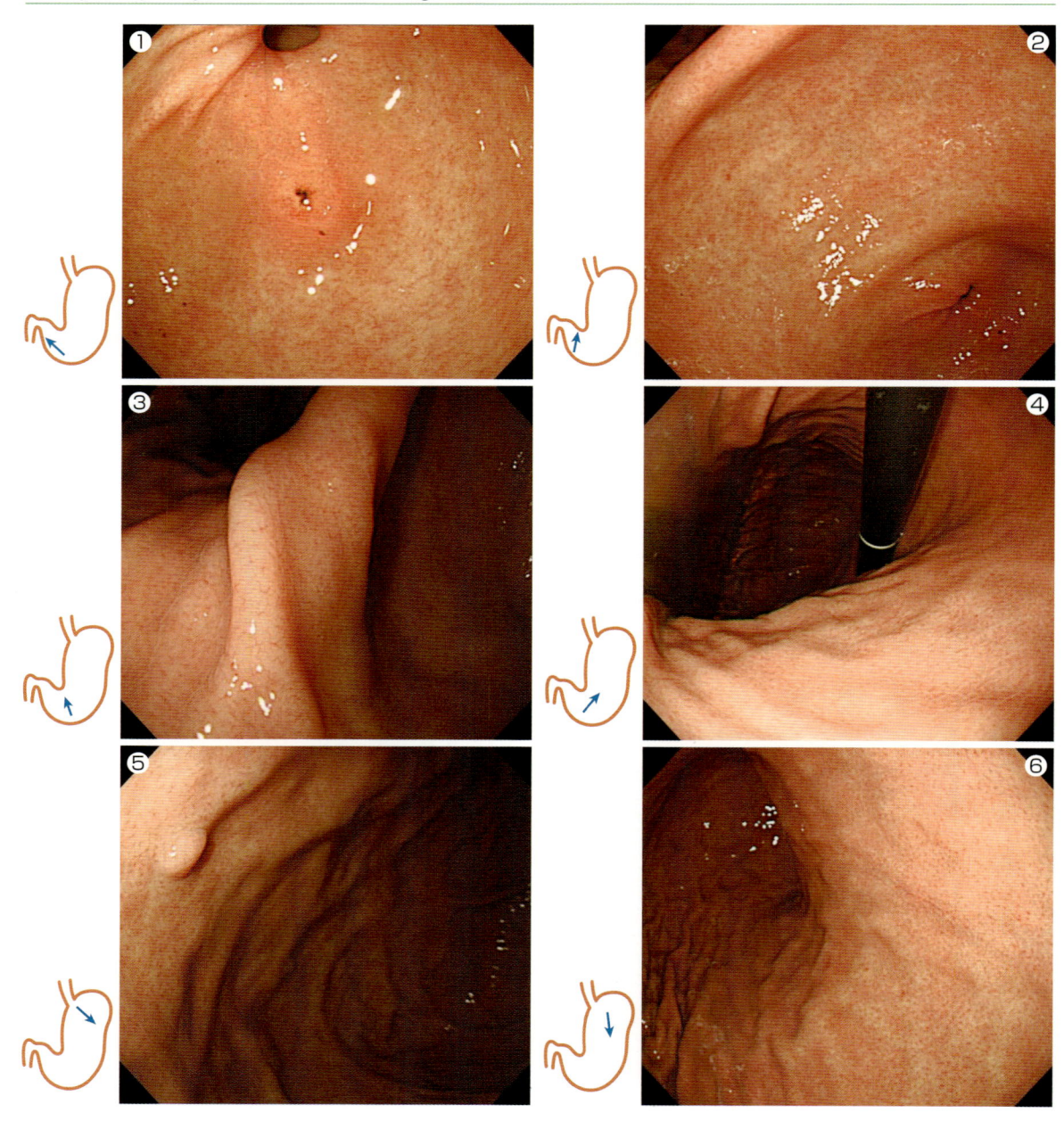

> **Hint** 💡   Pay attention to erosion that has occurred in a single location.

The answer and diagnosis are on page 131.

Screening endoscopy at the cancer screening center ⑥

▶ Male in his 40s.

▶ A screening endoscopy was performed at the Cancer Screening Center of the Cancer Institute Hospital.

Can you specify the location of the gastric cancer?

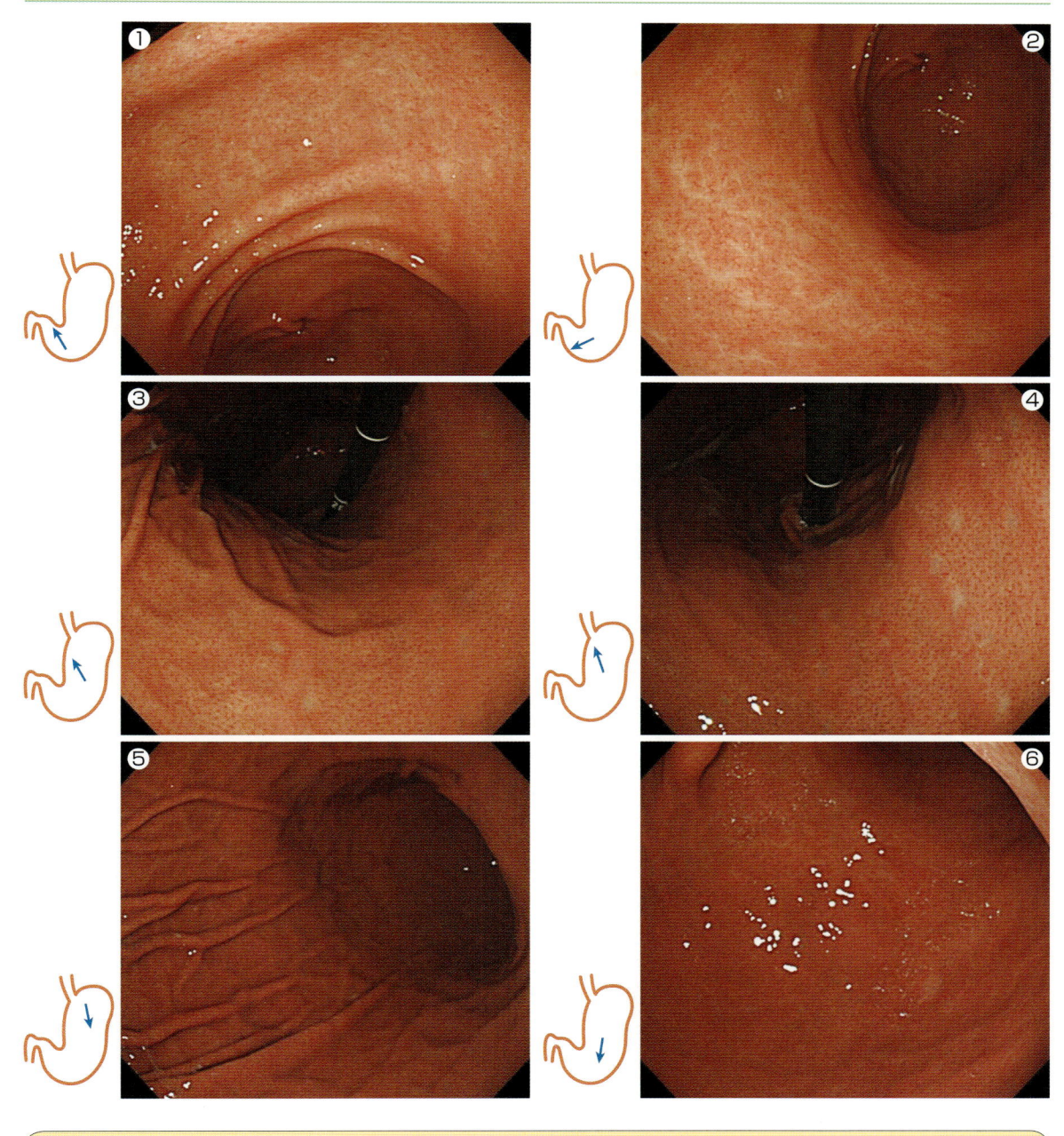

Hint 💡   Look for fading.

The answer and diagnosis are on page 132.

Screening endoscopy at the cancer screening center ⑦

▶ Female in her 50s.
▶ A screening endoscopy was performed at the Cancer Screening Center of the Cancer Institute Hospital.
▶ No history of *H. pylori* eradication, serum anti-*H. pylori* antibodies negative, urea breath test negative, serum pepsinogen test method negative.

Can you specify the location of the gastric cancer?

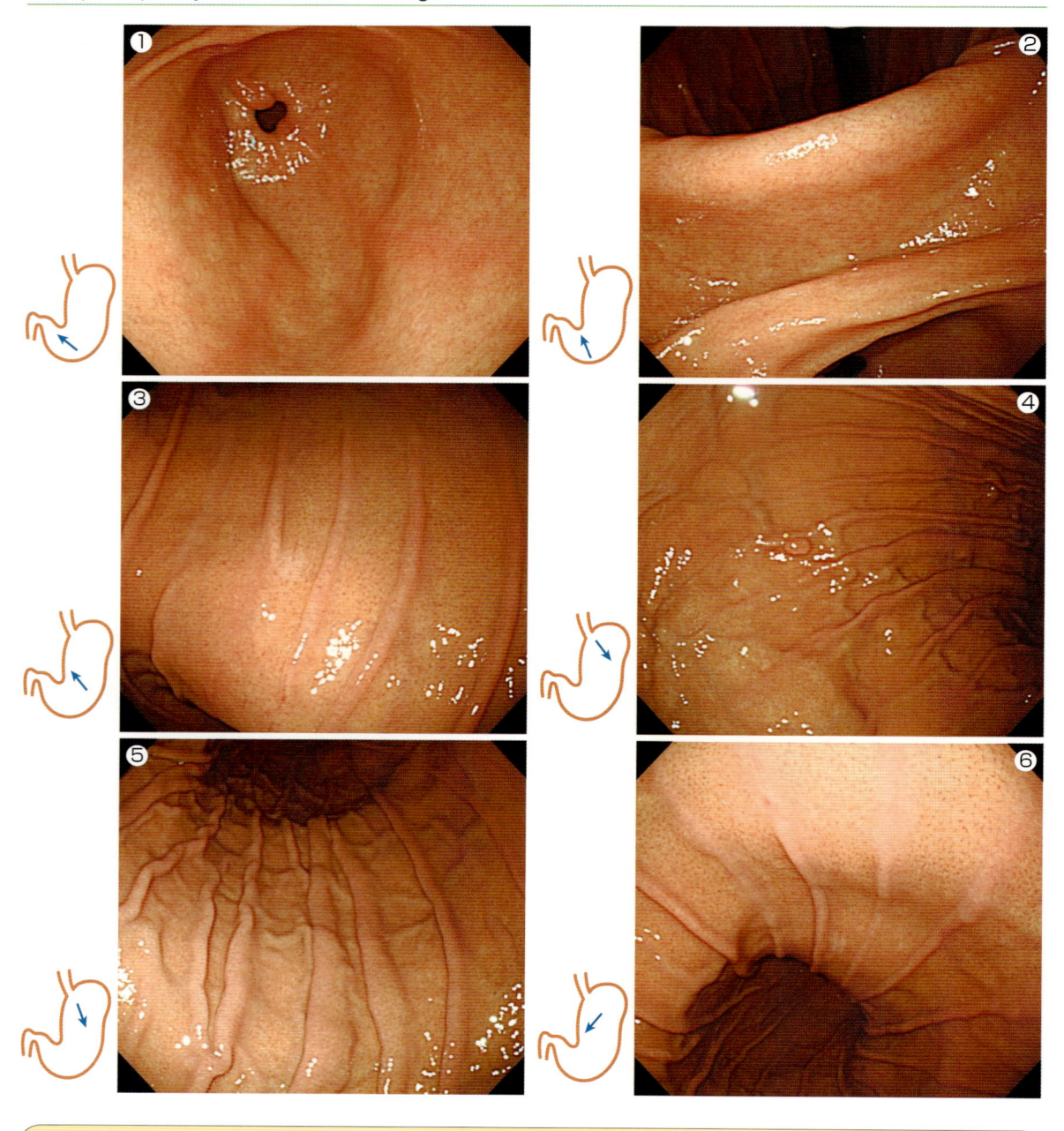

Hint 💡 Look for fading.

The answer and diagnosis are on page 133.

case 8

Screening endoscopy at the cancer screening center ⑧

- ▶ Male in his 60s.
- ▶ A screening endoscopy was performed at the Cancer Screening Center of the Cancer Institute Hospital.
- ▶ No history of *H. pylori* eradication, serum anti-*H. pylori* antibodies negative, urea breath test negative, serum pepsinogen test method negative.

Can you specify the location of the gastric cancer?

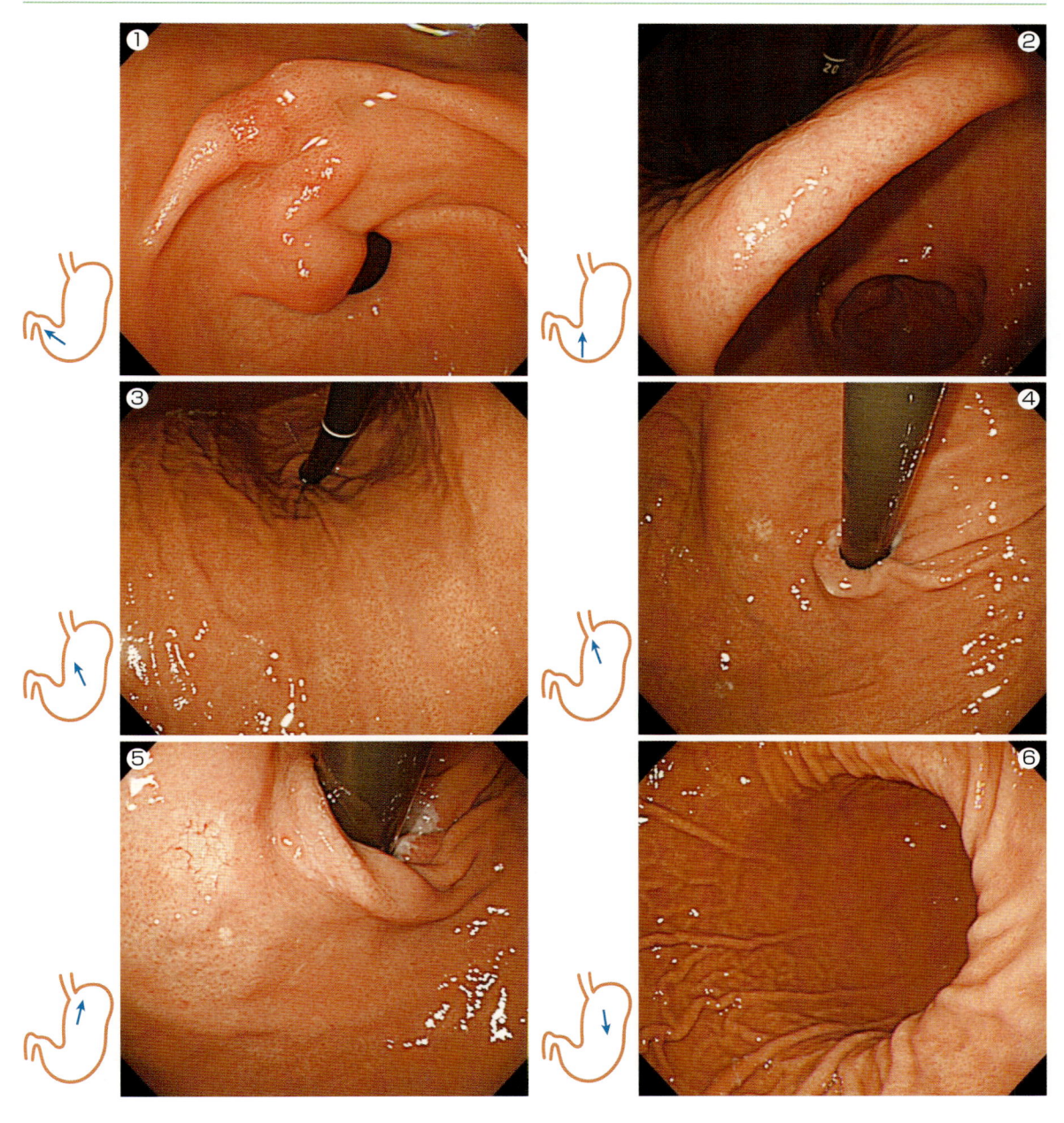

Hint    It's a special cancer.

The answer and diagnosis are on page 135.

Screening endoscopy at the cancer screening center ⑨

▶ Male in his 50s.

▶ A screening endoscopy was performed at the Cancer Screening Center of the Cancer Institute Hospital.

▶ No history of *H. pylori* eradication, serum anti-*H. pylori* antibodies negative, urea breath test negative, serum pepsinogen test method negative.

Can you specify the location of the gastric cancer?

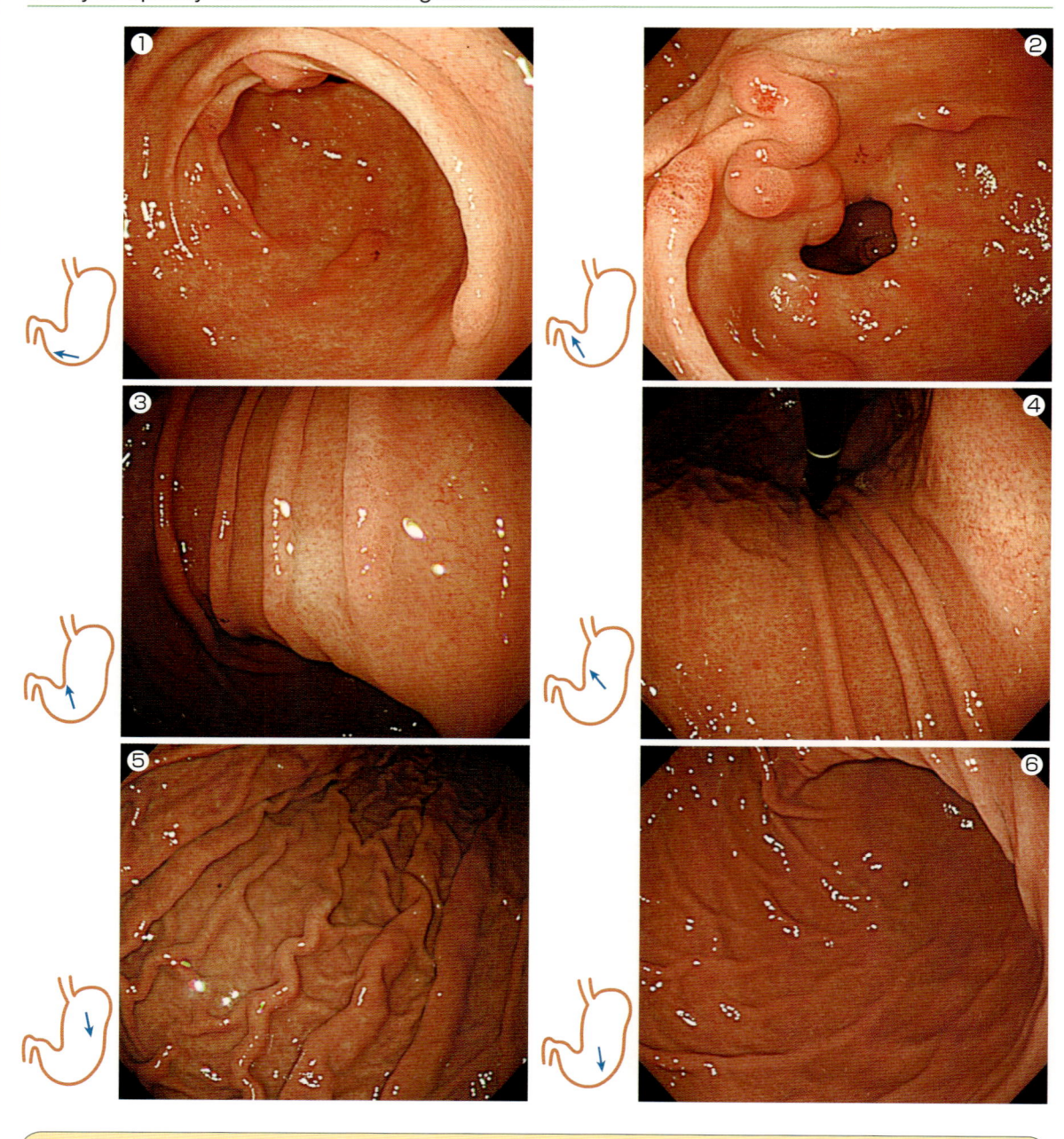

The answer and diagnosis are on page 138.

Hint 💡   Look for fading.

Screening endoscopy at the cancer screening center ⑩ :Young female with gastric cancer

▶ Female in her early 30s.
▶ A screening endoscopy was performed at the Cancer Screening Center of the Cancer Institute Hospital.

Can you specify the location of the gastric cancer?
What is the common histological type of gastric cancer found in young females?

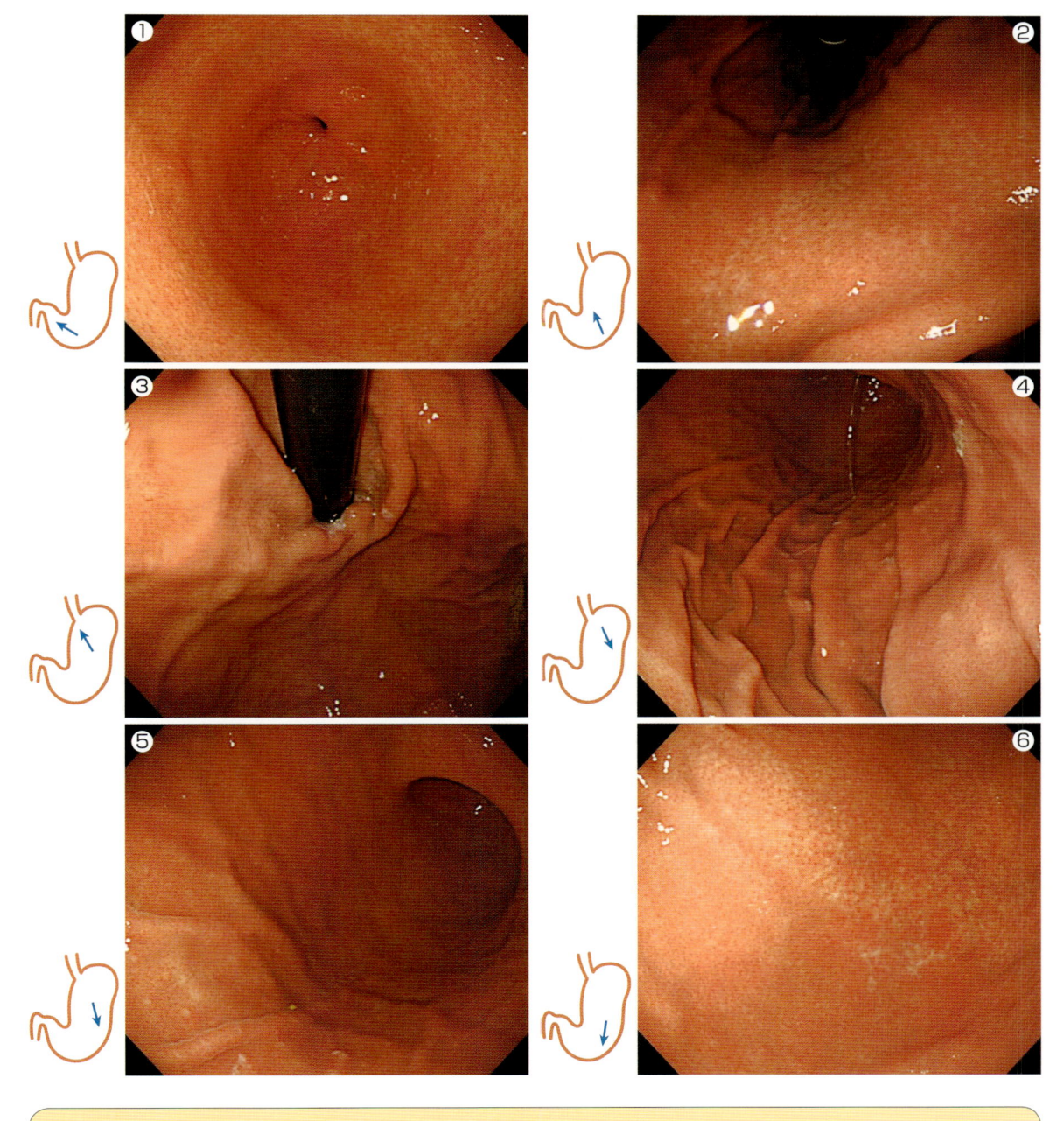

Hint Look for fading.

The answer and diagnosis are on page 139.

Screening endoscopy of chronic gastritis ①

▸ Male in his 60s.

▸ A screening endoscopy was performed for chronic gastritis.

▸ *H. pylori* had been eradicated 5 years previously.

Can you specify the location of the gastric cancer?

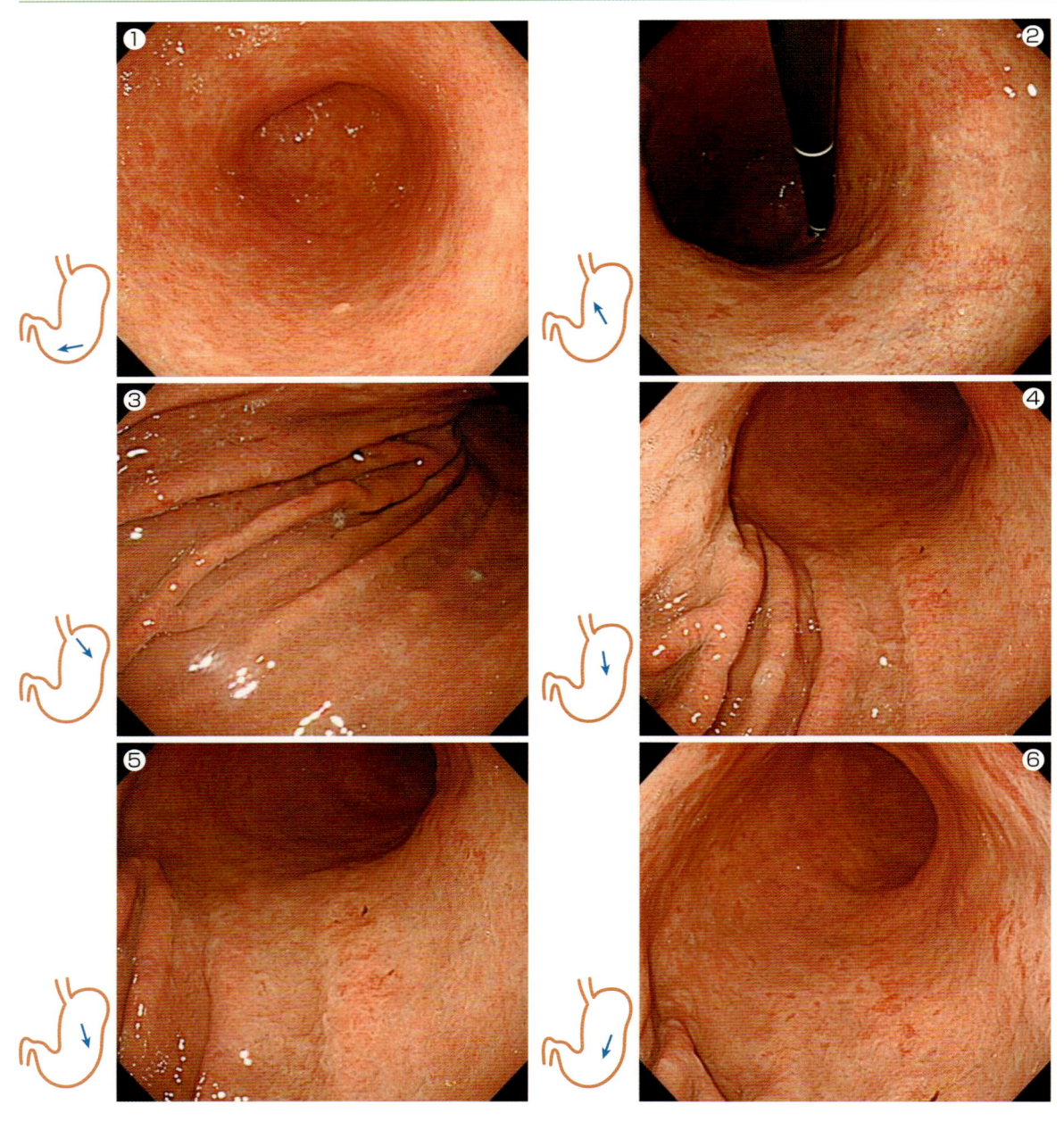

Hint 💡 The cancer is hidden among multiple erythematous depressions.

The answer and diagnosis are on page 141.

Screening endoscopy of chronic gastritis ②

- ▸ Female in her 80s.
- ▸ Screening endoscopies for chronic gastritis were performed each year.
- ▸ *H. pylori* had been eradicated 4 years previously.

Can you specify the locations of the 2 cancer lesions?

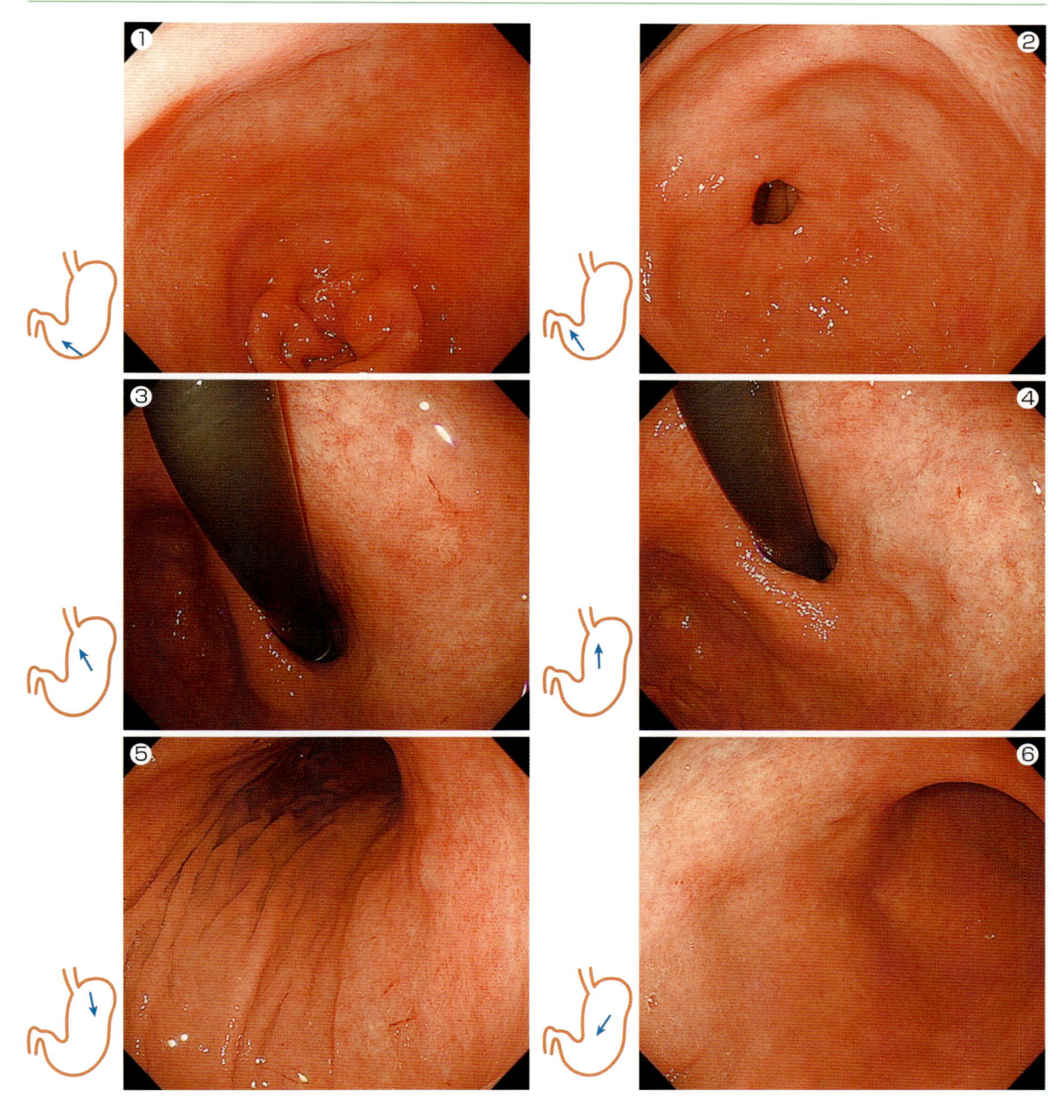

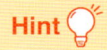 **Hint** 💡
- • Pay attention to subtle changes in color.
- • One of the lesions was missed in this examination.

The answer and diagnosis are on page 142.

Screening endoscopy of chronic gastritis ③

▸ Male in his 60s.

▸ A periodic screening endoscopy for chronic gastritis was performed.

Can you specify the location where a gastric tumor is suspected?

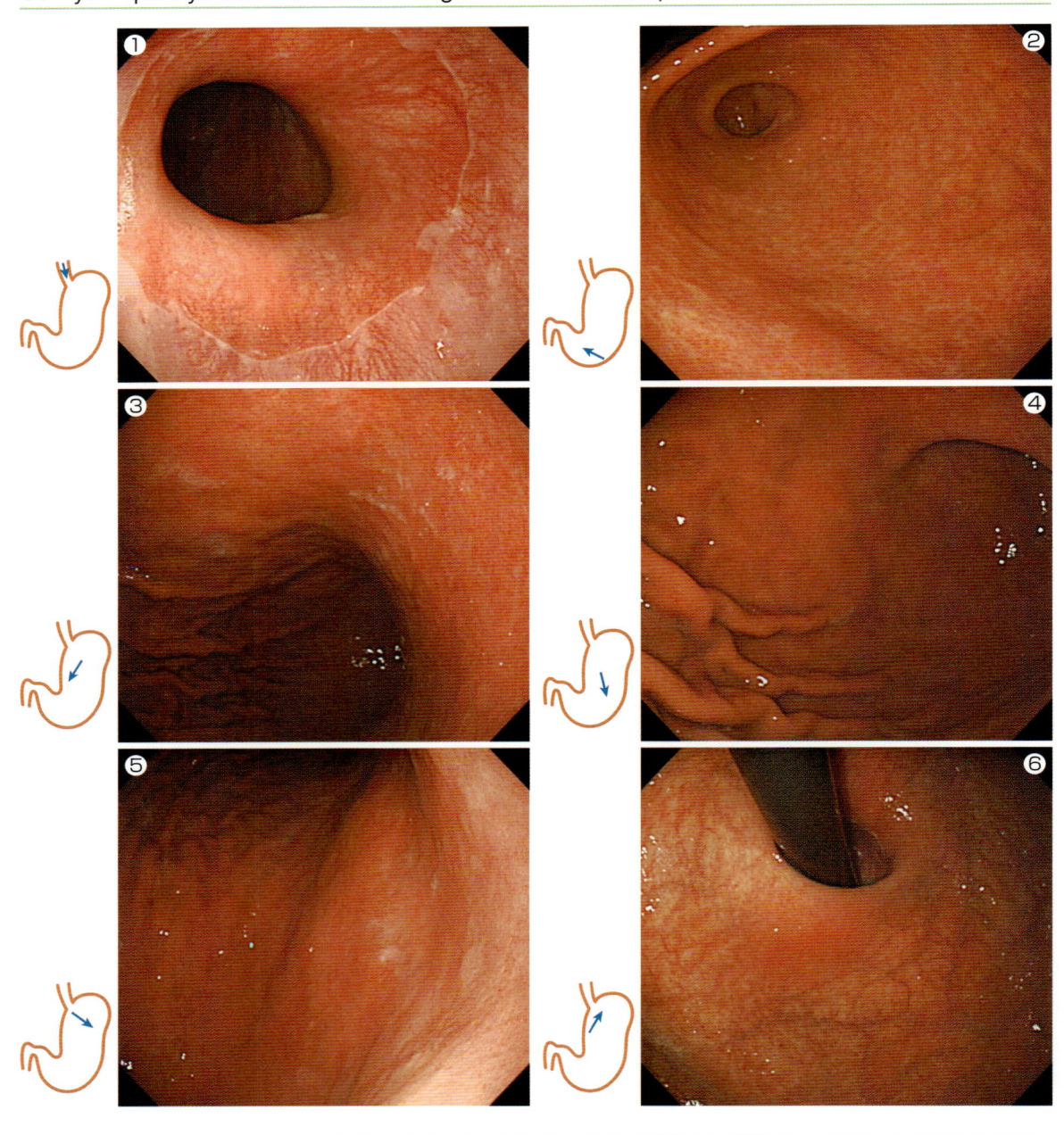

Hint 💡 Pay attention to disappearance of vascular patterns.

The answer and diagnosis are on page 144.

Screening endoscopy of chronic gastritis ④

- ▶ Male in his 50s.
- ▶ Chronic gastritis follow-up endoscopies were performed each year at the Cancer Screening Center of the Cancer Institute Hospital.
- ▶ *H. pylori* had been eradicated 5 years previously.

Can you specify the location of the gastric cancer?

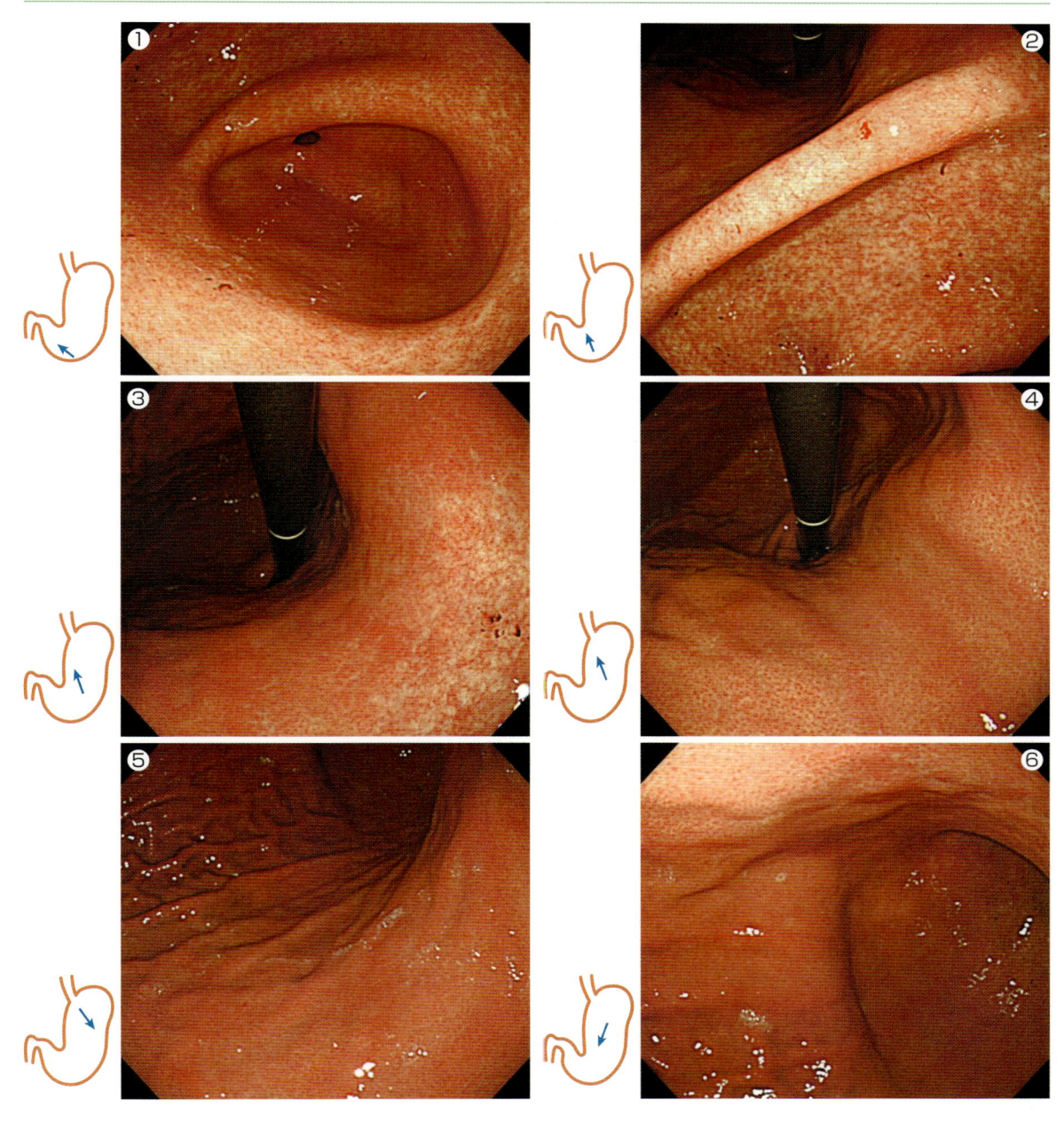

> **Hint** 💡 Look for findings that accompany gastric cancer.

The answer and diagnosis are on page 146.

Screening endoscopy of chronic gastritis ⑤

▸ Male in his 60s.

▸ He had a history of gastric ulcer. *H. pylori* had been eradicated a few years previously.

▸ A periodic screening endoscopy for chronic gastritis was performed.

Can you specify the location of the gastric cancer?

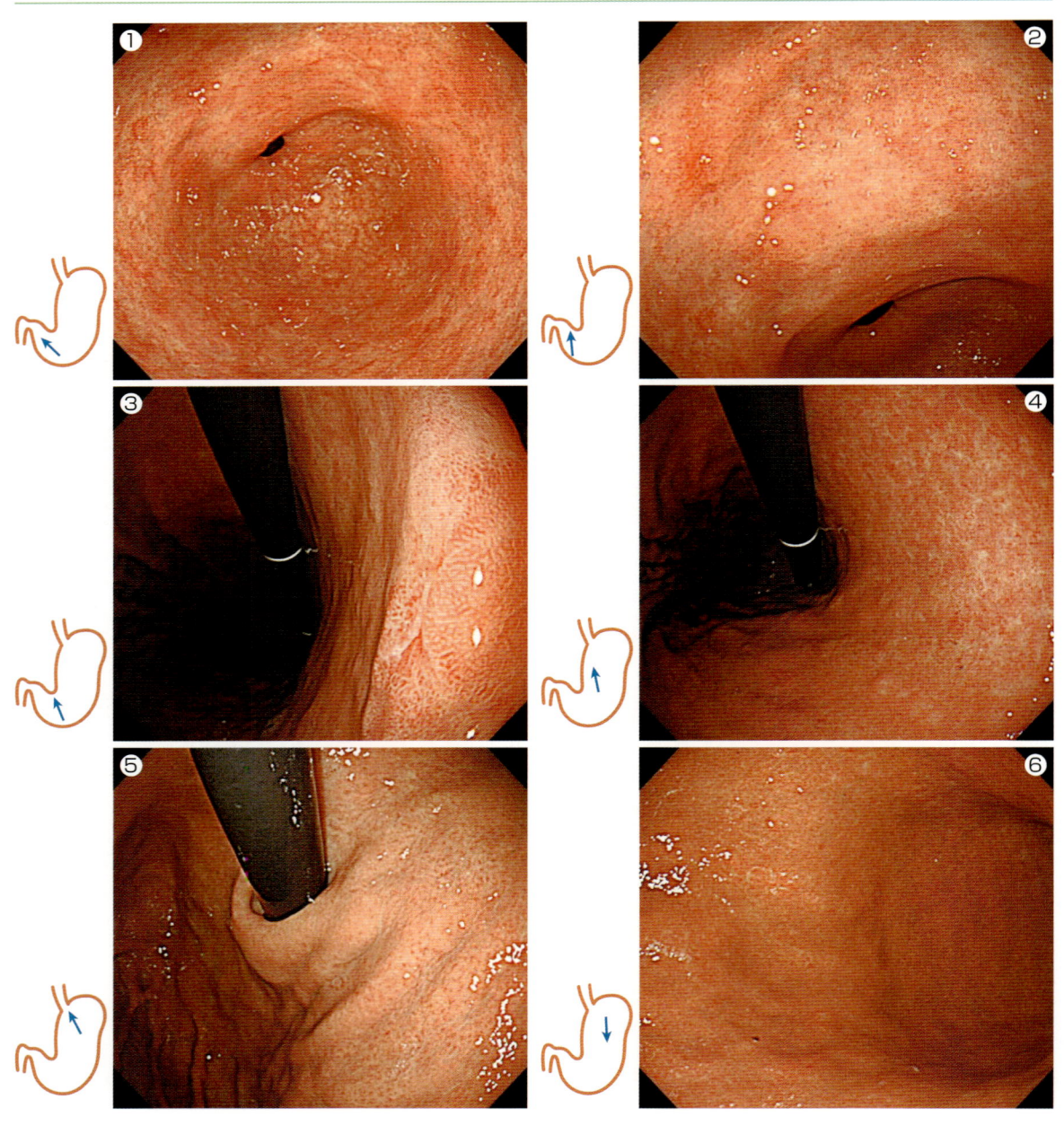

Hint 💡   Look for a conspicuous erythematous depression.

The answer and diagnosis are on page 148.

Patient complaining of stomach ache after eating

- ▶ Female in her 60s.
- ▶ An endoscopy was performed for detailed examination of stomach ache after eating.
- ▶ No history of *H. pylori* eradication, serum anti-*H. pylori* antibodies negative, urea breath test negative, serum pepsinogen test method negative.

Can you specify the location of the gastric cancer?

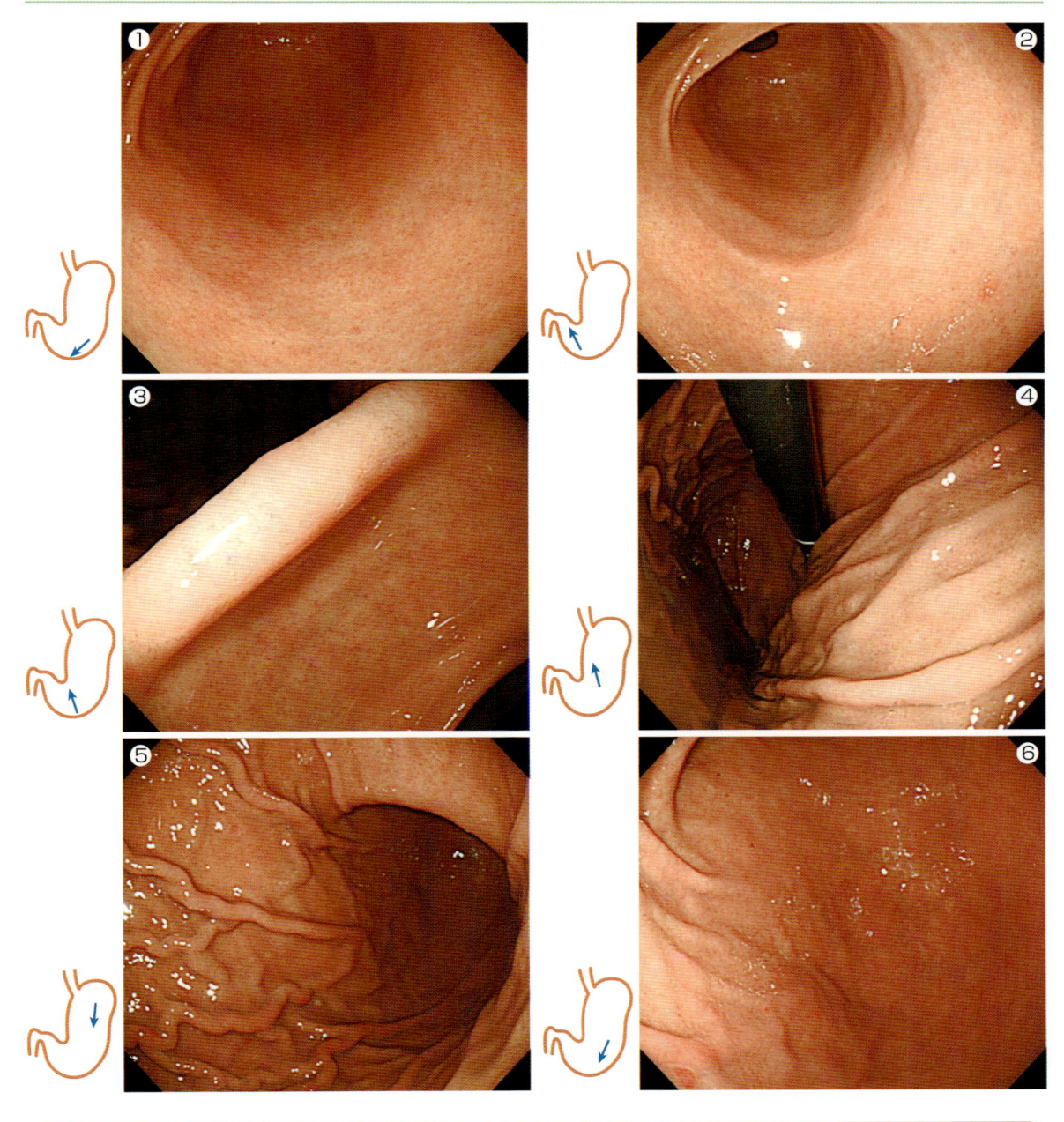

| Hint 💡 | Look for fading. |

The answer and diagnosis are on page 149.

17

Patient complaining of stomach discomfort

▶ Female in her 60s.

▶ The patient was complaining of stomach discomfort. An endoscopy was performed.

▶ No history of *H. pylori* eradication, serum anti-*H. pylori* antibodies negative, urea breath test negative, serum pepsinogen test method negative.

Can you specify the location of the gastric cancer?

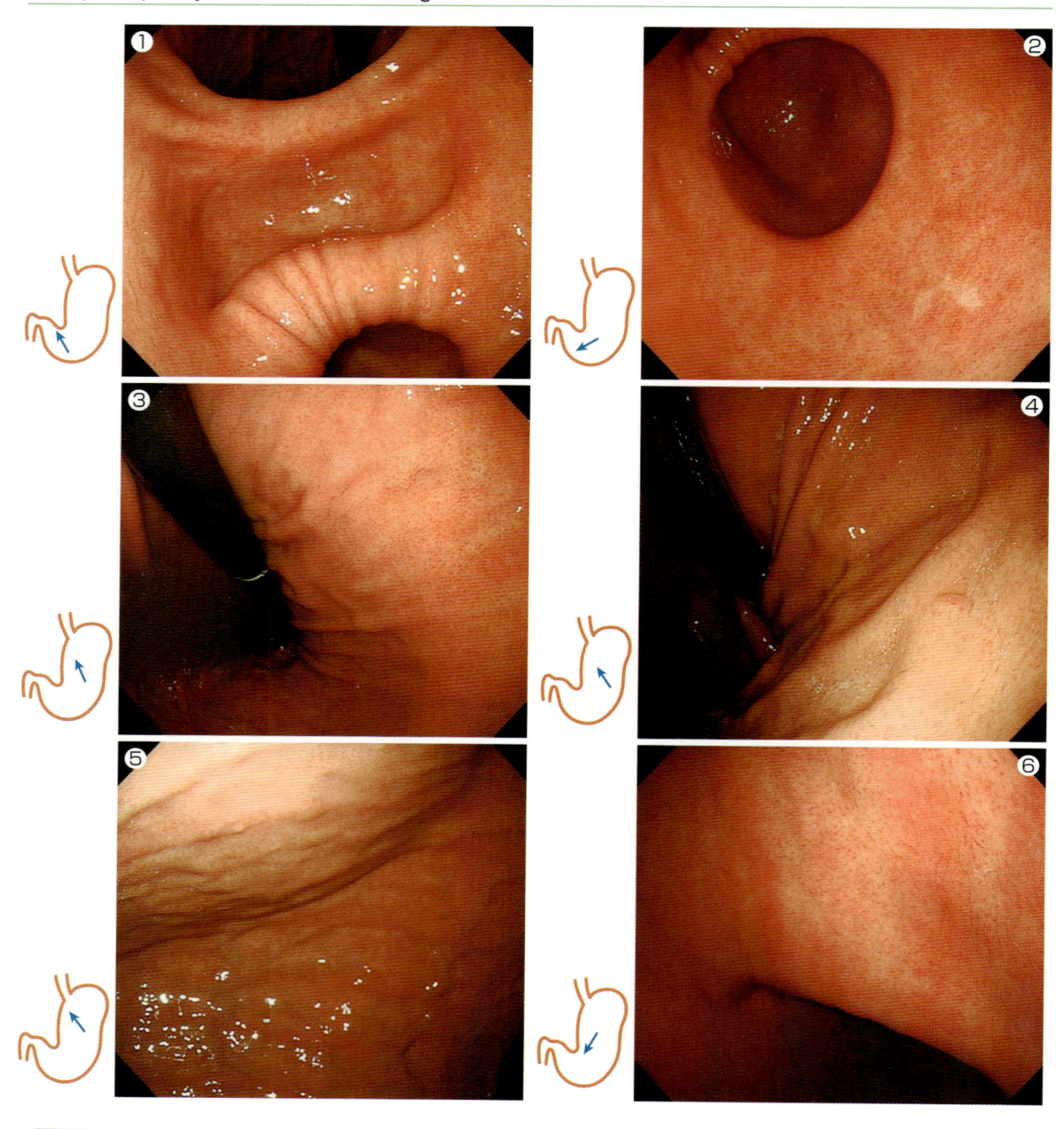

Hint 💡   Look for fading.

The answer and diagnosis are on page 150.

Patient complaining of heartburn

▶ Male in his 60s.

▶ A postoperative prostate cancer and lung cancer patient, he was complaining of heartburn.
An endoscopy was performed.

Can you find a malignant tumor?

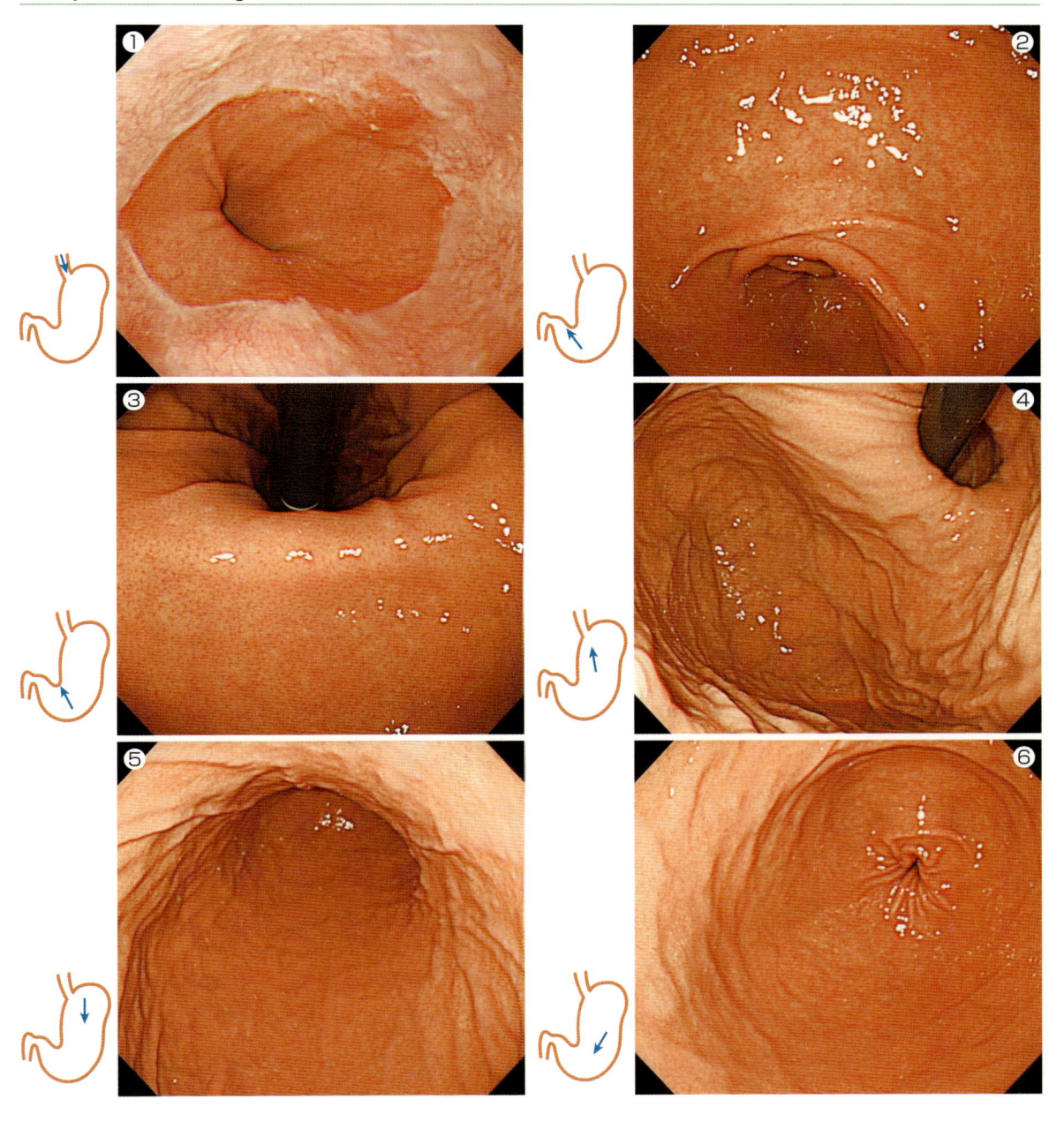

Hint 💡 Look for any redness.

The answer and diagnosis are on page 151.

Follow-up endoscopy for gastric adenoma

▸ Male in his 70s.

▸ A follow-up endoscopy was performed for gastric adenoma on the greater curvature of the antrum.

▸ *H. pylori* had been eradicated 5 years previously.

Can you find a lesion other than the adenoma on the greater curvature of the antrum?

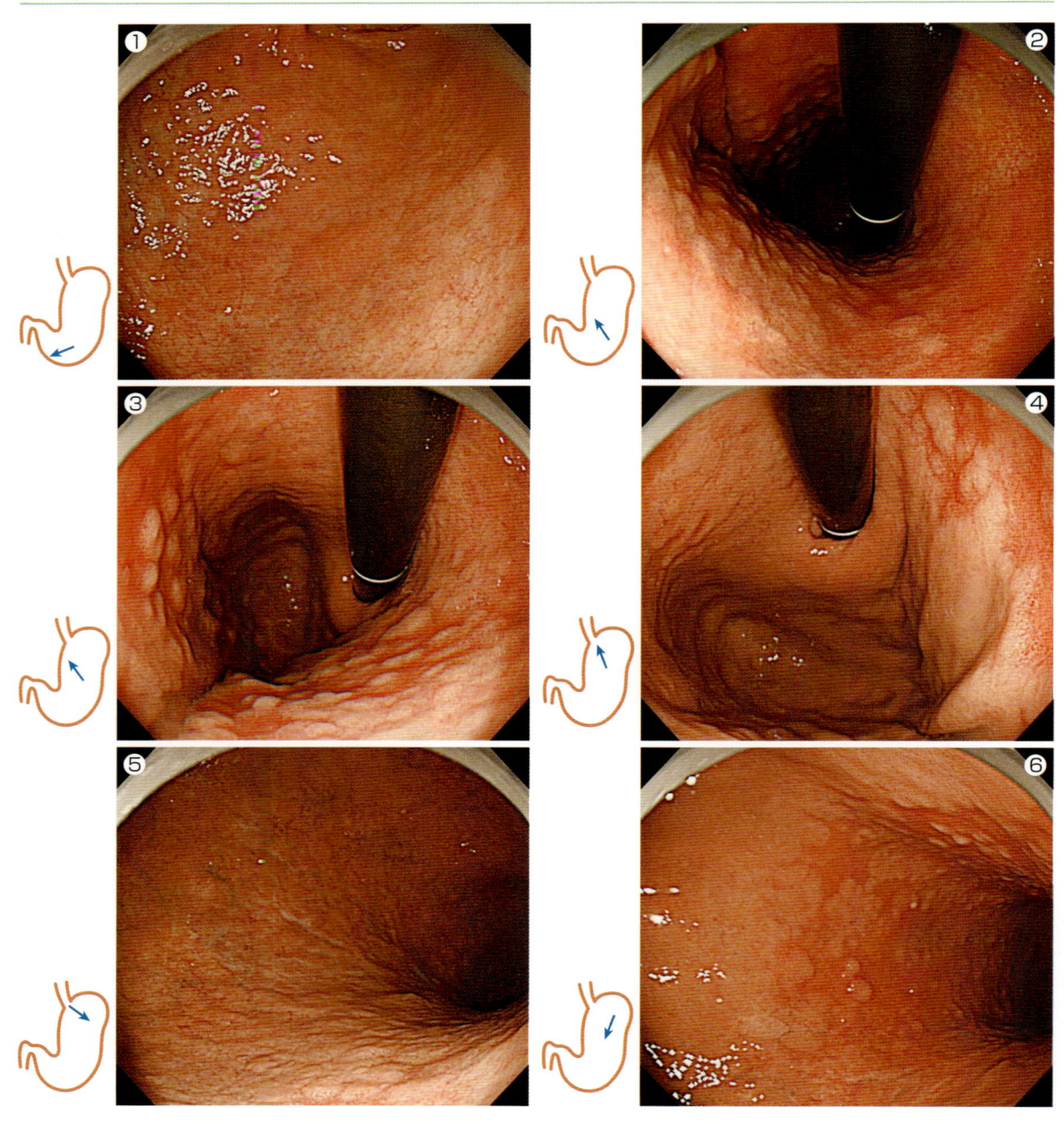

Hint 💡   Try to spot a lesion that is hidden in the gastritis.

The answer and diagnosis are on page 154.

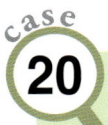

Patient referred to us after detection of superficial esophageal cancer

▶ Male in his 70s.
▶ Diagnosed with superficial esophageal cancer and referred to our hospital.

Can you specify the location of the gastric cancer? Also try to elaborate on the pathological findings of the gastric polyps.

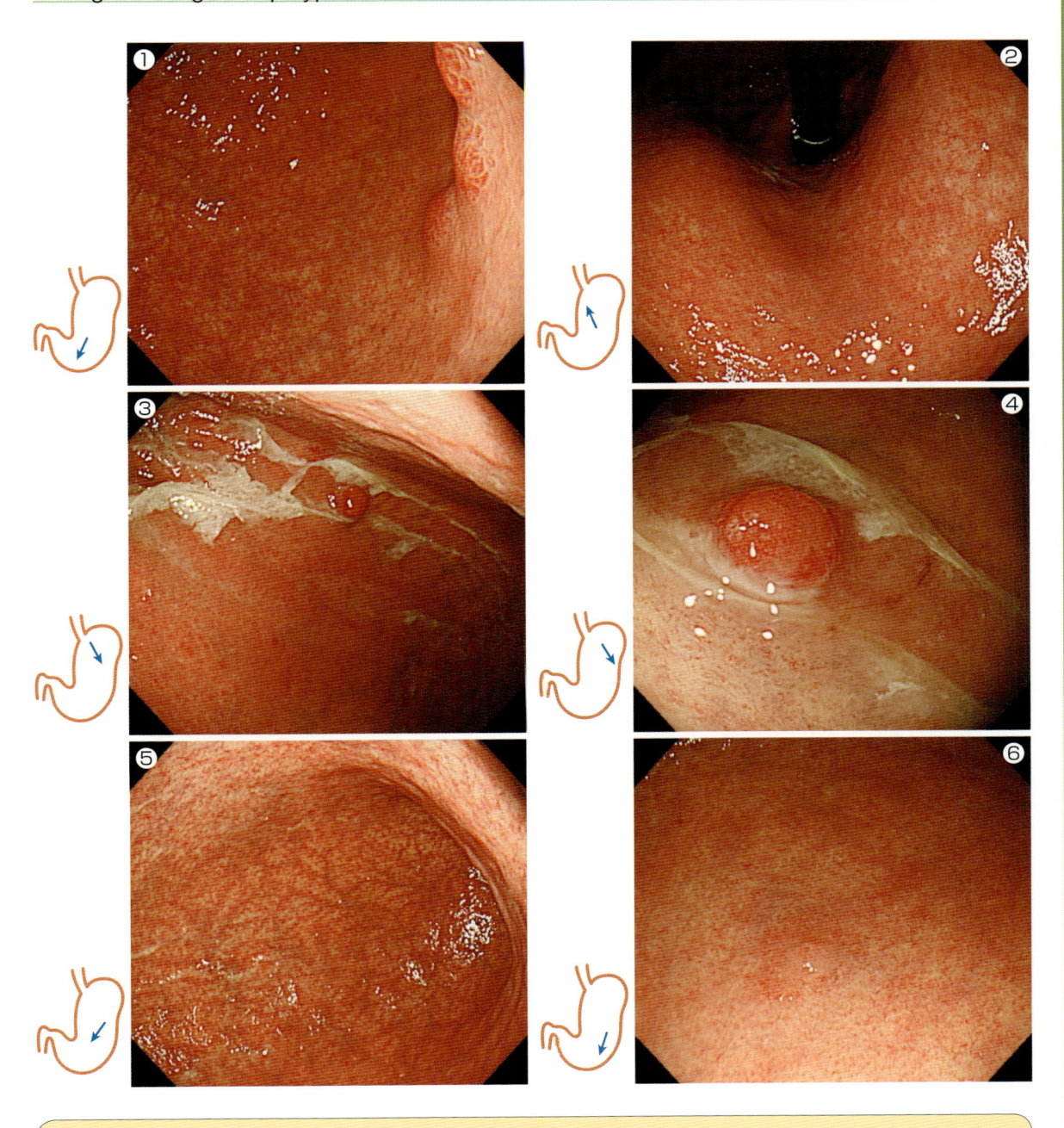

Hint 💡 • Look for redness.
• Compare the two polyps.

The answer and diagnosis are on page 156.

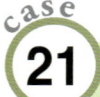

Patient referred to us due to suspected gastric cancer

case
21

▶ Male in his 70s.

▶ Gastric cancer on the posterior wall of the middle body suspected after an upper gastrointestinal series performed at a check-up. Patient was referred to our hospital.

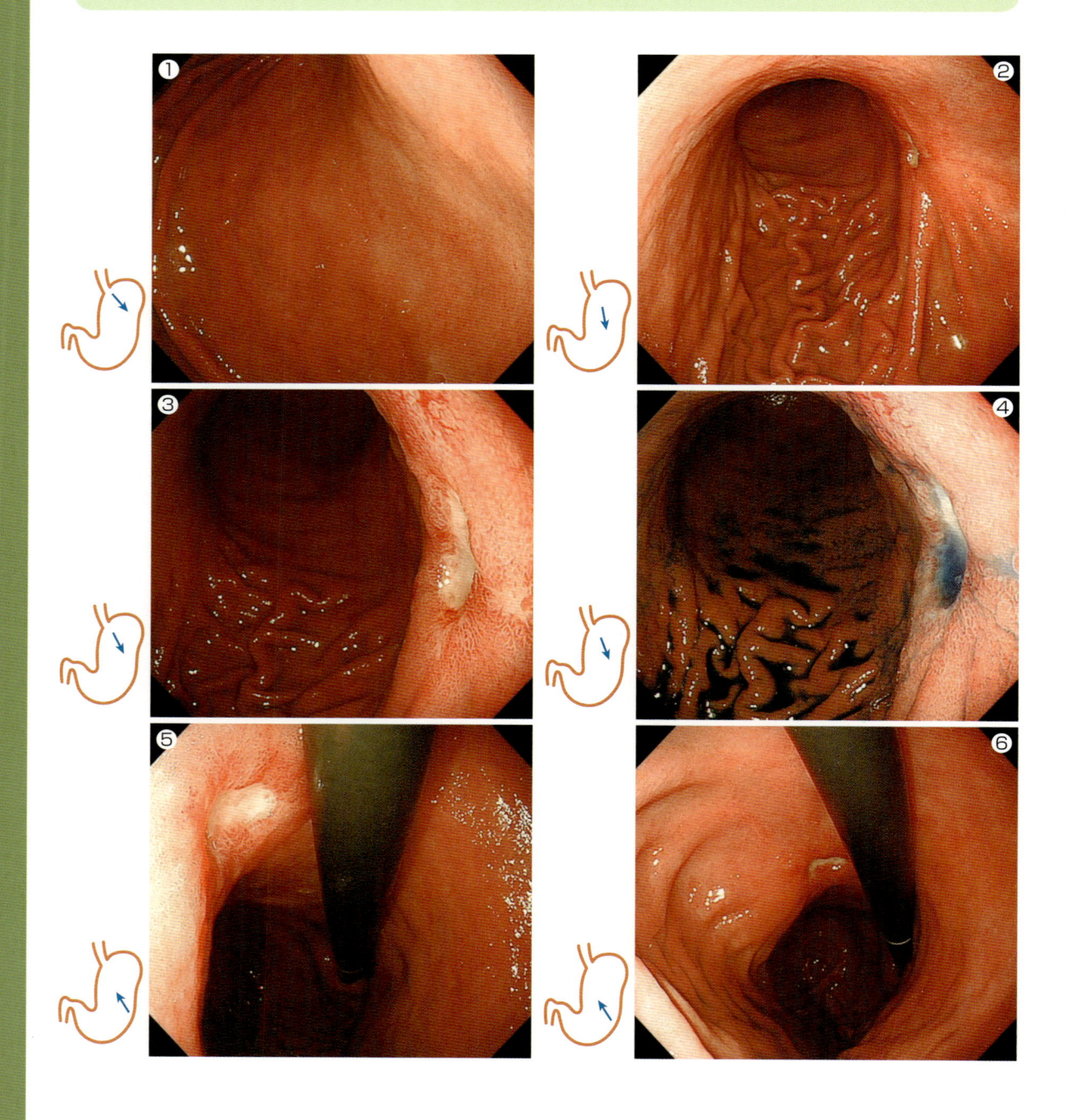

[1] Is the ulcer on the posterior wall of the middle body benign or malignant?
[2] Can you find any other lesion(s) that may be hidden?

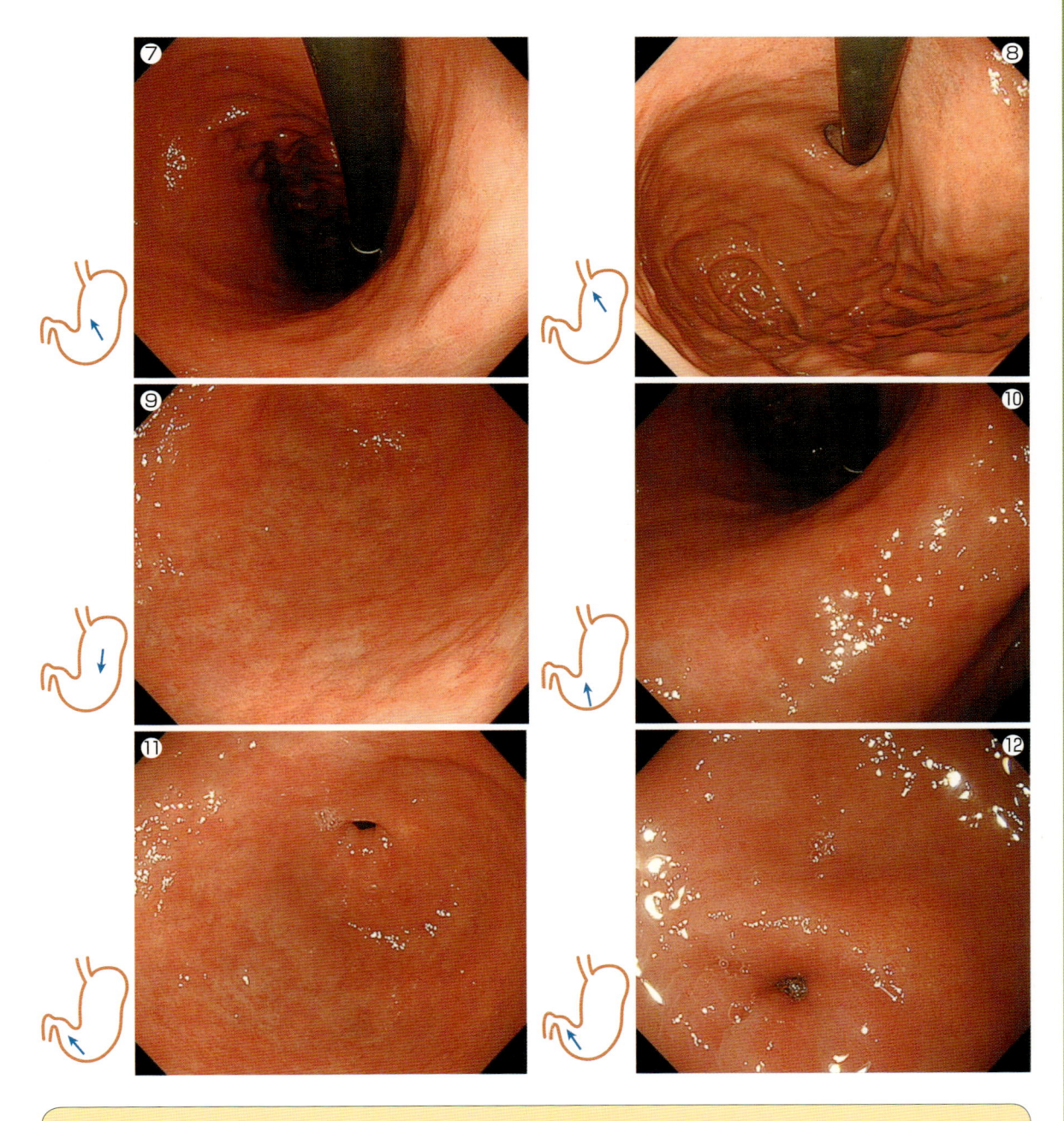

 Hint
- Pay attention to the property of the ulcer folds as well as the findings for the base and the boundaries of the ulcer.
- Pay attention to mucosa that is more yellowish than the surrounding area.

The answer and diagnosis are on page 159.

Patient referred to us after being diagnosed with gastric SMT

▸ Female in her 60s.
▸ Diagnosed with gastric SMT and referred to our hospital.

Can you specify the location of the gastric cancer?

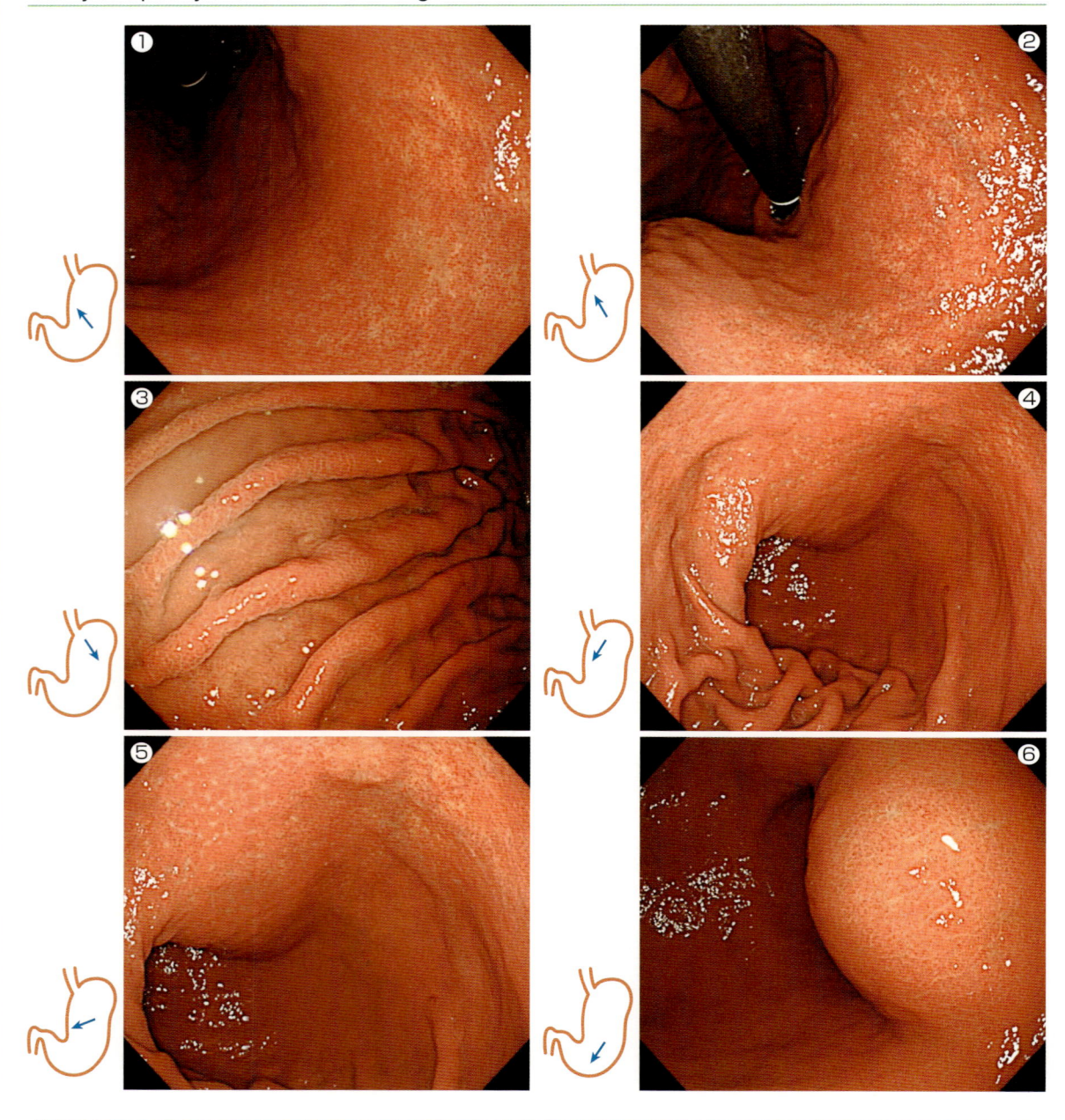

Hint Pay attention to any color changes that extend over a relatively large area.

The answer and diagnosis are on page 161.

Patient referred to us due to a high CA19-9 level

▶ Female in her 50s.

▶ After being referred to our hospital due to a slightly high CA19-9 level, she underwent screening endoscopy.

▶ No history of *H. pylori* eradication, serum anti-*H. pylori* antibodies negative, urea breath test negative, serum pepsinogen test method negative.

Can you specify the location of the malignant tumor?

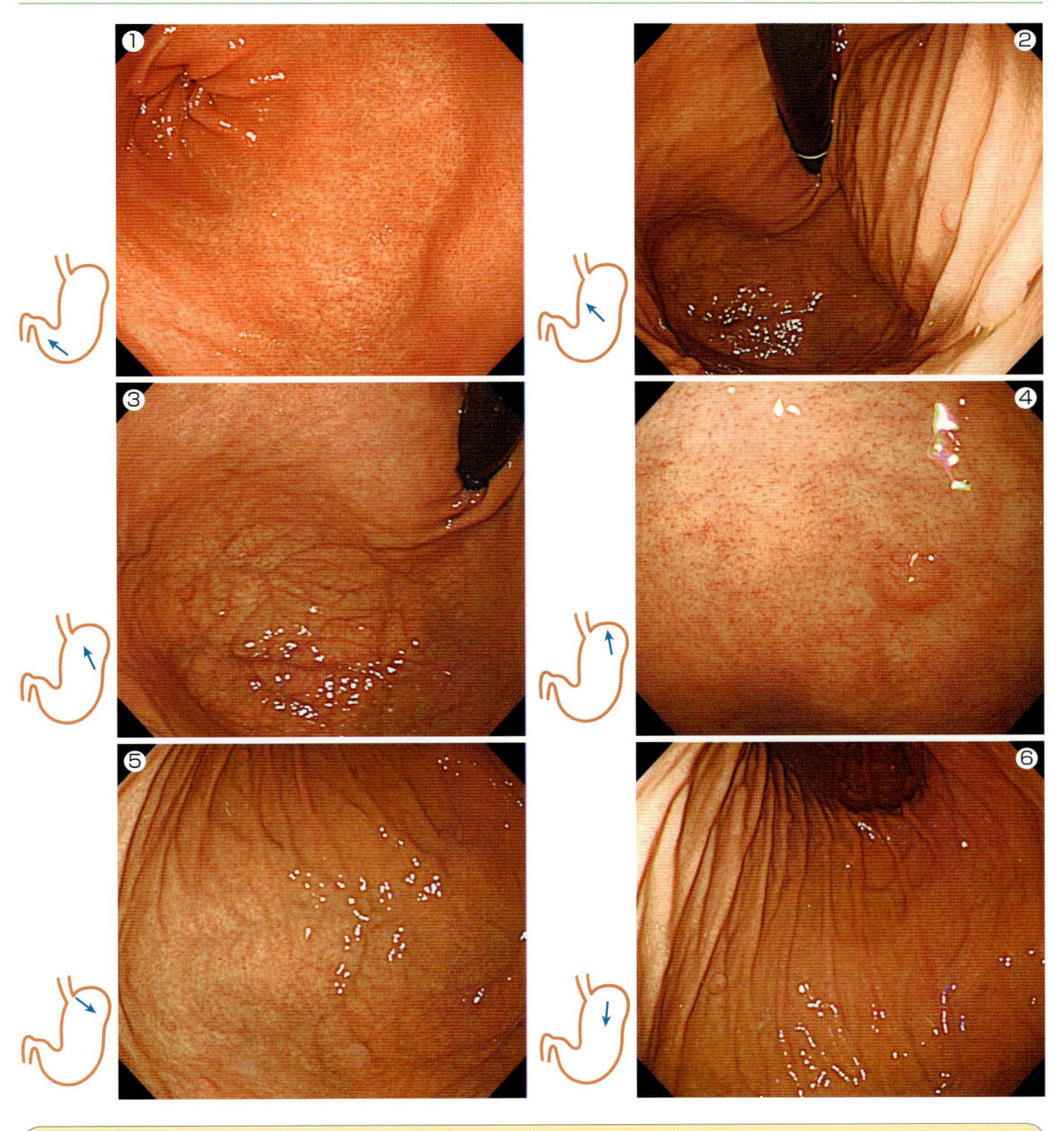

Hint Are all the polyps fundic gland polyps?

The answer and diagnosis are on page 163.

Synchronous multiple lesions found in detailed preoperative examination ①

▶ Female in her 40s.
▶ Her previous doctor found early gastric cancer, and she was referred to our hospital for surgery.

Try to spot the synchronous multiple lesions.

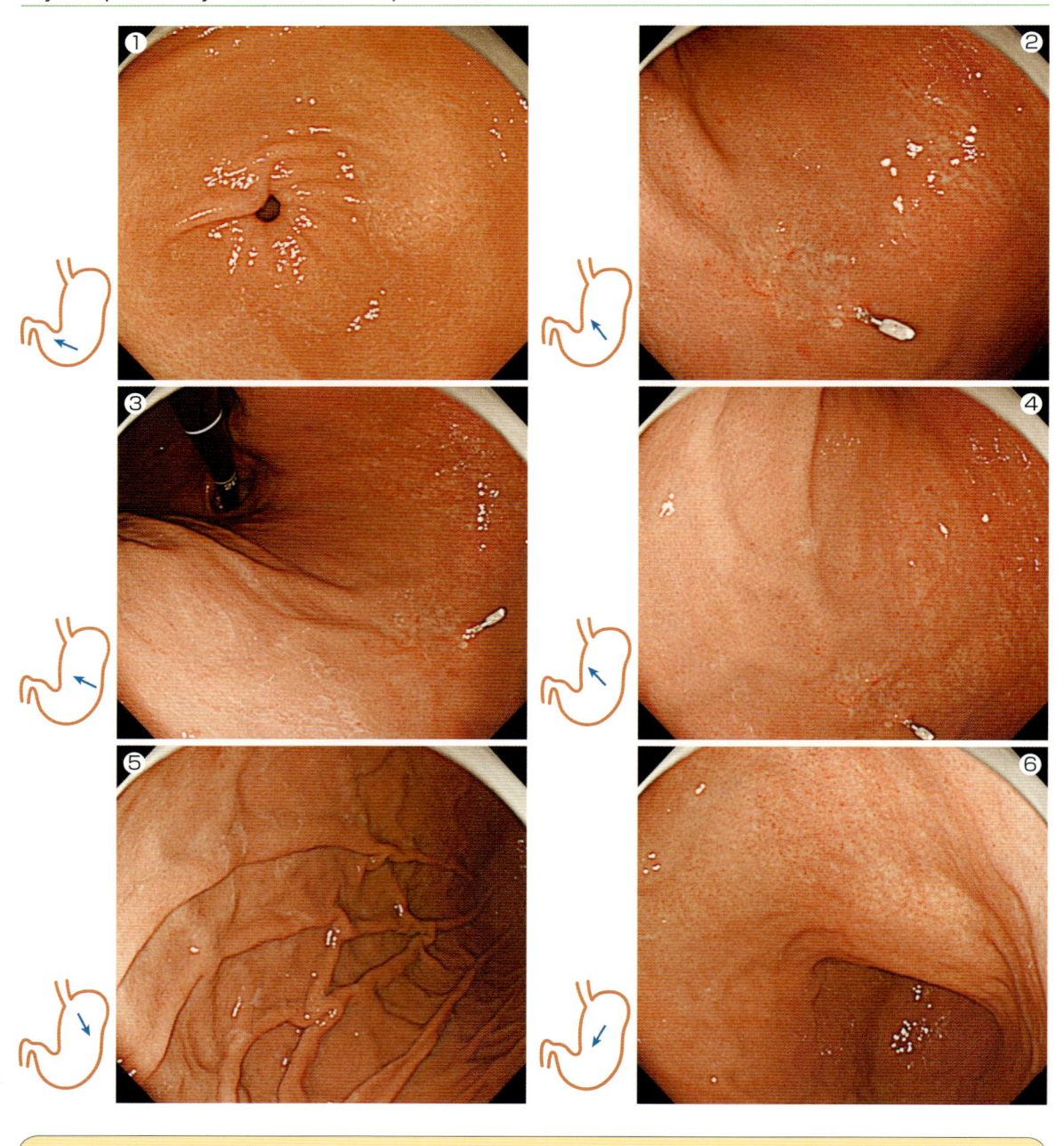

Hint 💡   Look for fading.

The answer and diagnosis are on page 166.

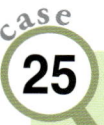

Synchronous multiple lesions found in detailed preoperative examination ②

▶ Male in his 70s.
▶ An early gastric cancer lesion was found on the posterior wall of the upper body, and the patient was referred to our hospital.

Try to spot another cancer lesion other than the one on the posterior wall of the upper body.

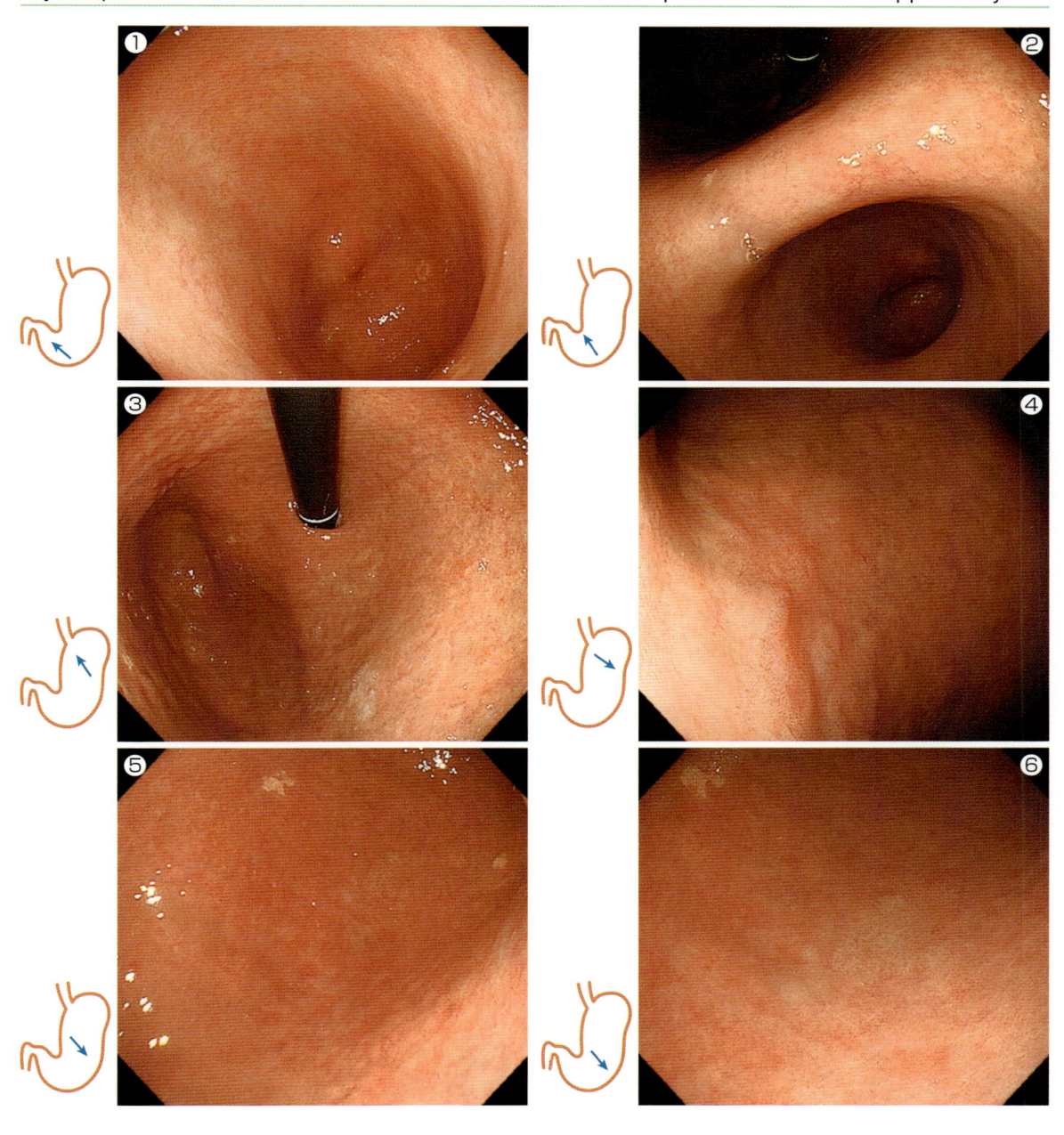

Hint 💡 Look for yellowish-white mucosa.

The answer and diagnosis are on page 167.

Synchronous multiple lesions found in detailed preoperative examination ③

▸ Male in his 60s.
▸ An early gastric cancer was found on the posterior wall of the middle body, and the patient was referred to our hospital.
▸ Although the patient was *H. pylori*-positive, he had a penicillin allergy and *H. pylori* had not been eradicated.

Can you see any synchronous multiple lesions other than the one on the posterior wall of the middle body?
There are two lesions in addition to the one found by his previous doctor.

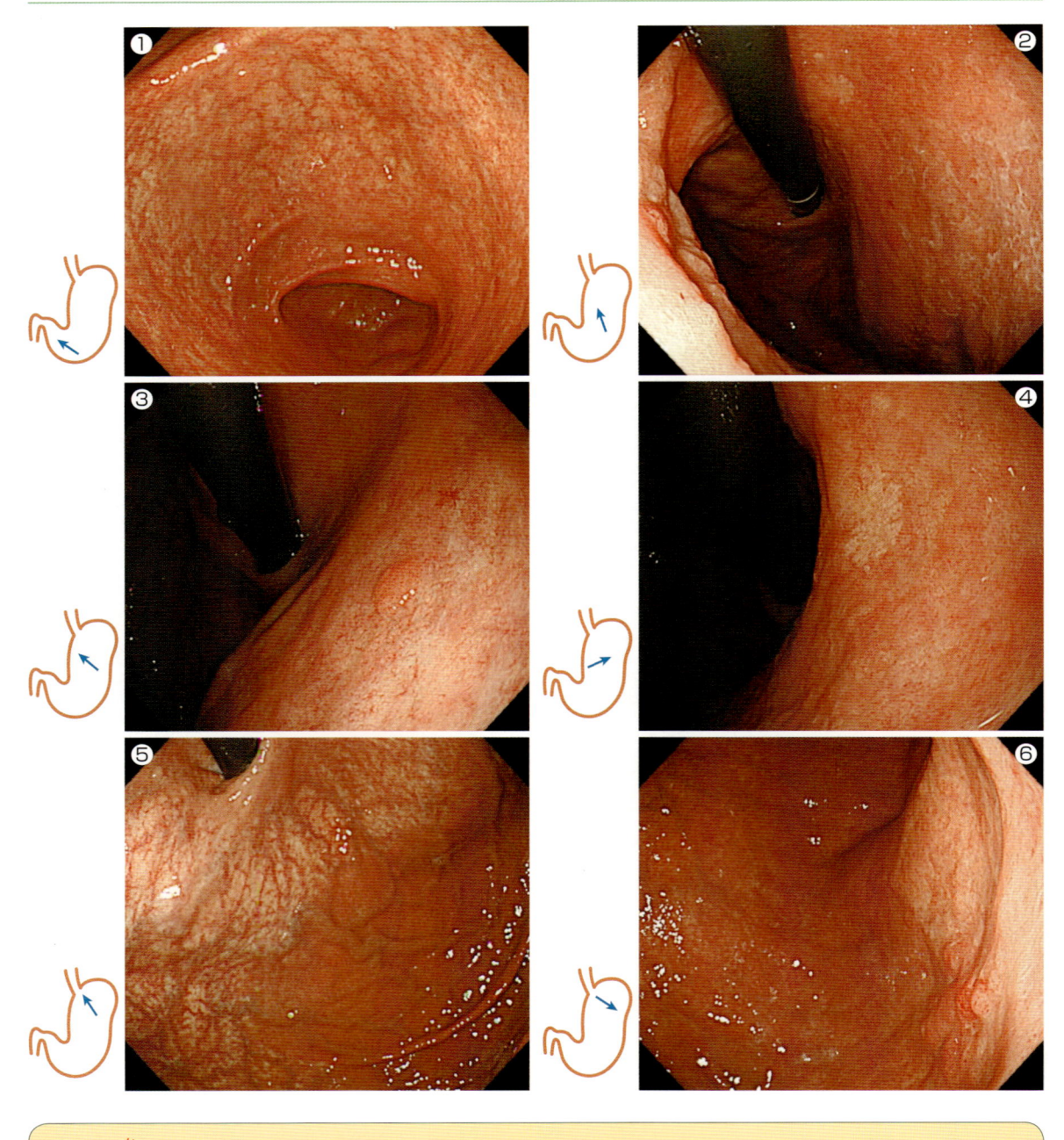

Hint 💡 Look for erythematous and whitish lesions.

The answer and diagnosis are on page 169.

Synchronous multiple lesions found in detailed preoperative examination ④

> ▶ Female in her 50s.
> ▶ An early gastric cancer was found on the greater curvature of the middle body and the patient was referred to our hospital.
> ▶ *H. pylori* had been eradicated 2 years previously.

Can you spot the synchronous multiple lesions?

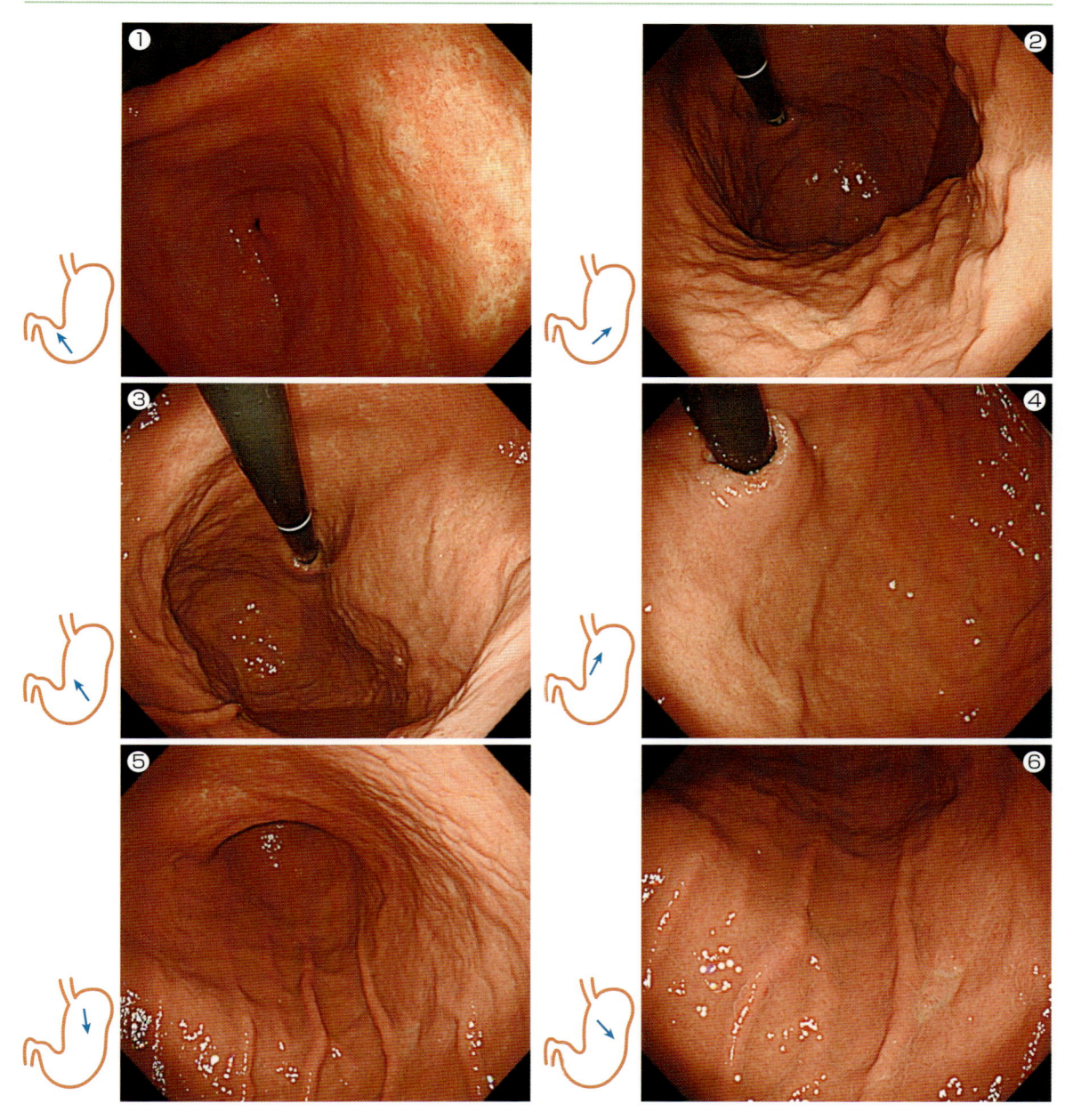

Hint 💡 The histological type of the cancer likely to occur differs depending on the background mucosa.

The answer and diagnosis are on page 172.

Synchronous multiple lesions found in detailed preoperative examination ⑤

- ▶ Male in his 70s.
- ▶ Diagnosed with early gastric cancer on the lesser curvature of the upper body and referred to our hospital.

Can you see any synchronous multiple lesions other than the one on the lesser curvature of the upper body?

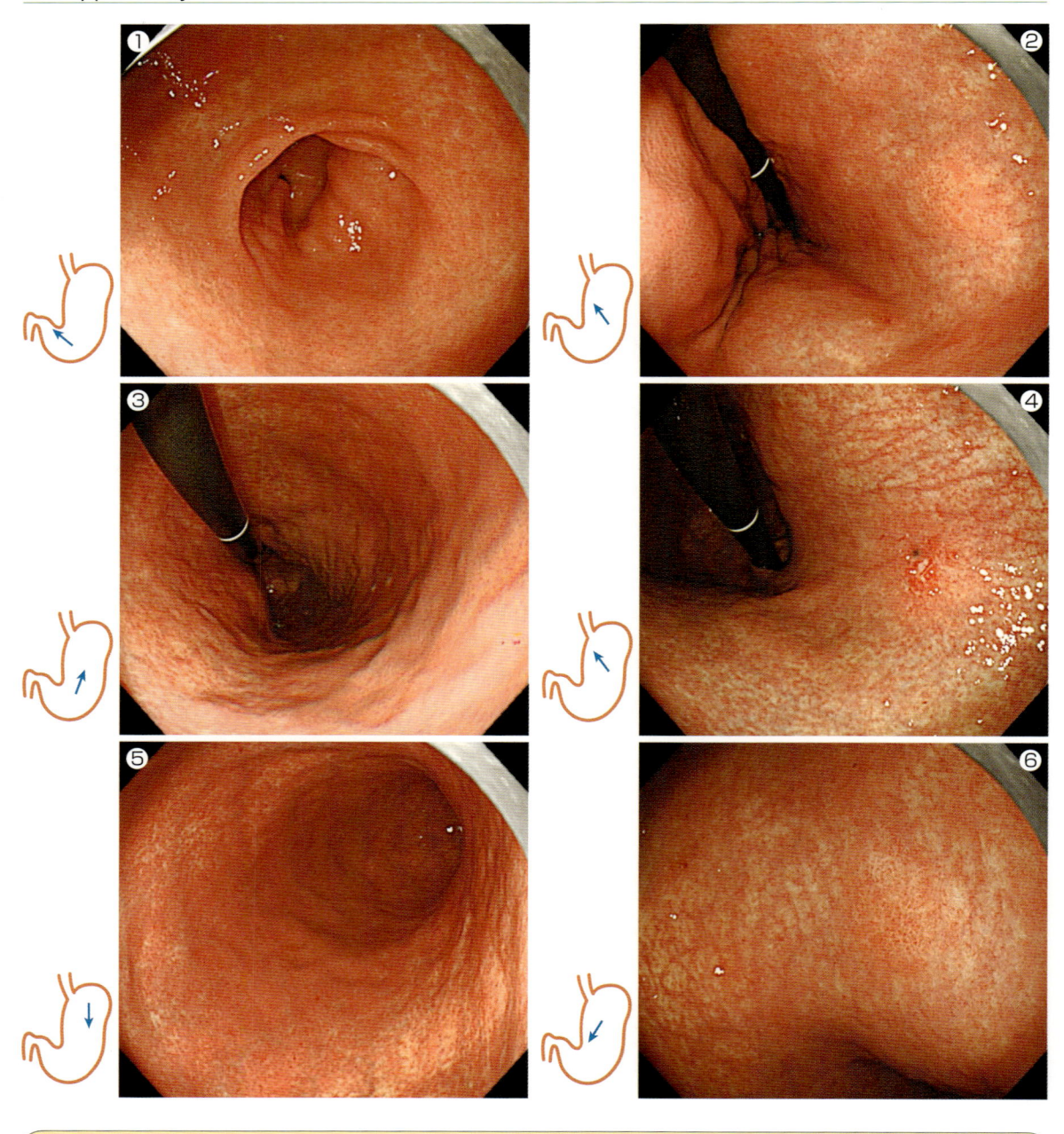

Hint 💡 Look for changes in color tone.

The answer and diagnosis are on page 174.

Synchronous multiple lesions found in detailed preoperative examination ⑥

▸ Male in his 60s.

▸ Gastric cancer was found in the cardia, and the patient was referred to our hospital.

▸ *H. pylori* had been eradicated a few years previously.

Can you see any gastric cancer lesions other than the one on the lesser curvature of the cardia?

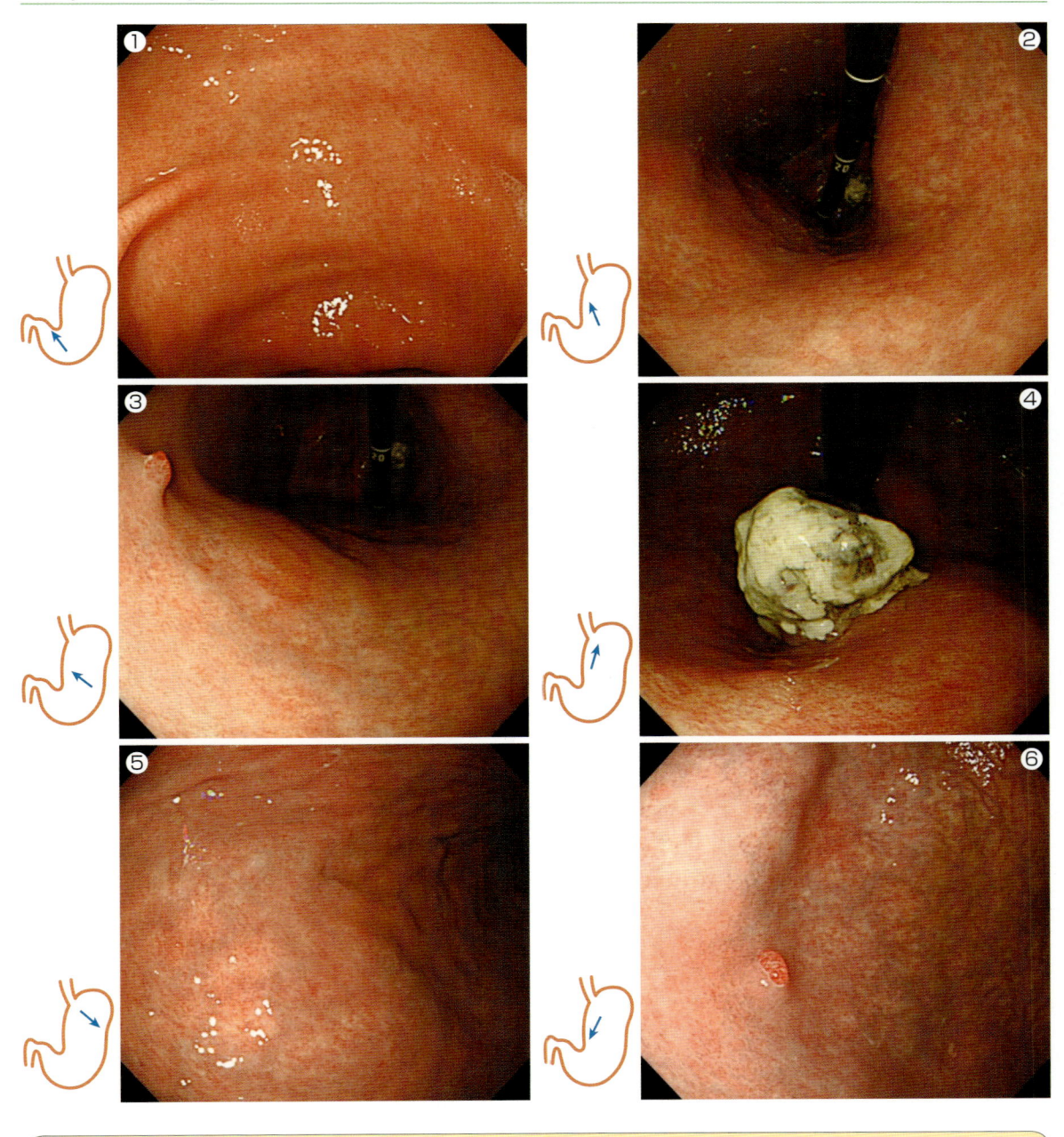

Hint 💡 Look for redness.

The answer and diagnosis are on page 176.

Synchronous multiple lesions found in detailed preoperative examination ⑦

▶ Male in his 70s.

▶ His previous doctor found early gastric cancer on the greater curvature of the antrum and referred him to our hospital.

Can you specify the location of the lesion found by the previous doctor as well as the locations of the synchronous multiple lesions?

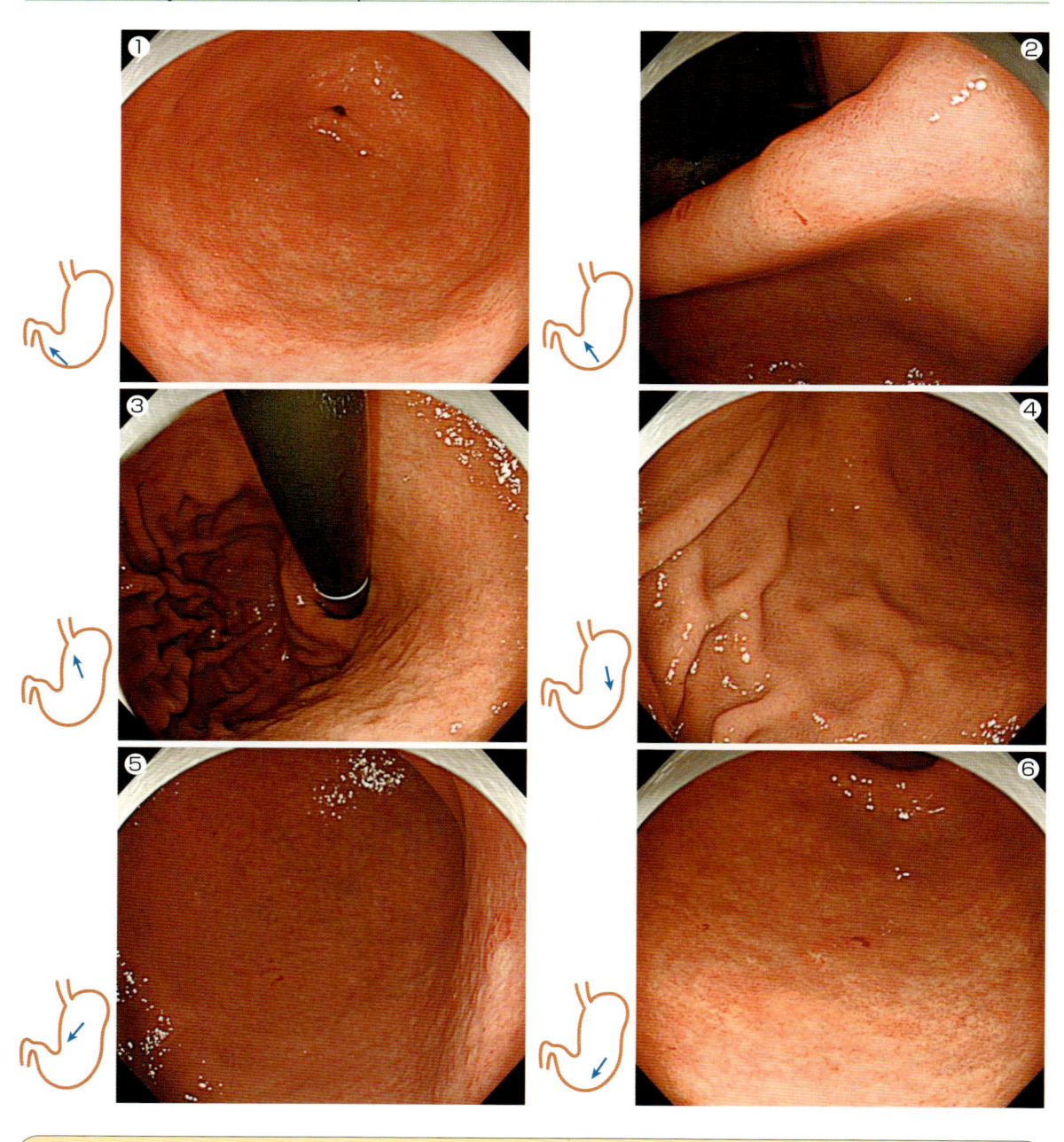

Hint 💡   Look for a biopsy scar and a flat elevated lesion.

The answer and diagnosis are on page 178.

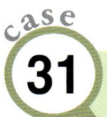
Periodic endoscopy after treatment of gastric ulcer

▶ Male in his 70s.

▶ History of gastric ulcer. *H. pylori* had been eradicated five years previously.

▶ A periodic endoscopy was performed.

Can you specify the location of gastric tumor?

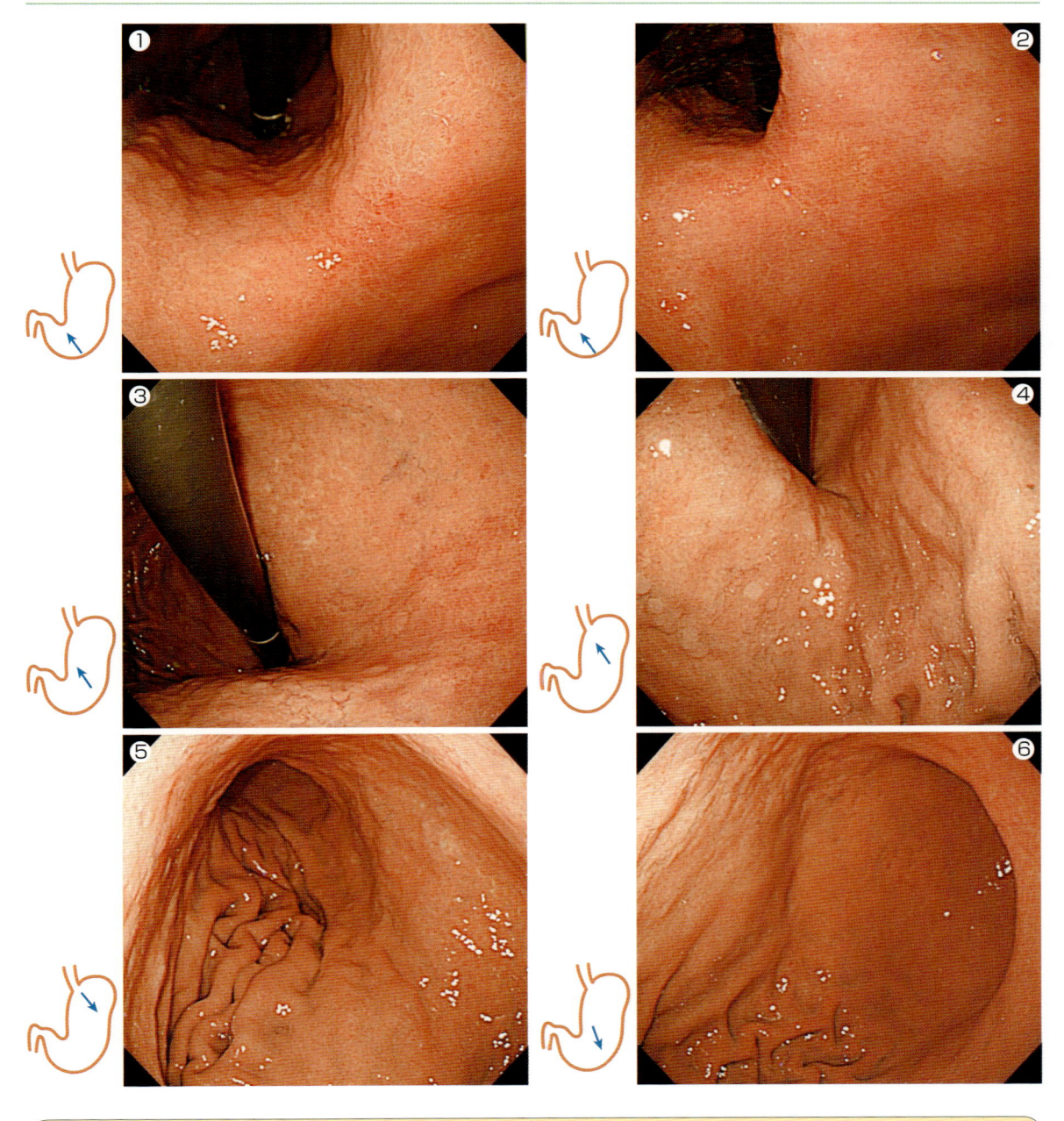

Hint 🔆   Look for yellowish mucosa.

The answer and diagnosis are on page 180.

Screening endoscopy after chemotherapy for gastric malignant lymphoma

▶ Male in his 70s.

▶ A screening endoscopy was performed after chemotherapy for gastric malignant lymphoma.

Can you specify the location of the gastric cancer?

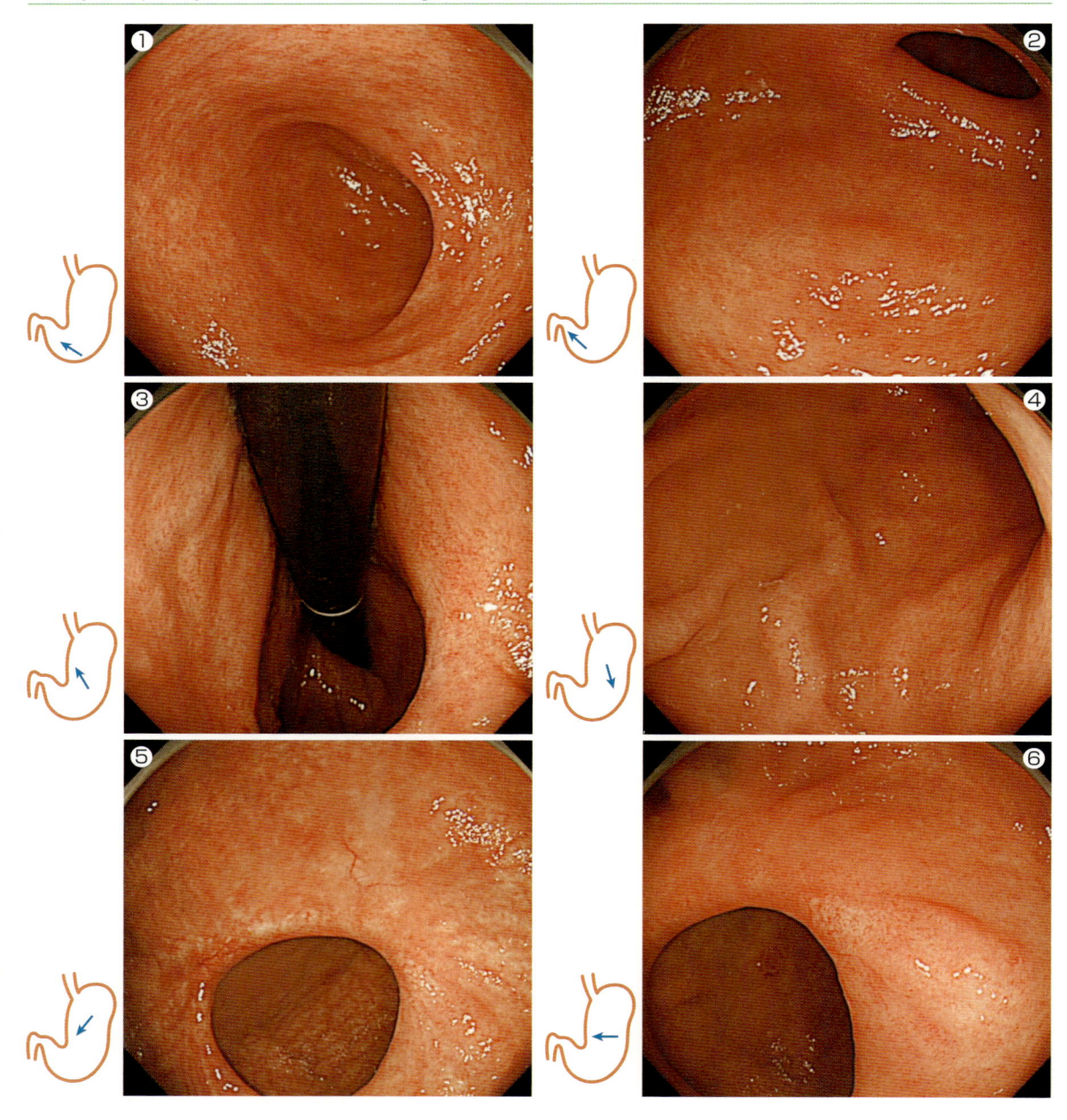

> **Hint** 💡   Look for yellowish-white mucosa.

The answer and diagnosis are on page 182.

Patient referred to us after uncurative ESD for gastric cancer

case
33

▸ Male in his 50s.
▸ ESD for early gastric cancer had been performed 1 month previously at another hospital. The ESD involved piecemeal resection, so he was referred to our hospital for additional treatment.

Can you specify the location of the gastric cancer?

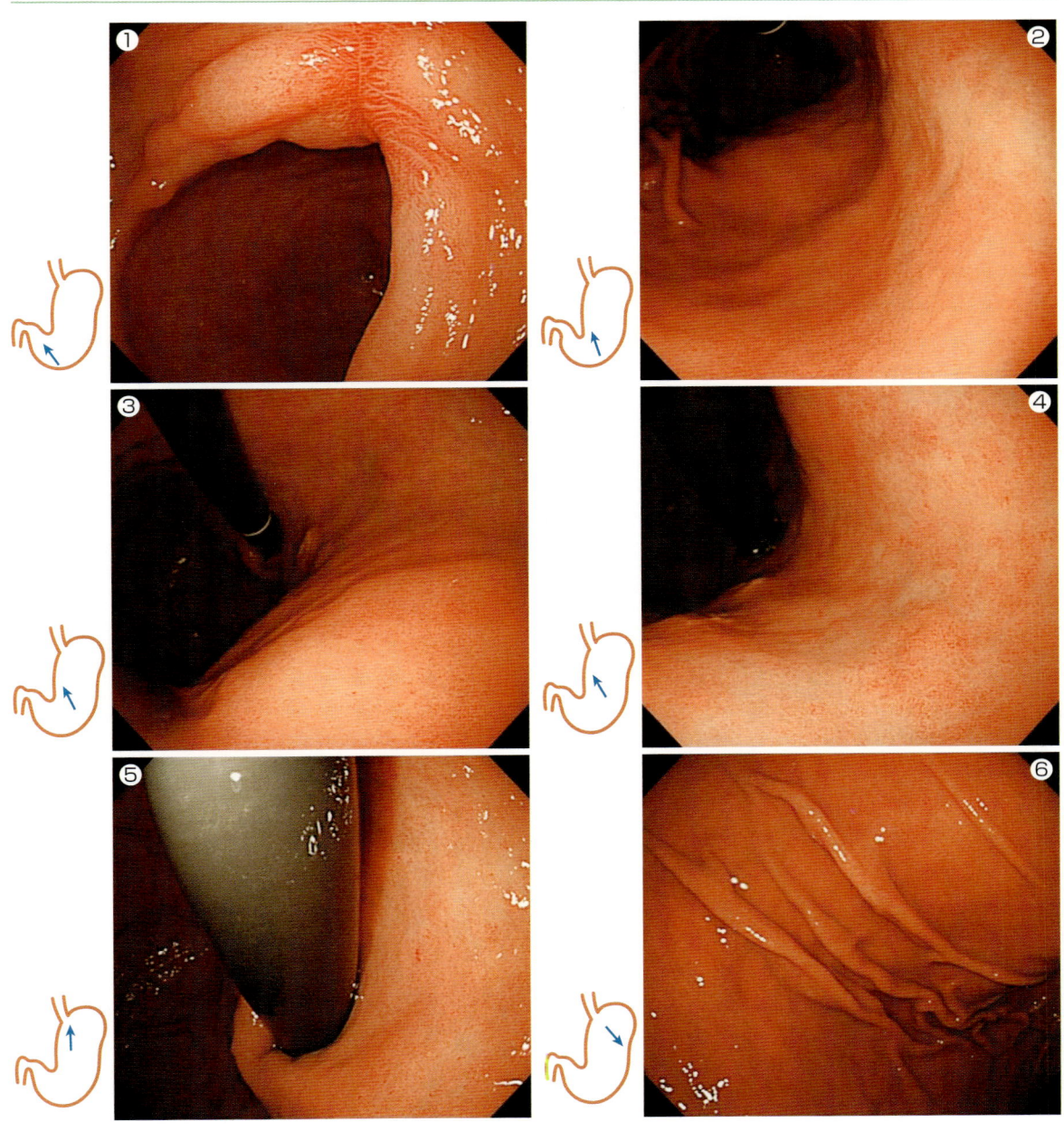

> **Hint** 💡   Look for surface irregularities on the mucosa.

The answer and diagnosis are on page 183.

Screening endoscopy after ESD for gastric cancer ①

▶ Male in his 50s.
▶ The patient had a history of ESD for 3 early gastric cancer lesions. We performed a follow-up endoscopy.
▶ *H. pylori* had been eradicated 5 years previously.

Can you specify the locations of the metachronous multiple lesions? There are two of them.

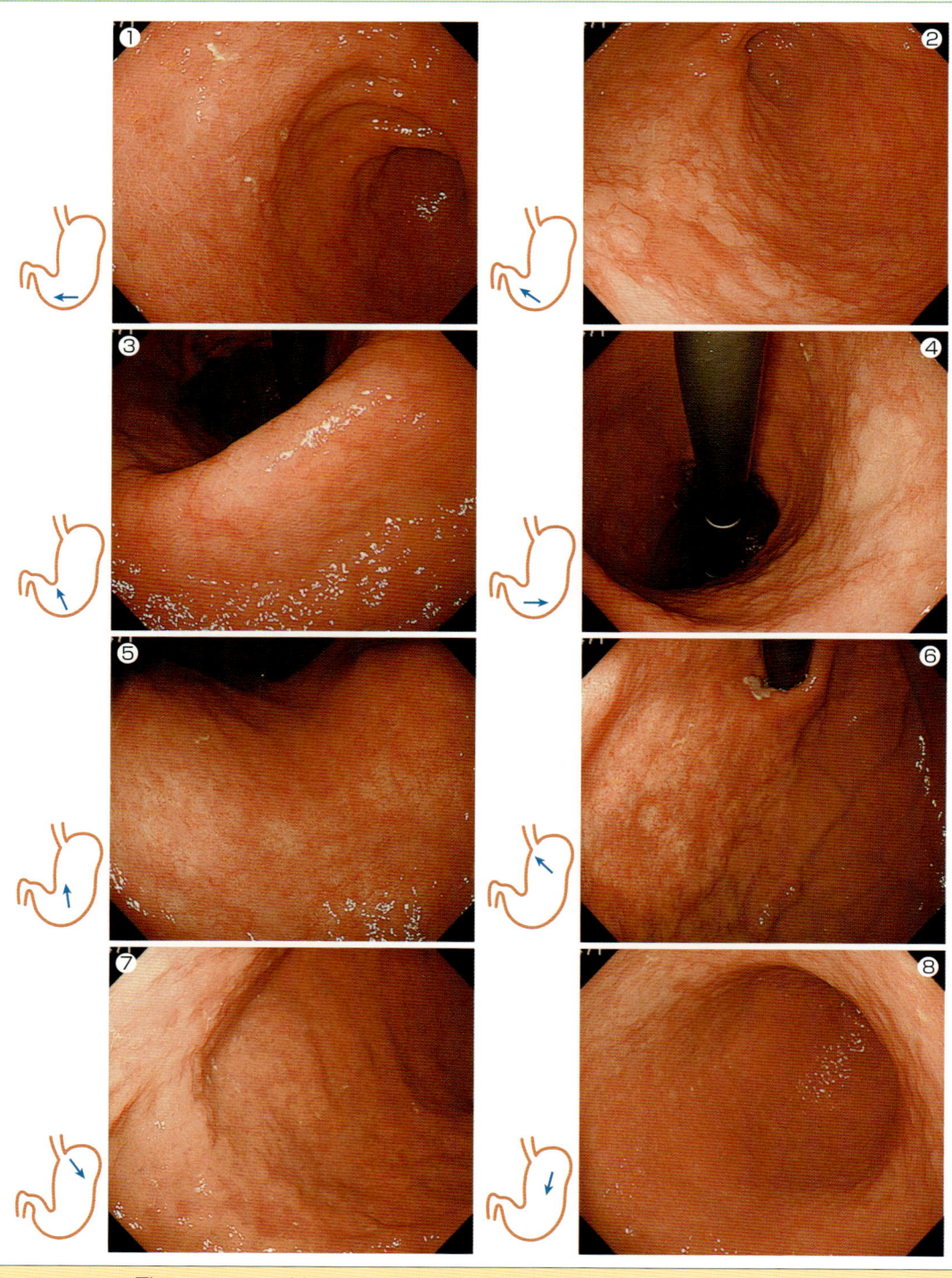

Hint 💡
· The tumors are hidden in intestinal metaplasia.
· Pay attention to any changes in color tone.

The answer and diagnosis are on page 184.

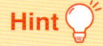

Screening endoscopy after ESD for gastric cancer ②

▶ Male in his 80s.

▶ ESD for gastric cancer had been performed 5 years previously. We performed a follow-up endoscopy.

▶ *H. pylori* had been eradicated 5 years previously.

Can you specify the location of the gastric cancer?

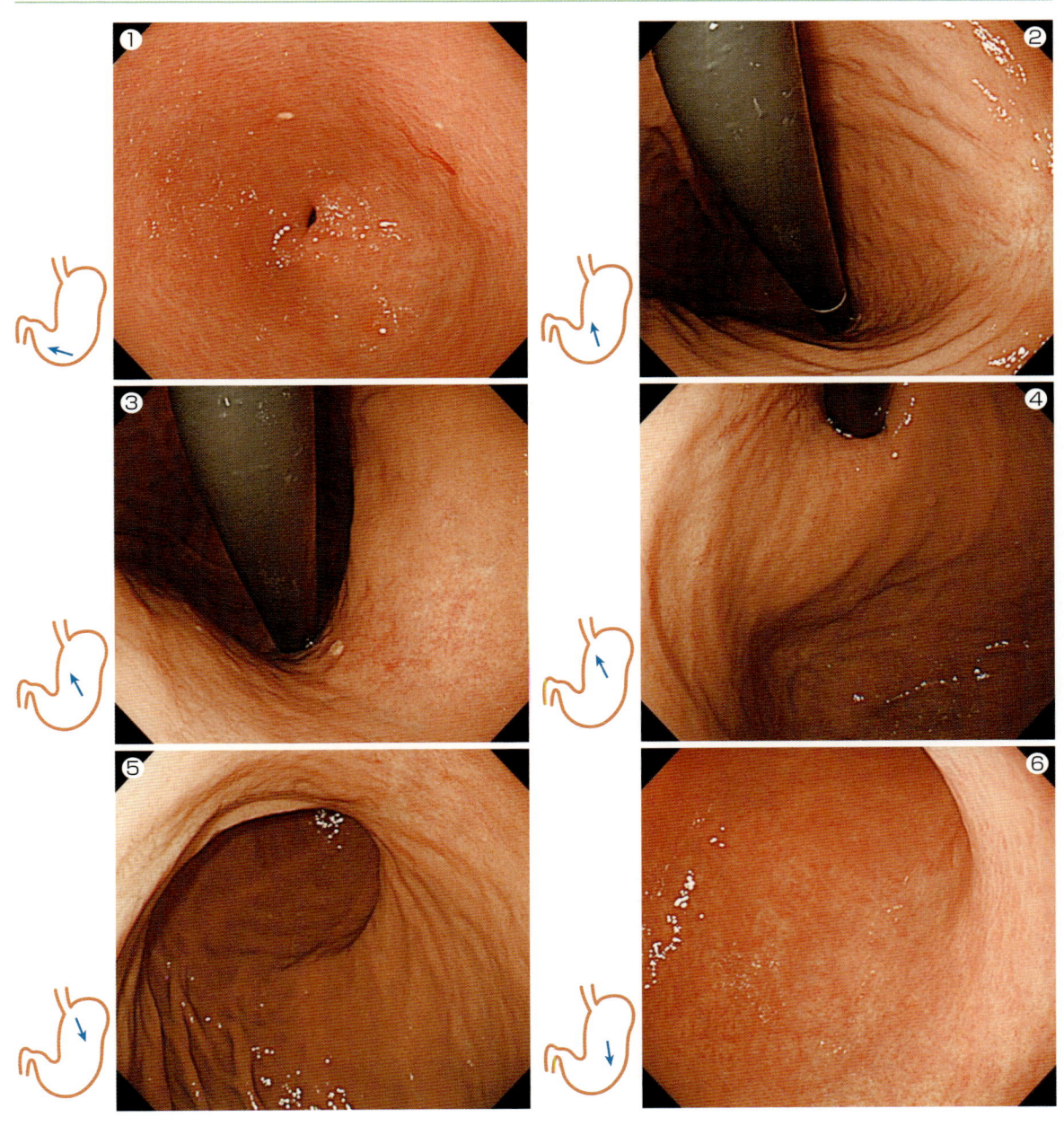

Hint 💡 Look for the finding(s) associated with cancer.

The answer and diagnosis are on page 186.

Screening endoscopy after ESD for gastric cancer ③

▶ Male in his 60s.
▶ ESD for gastric cancer had been performed 4 years previously and again 2 years previously. A follow-up endoscopy was performed at this time.
▶ *H. pylori* had been eradicated 4 years previously.

Can you specify the location of the gastric cancer?

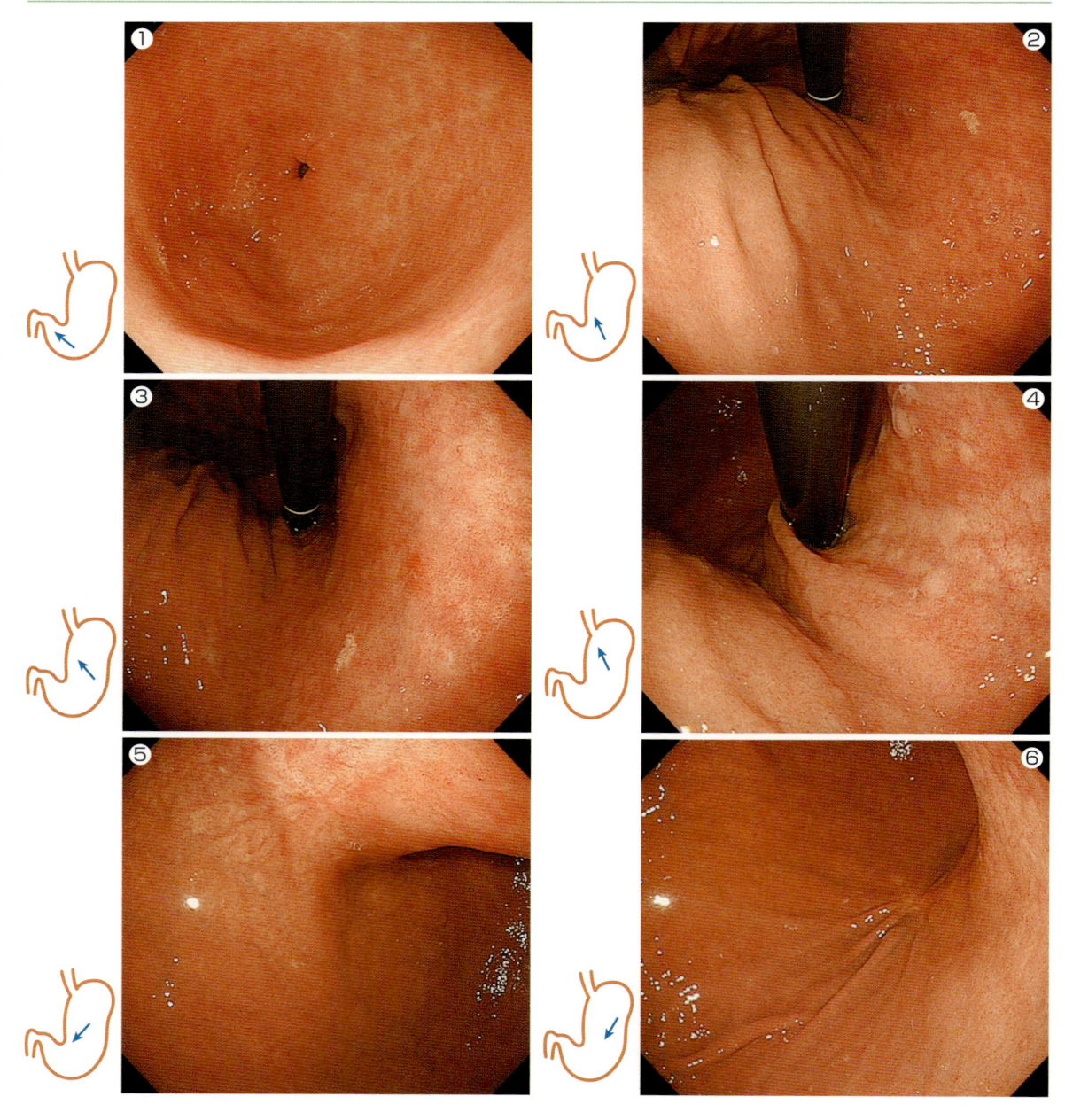

Hint 💡   Look for any redness.

The answer and diagnosis are on page 187.

case 37

Screening endoscopy after ESD for gastric cancer ④

- ▶ Female in her 70s.
- ▶ ESD for early gastric cancer had been performed 1 year previously. A follow-up endoscopy was performed at this time.
- ▶ *H. pylori* had been eradicated 1 year previously.

Can you specify the location of the gastric cancer?

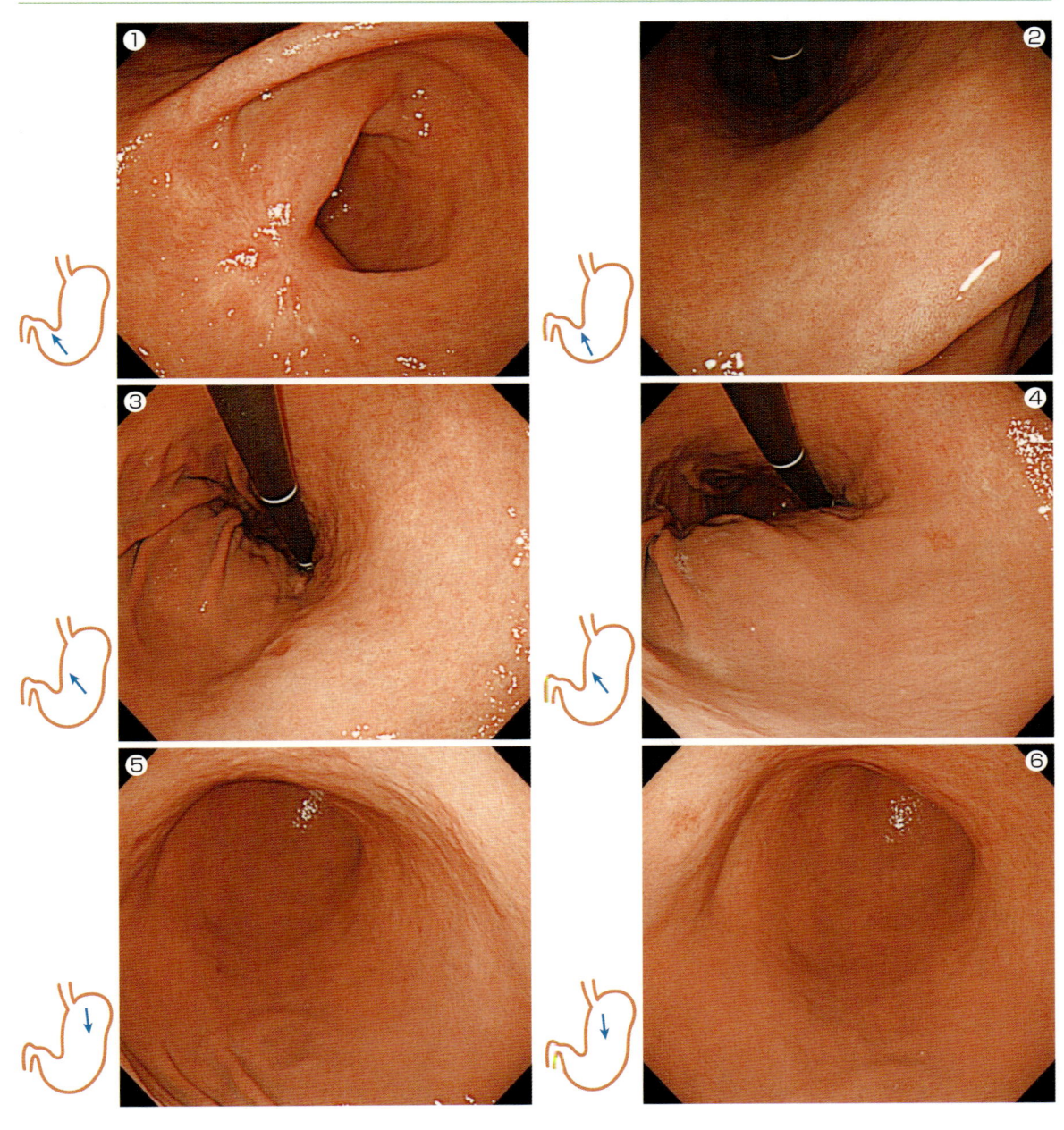

| Hint 💡 | Look for any redness. |

The answer and diagnosis are on page 189.

Screening endoscopy after ESD for gastric cancer ⑤

▶ Female in her 80s.

▶ ESD for early gastric cancer had been performed 1 year previously. A follow-up endoscopy was performed at this time.

▶ *H. pylori* had been eradicated 1 year previously.

Can you specify the location of the gastric cancer?

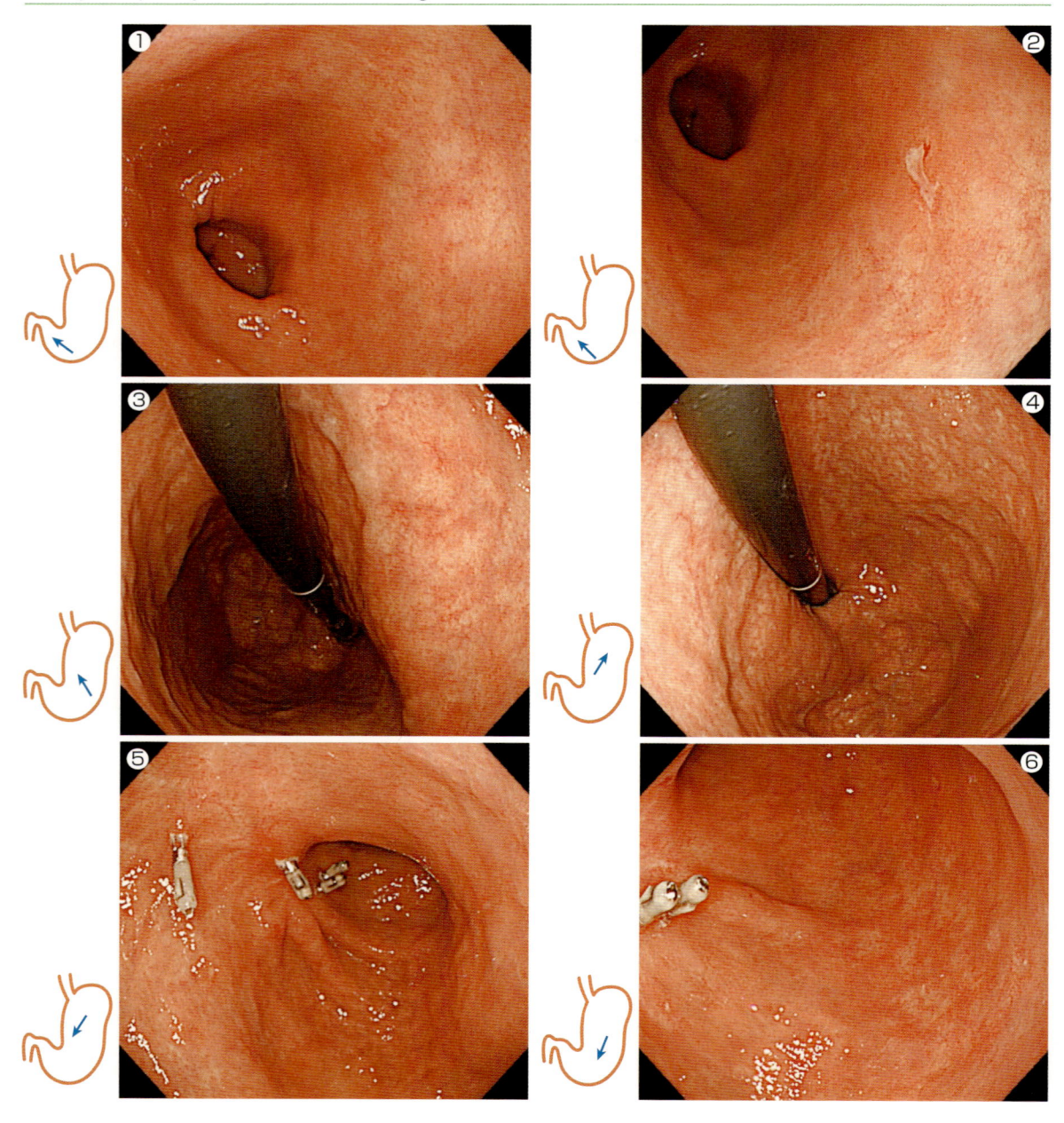

Hint 💡 Look for the finding(s) associated with cancer.

The answer and diagnosis are on page 191.

▶ Female in her 70s.
▶ ESD for 2 early gastric cancer lesions had been performed 3 years previously. A follow-up endoscopy was performed at this time.
▶ *H. pylori* had been eradicated 3 years previously.

Can you specify the location of the gastric cancer?

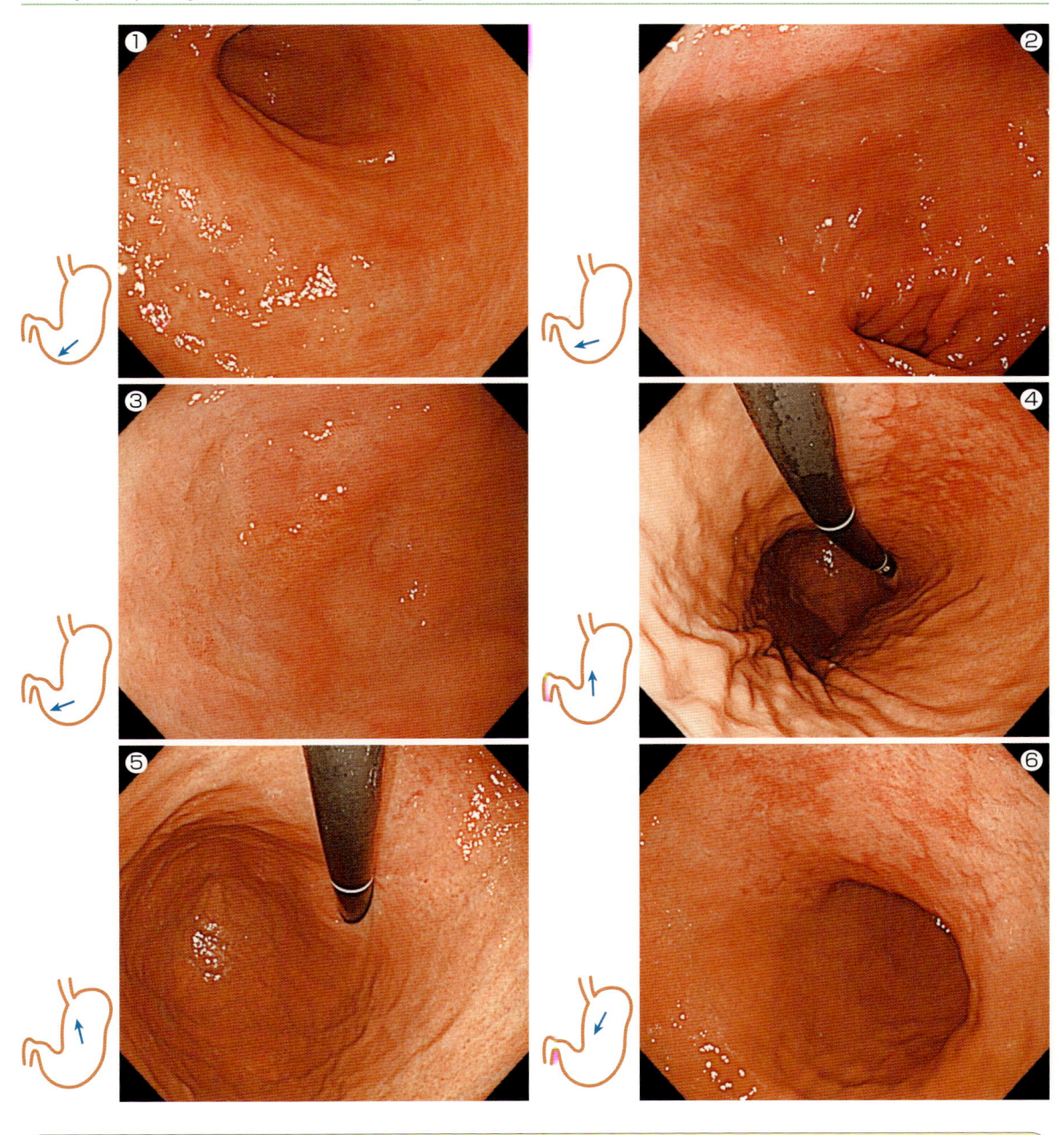

Hint 💡 Look for yellowish mucosa.

The answer and diagnosis are on page 192.

Screening endoscopy after ESD for gastric cancer ⑦

▶ Male in his 60s.

▶ ESD for gastric cancer had been performed 1 year previously. A follow-up endoscopy was performed at this time.

▶ *H. pylori* had been eradicated 5 years previously.

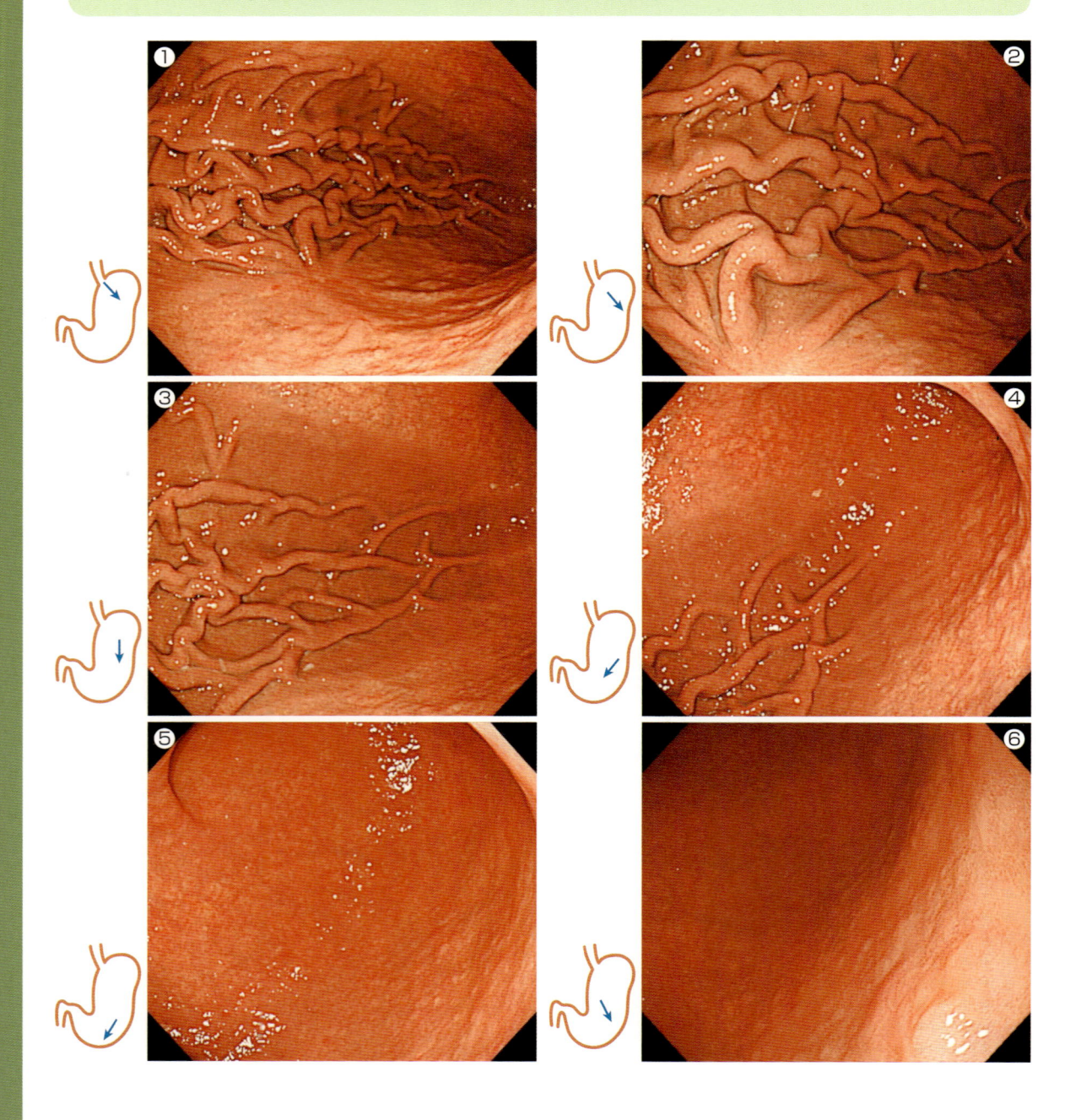

There are two extremely small hidden gastric cancer lesions.
Can you specify the locations that appear suspicous and should therefore be observed up close?

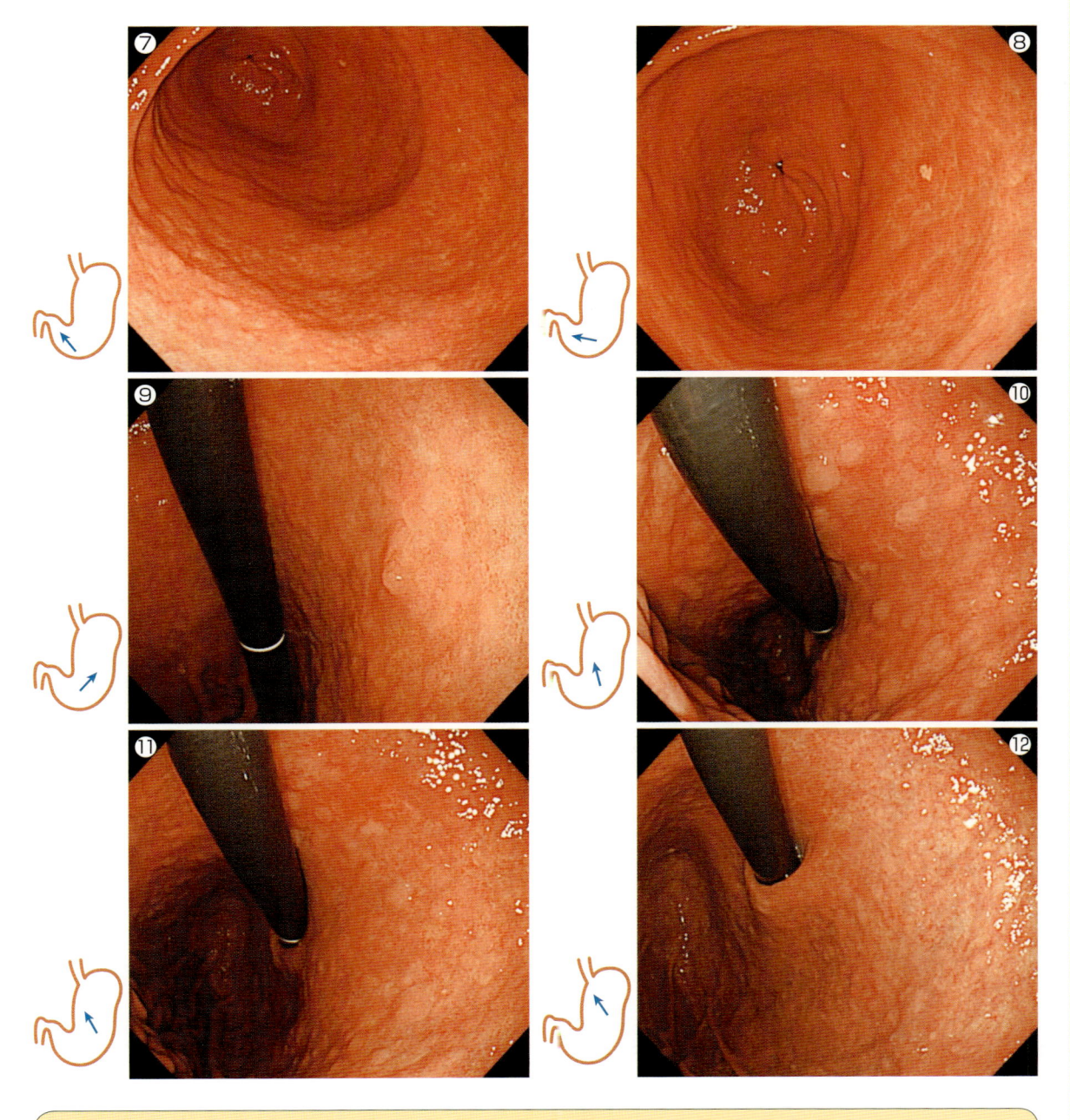

Hint 💡 Look for conspicuous surface irregularities, as well as yellowish mucosa.

The answer and diagnosis are on page 193.

Screening endoscopy after ESD for gastric cancer ⑧

▶ Male in his 50s.
▶ ESD for early gastric cancer had been performed 4 months previously. A follow-up endoscopy was performed at this time.
▶ *H. pylori* had been eradicated 2 years previously.

Can you specify the location of the gastric cancer?

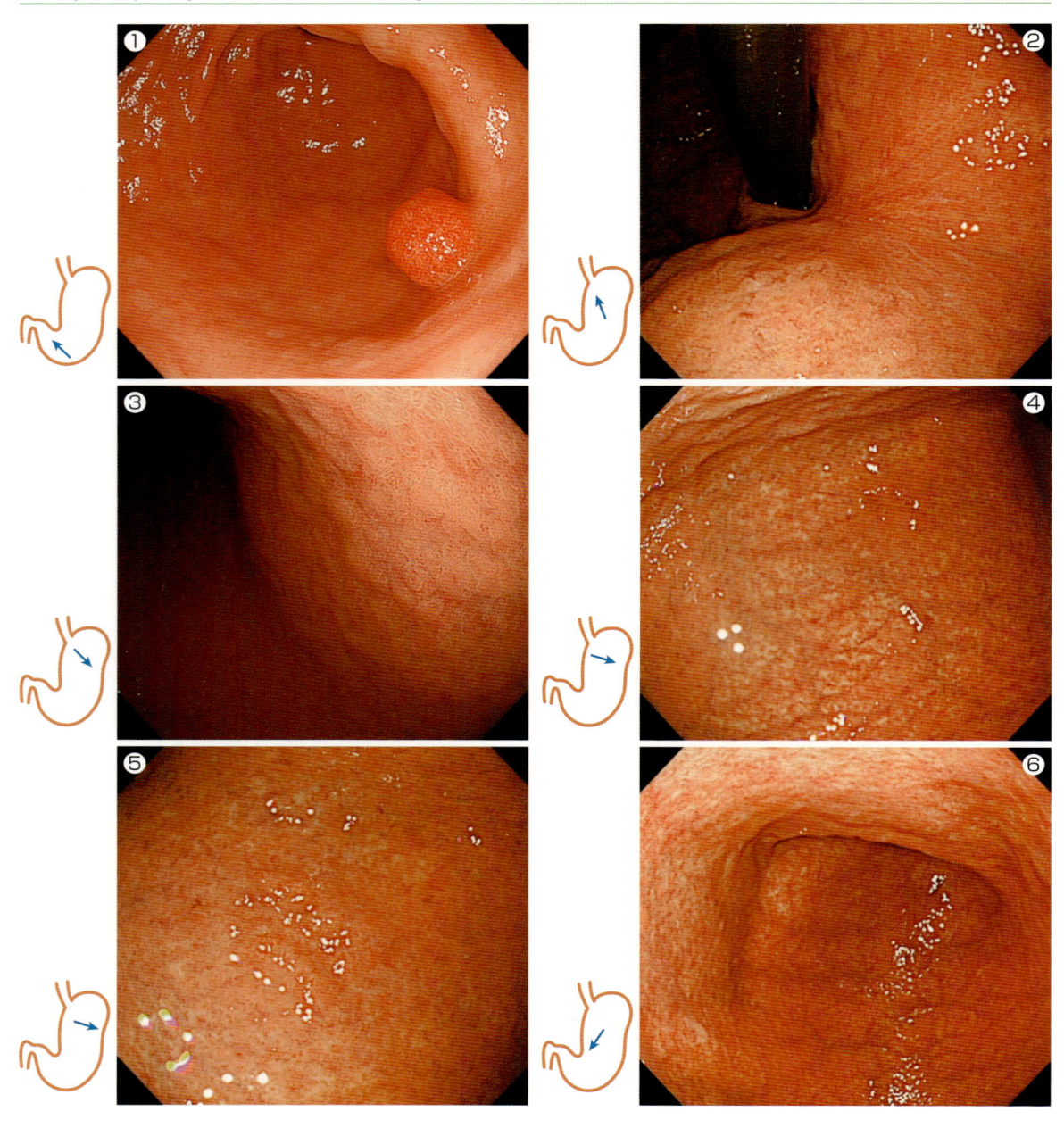

Hint ○ Look for surface irregularities on the mucosa.

The answer and diagnosis are on page 196.

Periodic screening endoscopy after gastrectomy ①

▶ Female in her 60s.

▶ Distal gastrectomy for undifferentiated-type gastric cancer had been performed 9 years previously. ESD for a 5-mm lesion of undifferentiated-type gastric cancer in the residual stomach had been performed a half year previously. A follow-up endoscopy was performed at this time.

▶ *H. pylori* had been eradicated a half year previously.

Can you specify the location of the gastric cancer?

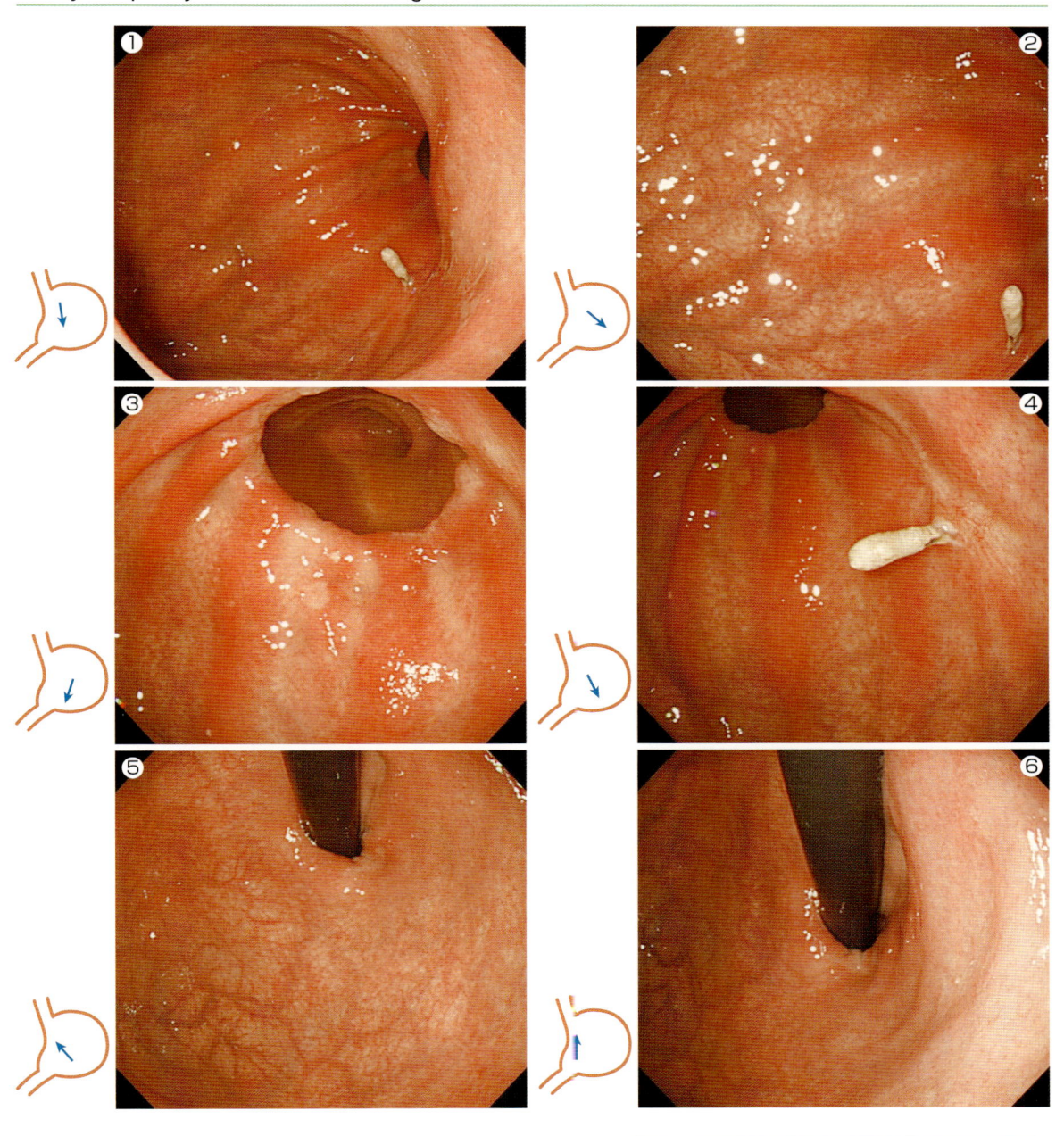

Hint 💡 When examining postoperative remnant stomach of undifferentiated-type gastric cancer, what kind of lesion should you expect to see?

The answer and diagnosis are on page 198.

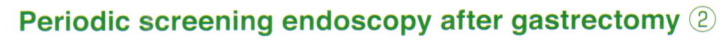

case

43

Periodic screening endoscopy after gastrectomy ②

▸ Female in her 60s.

▸ Distal gastrectomy for undifferentiated-type gastric cancer had been performed 19 years previously.

▸ A periodic screening endoscopy was performed at this time.

Can you specify the location of the gastric cancer?

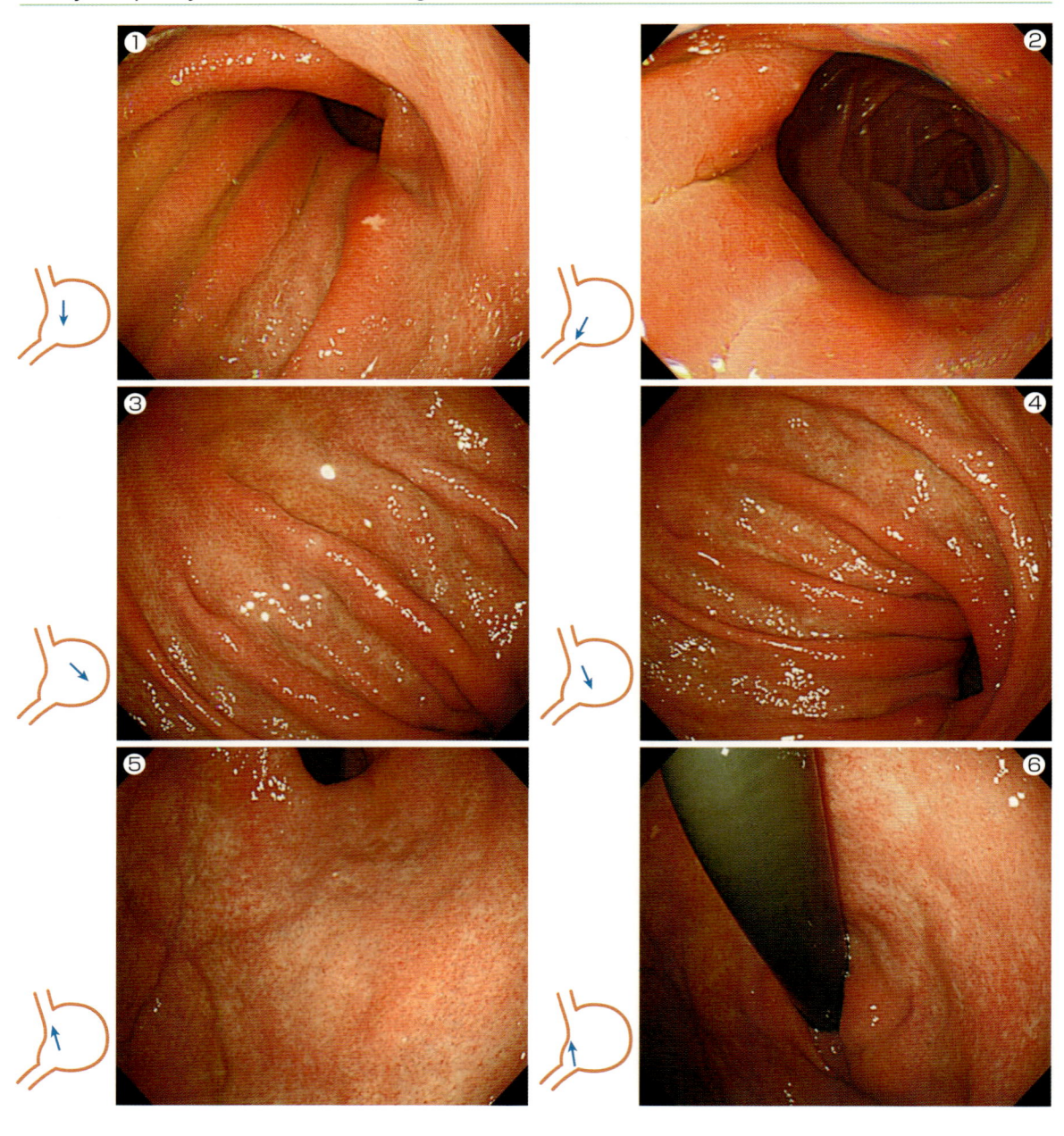

Hint 💡 Think about the histological type that's likely to occur after undifferentiated-type gastric cancer surgery.

The answer and diagnosis are on page 200.

Screening endoscopy before tongue cancer surgery

▶ Male in his 70s.

▶ Screening endoscopy for patient with tongue cancer was performed.

Can you specify the location of the gastric cancer?

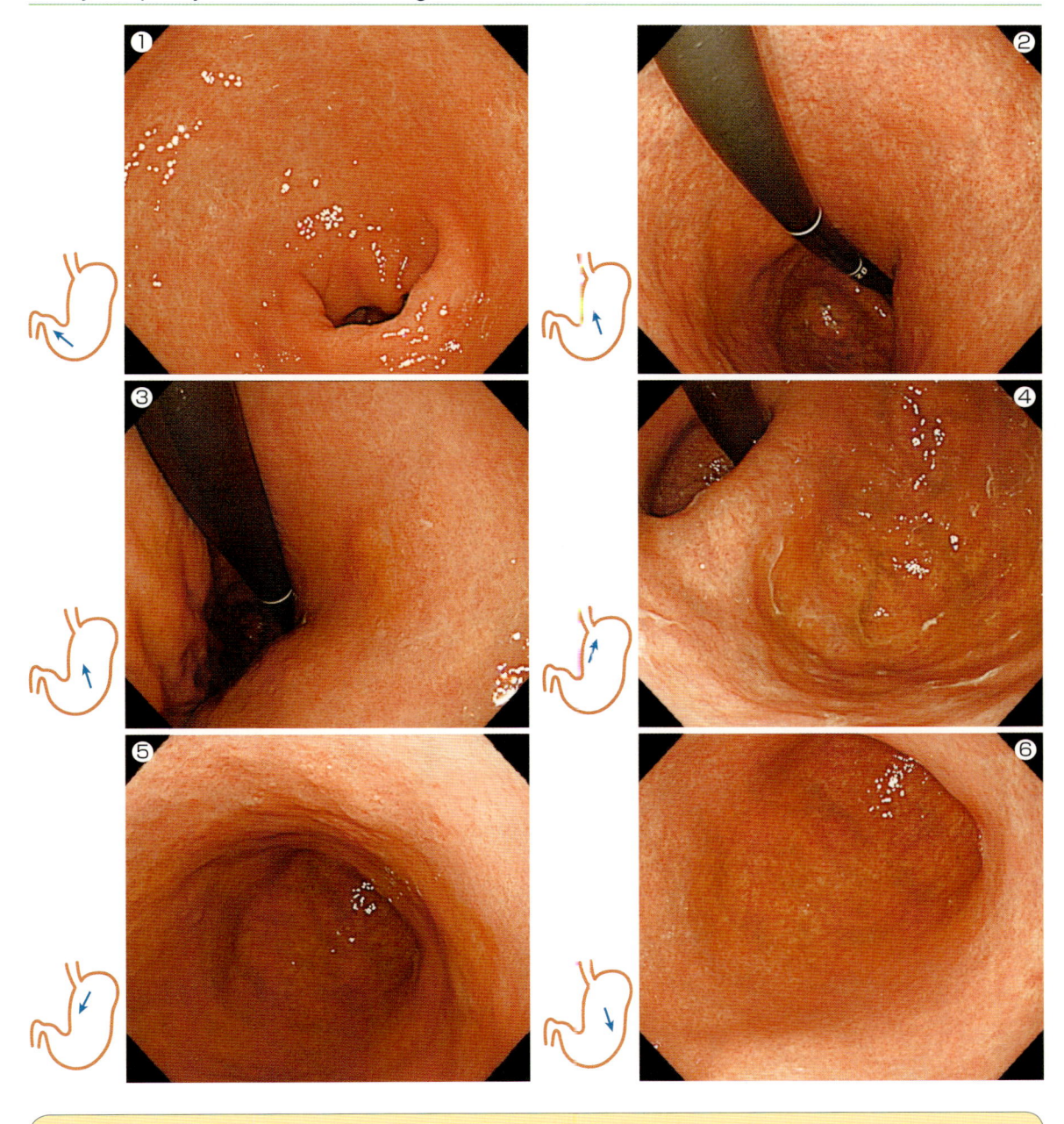

Hint 💡   Look for small white spots.

The answer and diagnosis are on page 202.

Screening endoscopy after floor of mouth cancer surgery

▸ Male in his 50s.
▸ A screening endoscopy was performed after floor of mouth cancer surgery.
▸ No history of *H. pylori* eradication, serum anti-*H. pylori* antibodies negative, urea breath test negative, serum pepsinogen test method negative.

Can you specify the location of the gastric cancer?

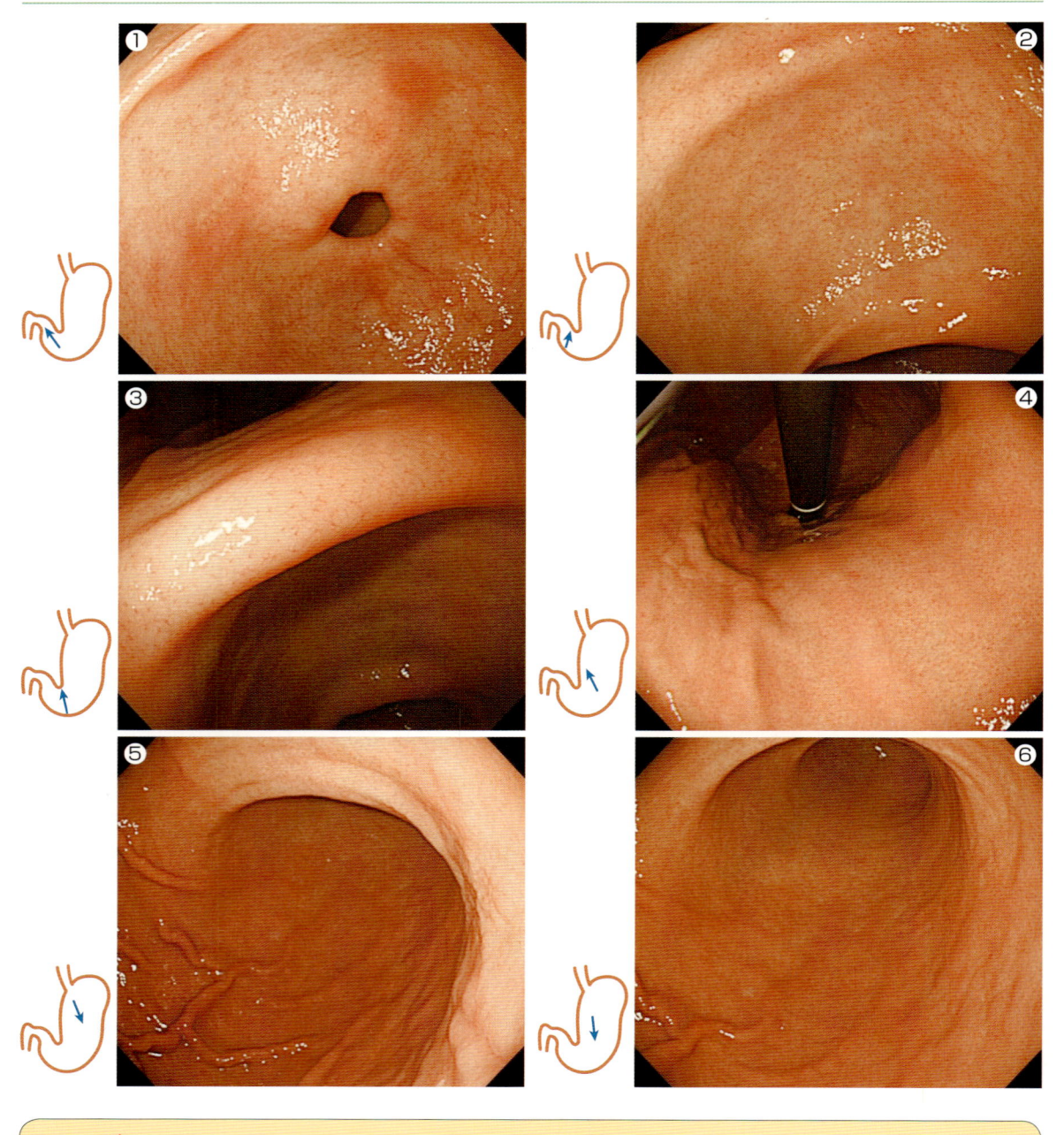

Hint 🔆 Look for fading.

The answer and diagnosis are on page 204.

Screening endoscopy for double cancer after hypopharyngeal cancer surgery

▶ Male in his 60s.
▶ A screening endoscopy was performed after hypopharyngeal cancer surgery to check for double cancer.

Can you specify the location of the gastric cancer?

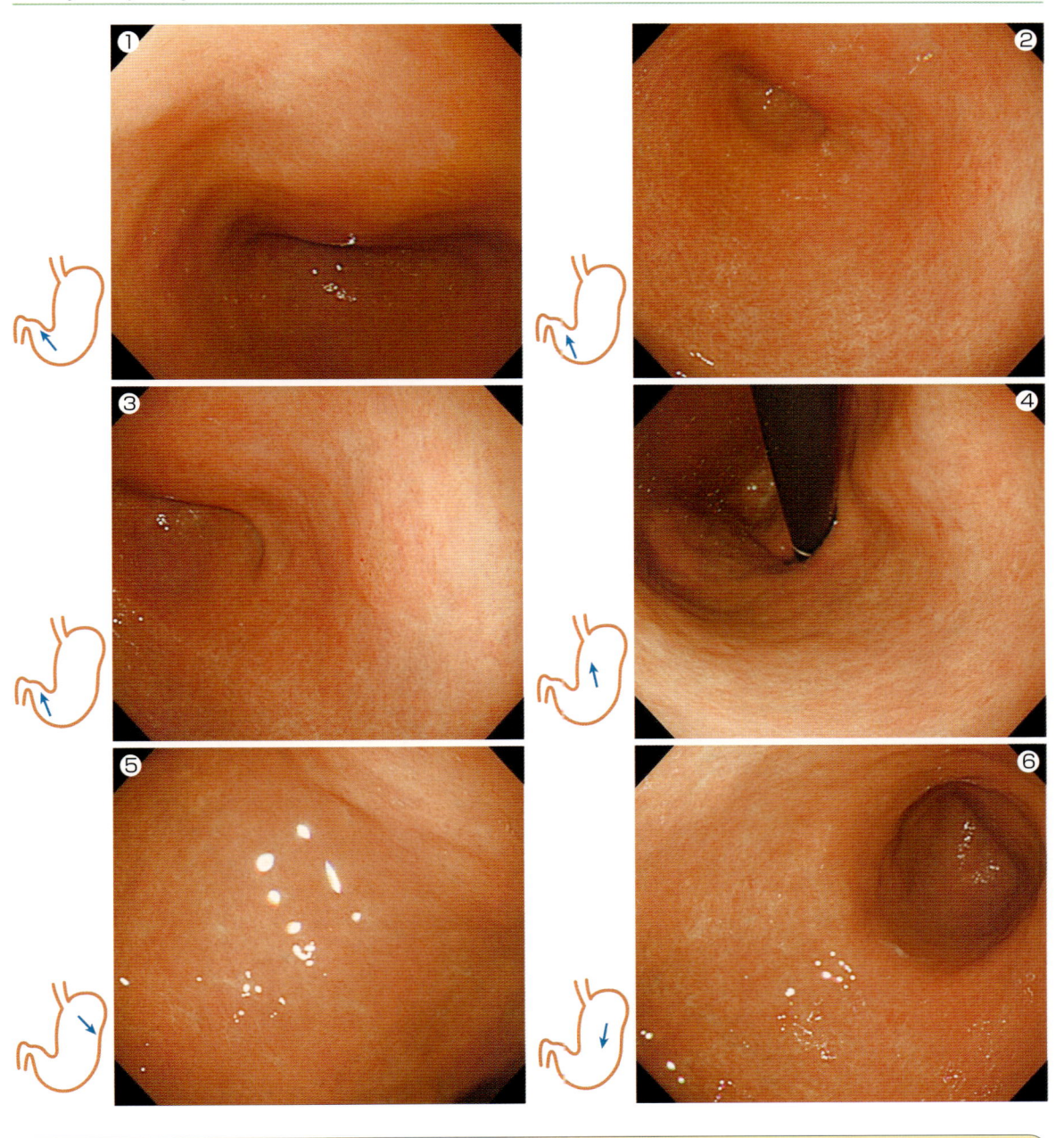

Hint 💡 Look for a yellowish-white lesion.

The answer and diagnosis are on page 205.

Screening endoscopy before surgery for colon cancer ①

▸ Female in her 70s.
▸ A screening endoscopy was performed before surgery for advanced colon cancer.

Can you specify the location of the gastric cancer?

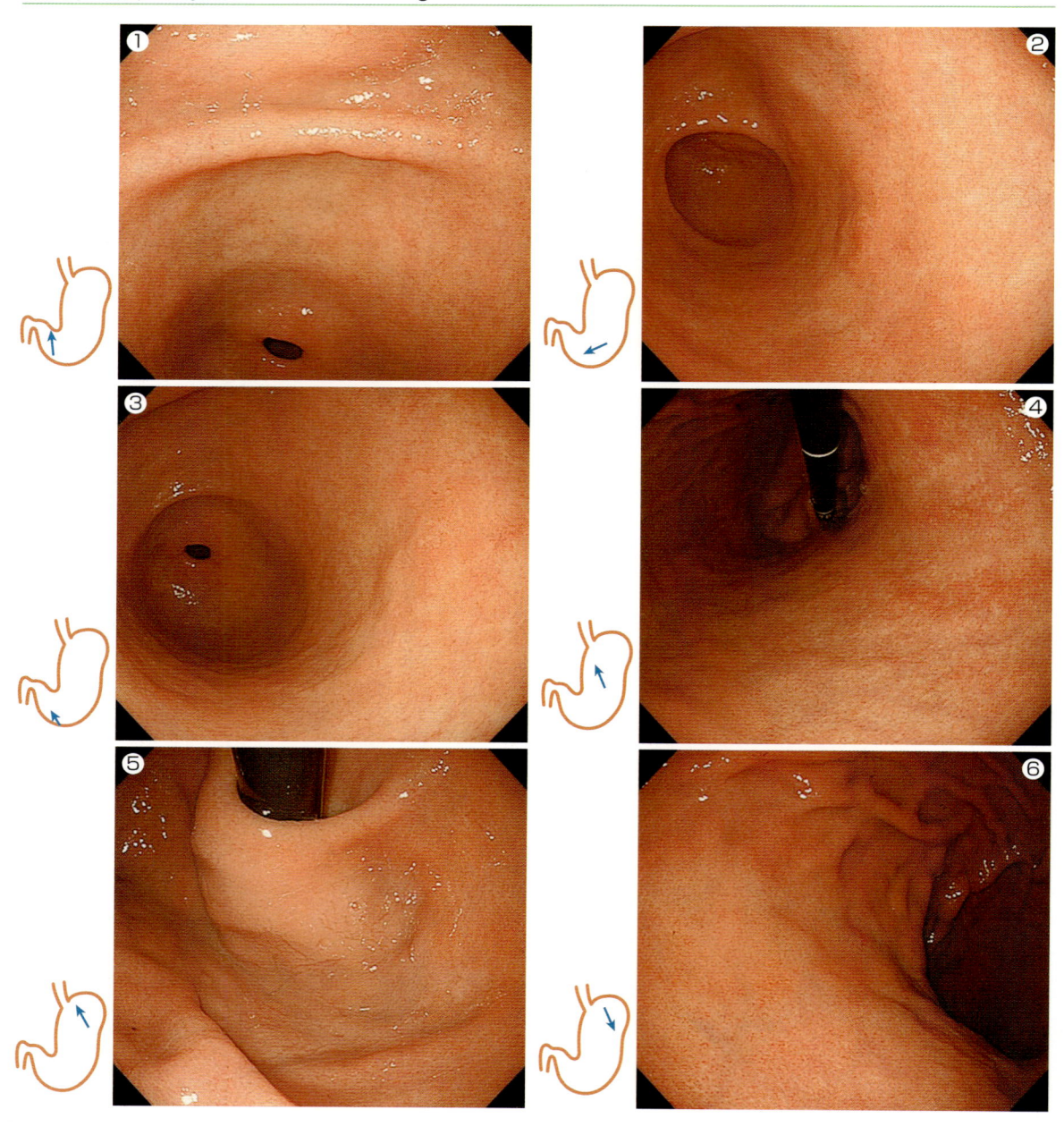

Hint 💡 Look for surface irregularities and color changes in the mucosa.

The answer and diagnosis are on page 206.

Screening endoscopy before surgery for colon cancer ②

▸ Male in his 60s.
▸ A screening endoscopy was performed before surgery for colon cancer.
▸ *H. pylori* had been eradicated 2 years previously.

Can you specify the location of the gastric cancer?

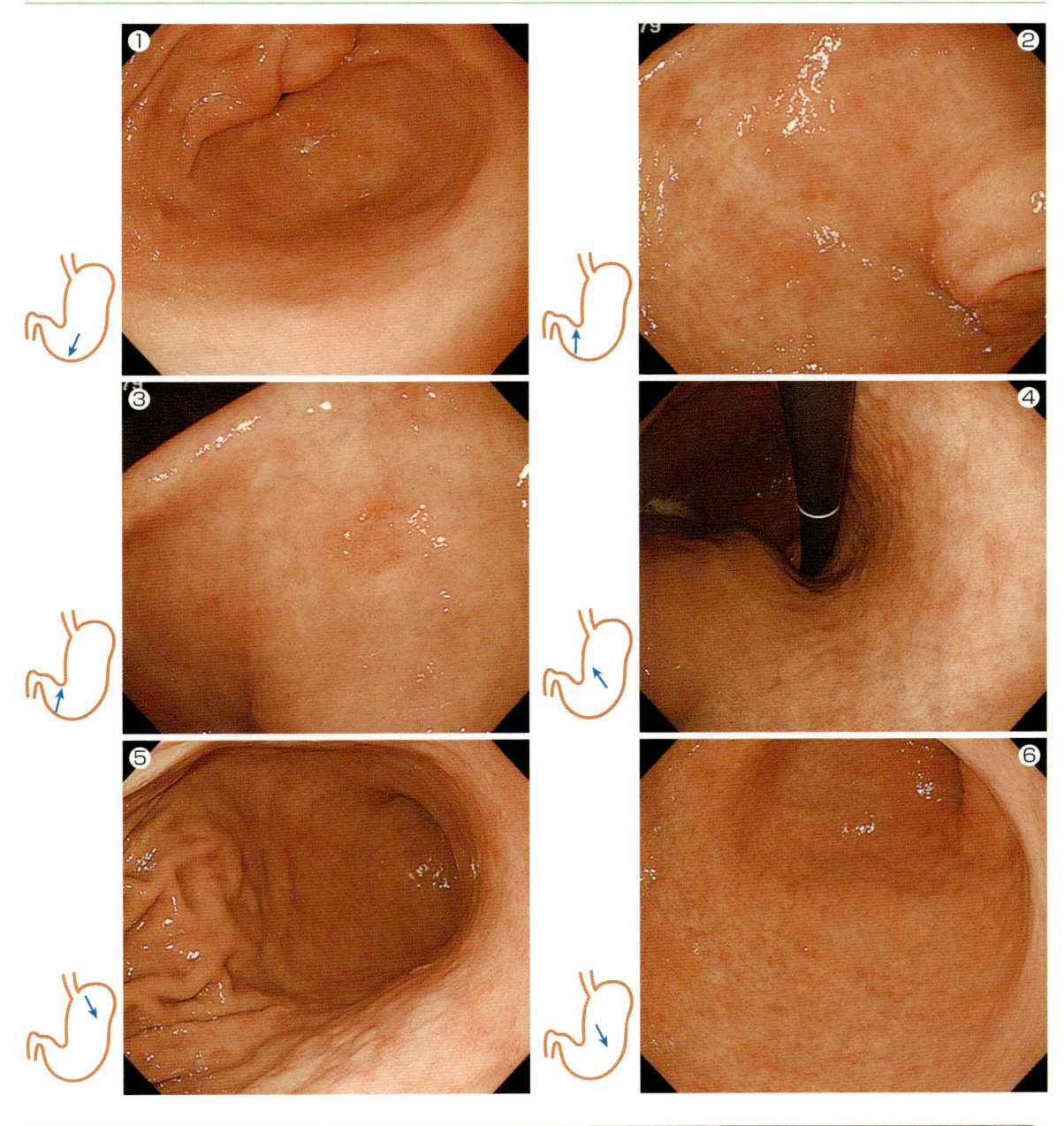

> **Hint** 💡 Look for any redness.

The answer and diagnosis are on page 207.

Screening endoscopy before surgery for colon cancer ③

▶ Female in her 60s.
▶ A screening endoscopy was performed before surgery for colon cancer.

Can you specify the location of the gastric cancer?

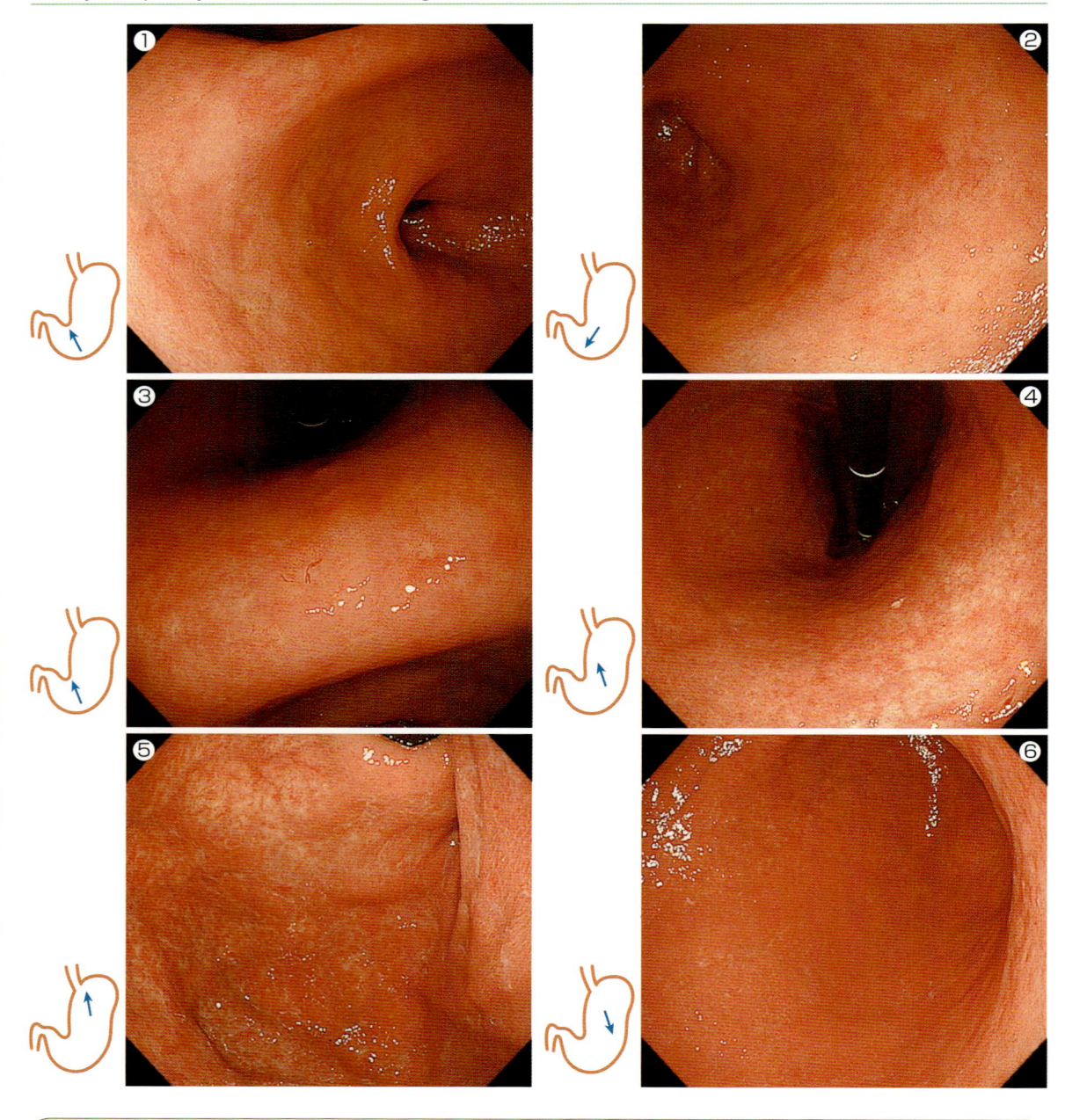

Hint 💡   Look for the finding(s) associated with cancer.

The answer and diagnosis are on page 208.

Screening endoscopy before surgery for colon cancer ④

▶ Male in his 60s.
▶ A screening endoscopy was performed before surgery for colon cancer.

Can you specify the location of the gastric cancer?

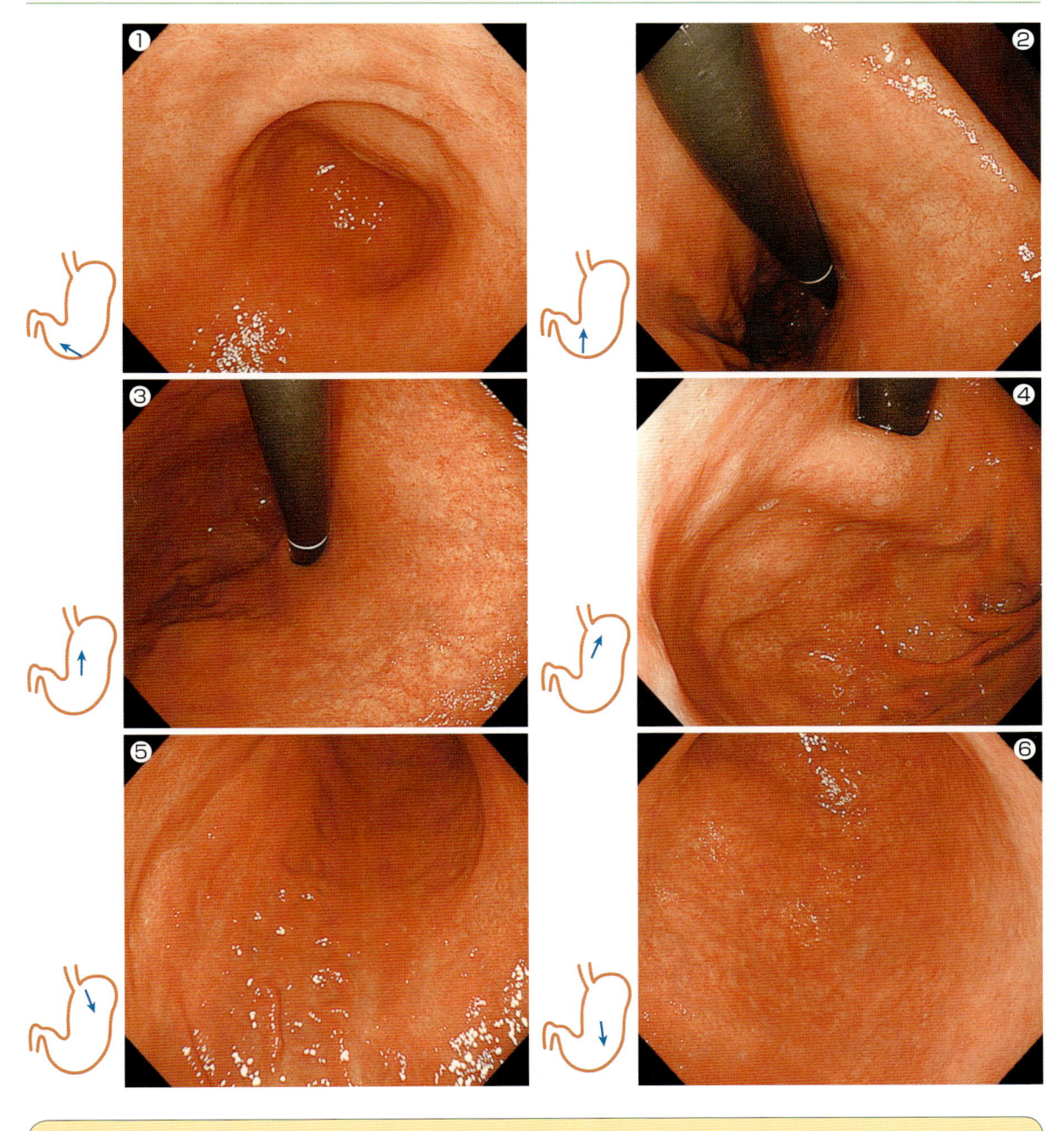

Hint 💡 Look for whitish mucosa.

The answer and diagnosis are on page 209.

case 51

Screening endoscopy after endoscopic treatment of colon cancer

▸ Male in his 70s.
▸ A screening endoscopy was performed after endoscopic treatment of colon cancer.

Can you specify the location of gastric tumor?

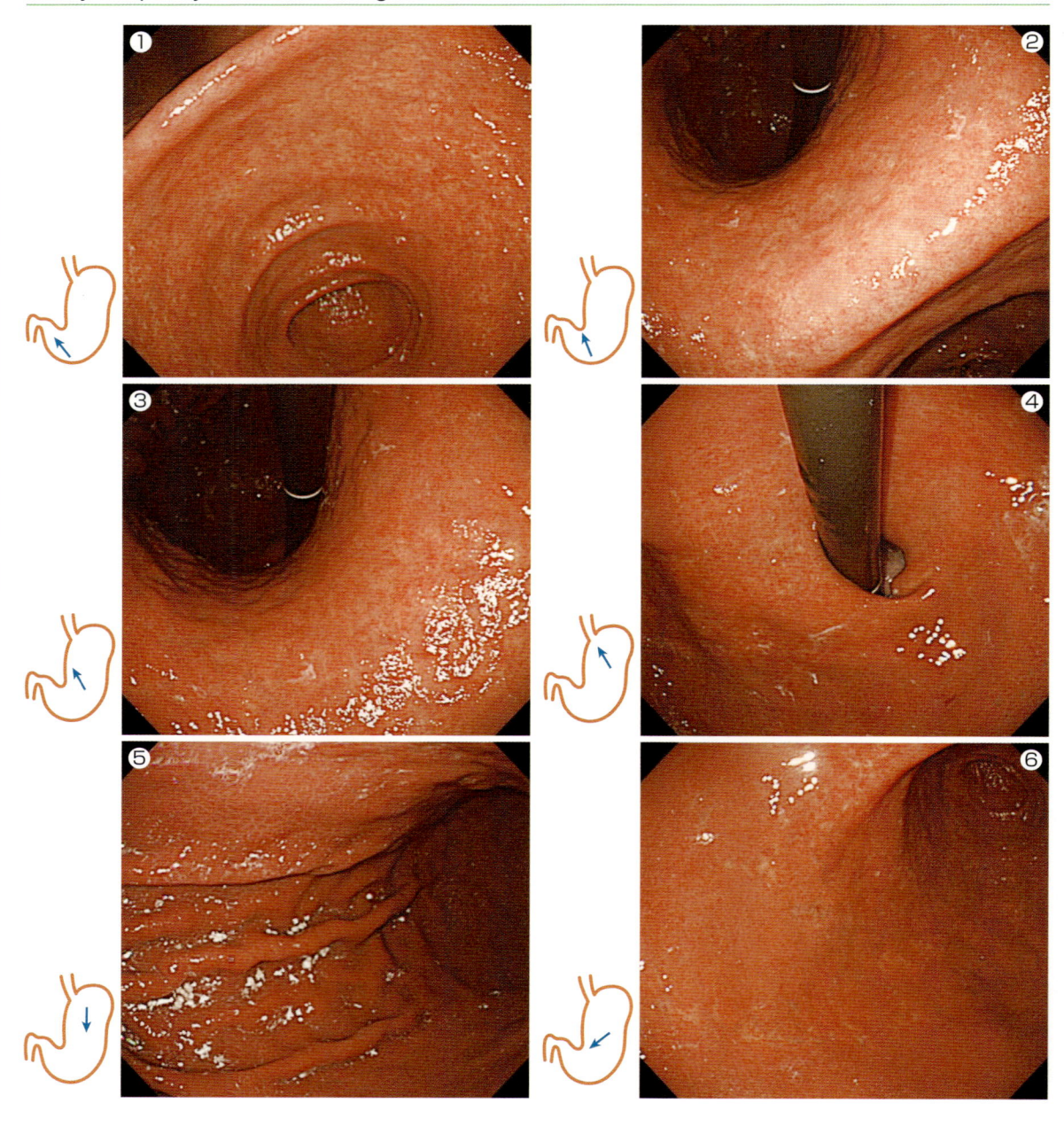

Hint 💡 Look for a depression with a different color tone.

The answer and diagnosis are on page 211.

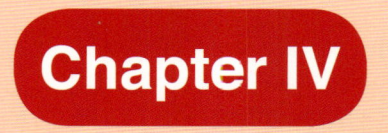

Did You Find the Gastric Cancer?
— Answers and Diagnoses —

Screening endoscopy at the cancer screening center ①

〔Gastric cancer with active *H. pylori* infection〕

Answer The gastric cancer is imaged in ① .

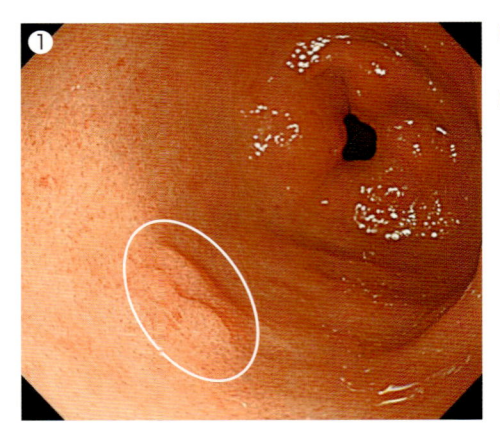

▶ O-1 atrophy is recognized in the background muco-sa.

▶ An elevation with a depression in its center is recognized near the anterior wall of the greater curvature of the antrum. At this point, you should suspect a 0-IIc lesion accompanied by a reactive elevation.

Close-up images

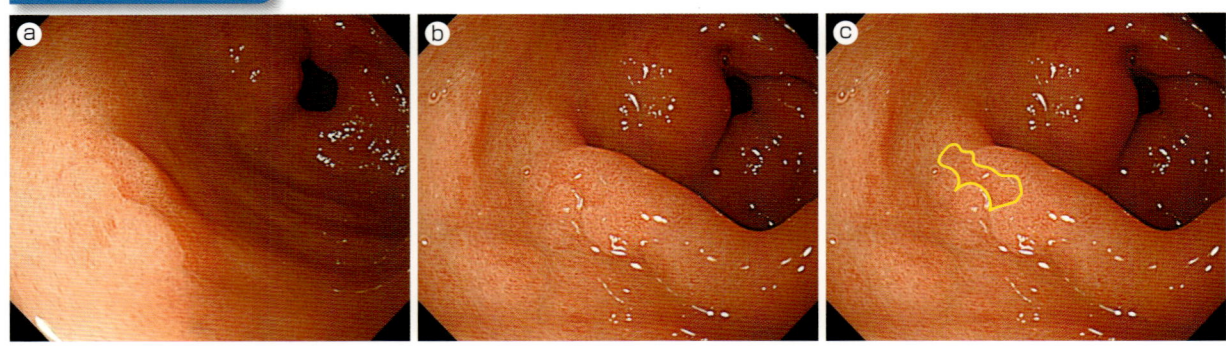

▶ a : In closed-up view, the depressed surface and surrounding elevation are clearly visible.

▶ b, c : When the lesion is viewed from the right front due to peristalsis, an encroachment (thorn-like intrusion to the sur-roundings) can be seen (outlined in yellow), presenting a strong likelihood of differentiated-type gastric cancer.

Indigo carmine sprayed images

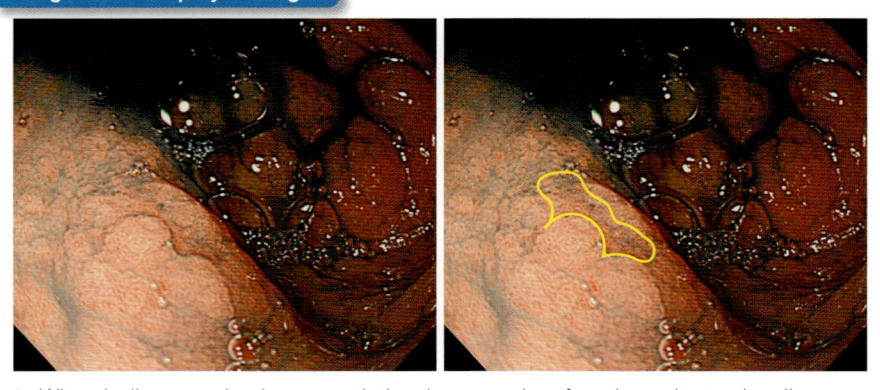

▶ When indigo carmine is sprayed, the depressed surface is easier to visualize.

▶ The elevation that surrounds the depression has the same mucosal structure as that of the background mucosa. This region has a reactive elevation and non-cancerous mucosa.

Tips

- Confirm the presence/absence of *H. pylori* infection from the background mucosa.
- Check reactive elevation to see if there is gastric cancer.
- Suspect gastric cancer if there is encroachment.

What's can be seen in the other pictures?

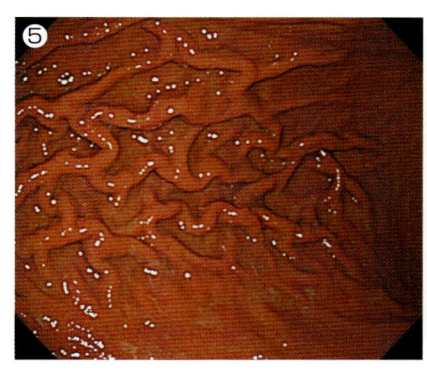
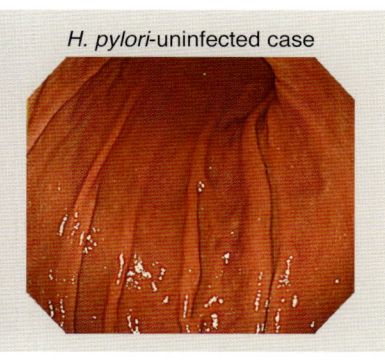

H. pylori-uninfected case

- Uniform erythematous mucosa extends throughout the body, manifesting as diffuse redness. The folds on the greater curvature of the body are enlarged and tortuous. Sticky mucus that cannot be washed away easily is attached.
- These findings indicate active *H. pylori* infection. When these findings are compared with the findings of *H. pylori*-uninfected cases, it is obvious that the color is different and the folds are larger and more tortuous.

Side Note   Transient parotitis after upper gastrointestinal endoscopy

"The patient is complaining of pain under his left ear!" A nurse told me in an endoscopy recovery area one day. When I went to take a look, the region that corresponded to the left parotid gland was red, swollen, and a little tender. I had performed endoscopy on him using pharyngeal anesthesia with ordinary Xylocaine Viscous and sedation with midazolam. Everything went smoothly so I was surprised by the appearance of symptoms I had never seen before. I ran a quick search on PubMed with "parotitis" and "endoscopy" and found that there was already a report on post-endoscopy transient parotitis[a]. Possible causes for this are believed to be increased secretion from the parotid gland after endoscopy, as well as transient occlusion of the duct due to a dilated vein in the parotid gland. Similar complications have been reported following bronchoscopy and endotracheal intubation. This patient's symptoms were transient and were managed conservatively.

Although I have performed many endoscopies, there are still many things that I don't know. This incident made me think that I should run a search on PubMed or other databases every time I encounter something I don't know.

a) Vadivel Kumaran S, Sumathi B Nirmala Natarajan D. Transient parotitis after upper gastrointestinal endoscopy. Endoscopy 2013 ; 45(Suppl. 2 UCTN) : E424–E425.

Screening endoscopy at the cancer screening center ②
[Gastric cancer with active *H. pylori* infection]

Answer The gastric cancer is imaged in ③ and ⑥ .

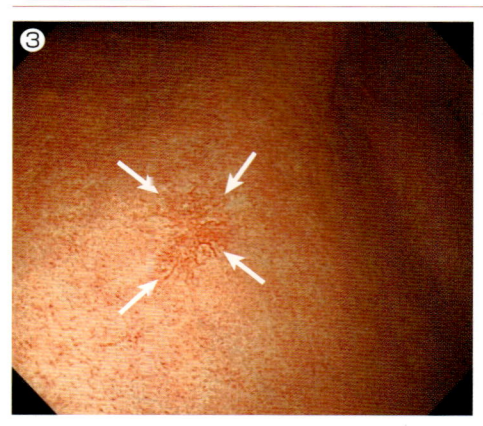

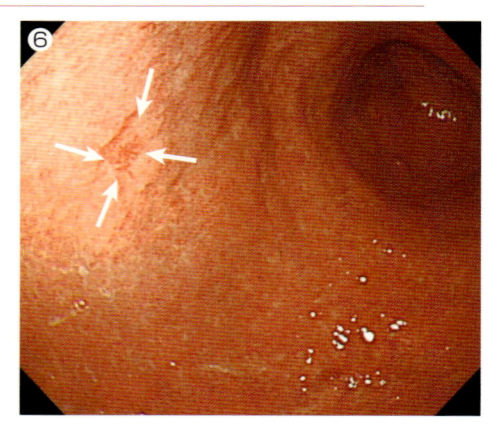

▶ O-3 atrophy, intestinal metaplasia, and diffuse redness can be seen on the background mucosa. Erythematous mucosa accompanied by dilated capillaries is visible on the anterior wall of the lower body. Although dilated capillaries are not necessarily indicative of cancer, they are sometimes seen with cancer and therefore must be observed in detail. When the site is observed from the right front, surface irregularities are difficult to recognize.

▶ When the site is observed tangentially, it appears as a reddish depressed lesion.

Non-magnifying NBI image

Indigo carmine sprayed images

Suctioned, in tangential direction

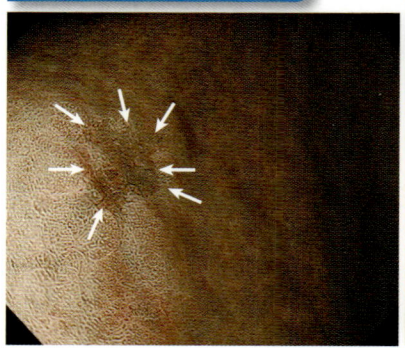

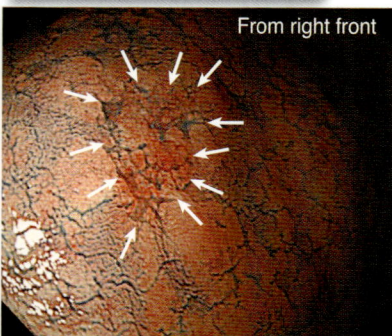
From right front

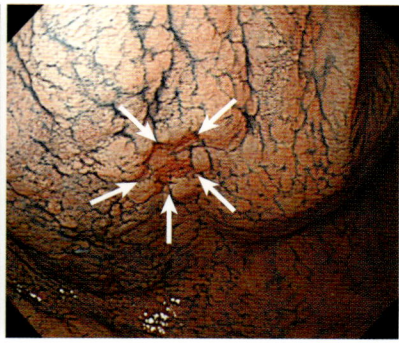

▶ In the non-magnifying NBI image, the depressed lesion appears brownish.

▶ When the lesion is observed from the right front after indigo carmine is sprayed, an unclear areae gastricae pattern can be seen on the depressed surface and the lesion's margins stand out clearly.

▶ When the stomach is suctioned and the lesion is observed tangentially, the depression is more noticeable, but detailed observation of the depressed surface is not possible.

Diagnosis Anterior wall of the lower body, 0–IIc, 10 mm, tub1, T1a (M), UL (–)

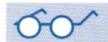 What's imaged in the other pictures?

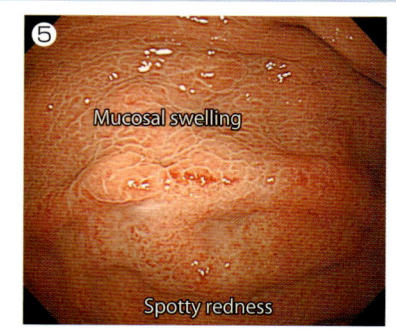
Mucosal swelling
Spotty redness

Tips

- Carefully observe the lesion while changing the distance, amount of air, and observation direction.
- Cancer should also be considered a possibility when a depression accompanied by dilated capillaries is observed.

- The areae gastricae is stretched and enlarged near the anterior wall of the greater curvature of the upper body — which is a finding that indicates mucosal swelling. On the greater curvature of the upper body, spotty redness is conspicuous. These findings indicate an active *H. pylori* infection.

Answer   The gastric cancer is imaged in ② .

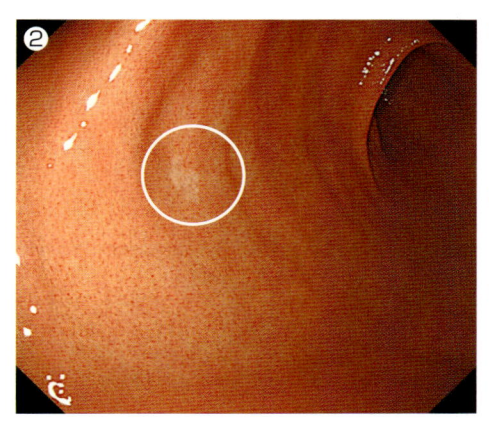

▶ The gastric mucosa is smooth and glossy in general, and no atrophy is found. In addition, numerous small red dots are arrayed in an orderly fashion. This is called RAC. These findings indicate that the gastric mucosa is normal and *H. pylori*-uninfected.

▶ Slightly faded mucosa (circled) can be seen near the anterior wall of the lesser curvature of the antrum.

▶ Faded mucosa in the fundic gland area without atrophy suggests the possibility of signet ring cell carcinoma.

| Close-up image | Non-magnifying NBI image | Indigo carmine sprayed image |

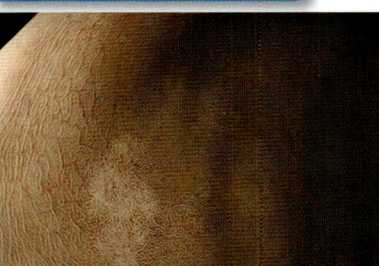
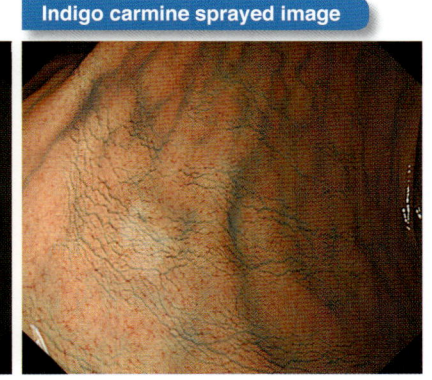

▶ Even when the lesion is observed in detail from up close, with NBI (non-magnifying), and with indigo carmine sprayed, changes on the mucosal surface are hard to detect except for color tone. In the early stage of undifferentiated-type gastric cancer, a IIb lesion without surface irregularities like this is often seen. As the tumor grows bigger, however, a depression starts to appear.

▶ According to a study of undifferentiated-type gastric cancer at our hospital, 36% of tumors with 10-mm-or-less diameter were 0–IIb and 64% were 0–IIc, while 6% of those with diameters of 11 to 20 mm were 0–IIb and 94% were 0–IIc[39].

Histological images of ESD-resected specimen

a : HE-stained, low-magnification image. A tumor can be seen in the area shown under the red line. The surrounding mucosa is non-atrophic fundic gland mucosa with no significant inflammation. There is no difference between the level of the cancerous and noncancerous areas. This is a 0–IIb lesion.

b : HE-stained, high-magnification image. A signet-ring cell carcinoma cluster that indicates uneven distribution of nuclei can be seen on the border between the foveolar epithelium and the proper gastric glands (neck of glands) in the middle layer of the mucosa. The cancer cells are not exposed on the surface of the mucosa, and the foveolar epithelium looks no different than noncancerous mucosa.

c : PAS-stained, high-magnification image. The signet-ring cell carcinoma cytoplasm shows as PAS-positive (the same region as b).

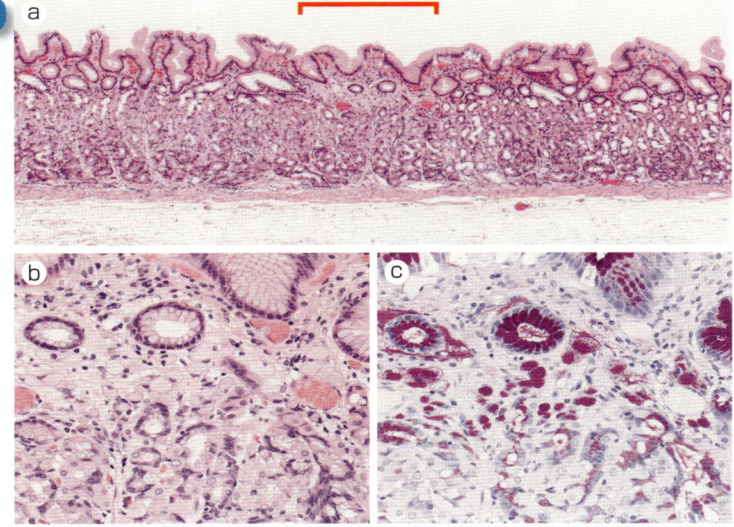

Diagnosis Anterior wall of the antrum, 0–IIb, 3 mm, sig, T1a (M), UL (–)

Tips

- A RAC-positive finding indicates *H. pylori*-uninfected condition.
- When there is no *H. pylori* infection, you should look for undifferentiated-type gastric cancer.
- Undifferentiated-type gastric cancer frequently exhibits fading.
- The only sign of early undifferentiated-type gastric cancer is a change in color tone. It is not accompanied by any change in surface irregularities.

Additional Info *H. pylori*-uninfected gastric cancer

- It has been reported that *H. pylori*-uninfected gastric cancer accounts for roughly 1 to 3% of gastric cancer cases. However, it has not been clearly defined and it is difficult to confirm whether or not it really is *H. pylori*-uninfected.
- To accurately determine whether or not there is or has been an *H. pylori* infection, we defined a case as *H. pylori*-uninfected condition only when all of the following six conditions are met: ① no history of eradication, ② no history of gastric surgery, ③ no endoscopic finding of atrophy, ④ pepsinogen method negative, ⑤ serum anti-*H. pylori* antibodies negative, and ⑥ urea breath test negative. Then, we examined ESD-resected specimens from 1,636 cases and found that 20 of them (1.2%) were *H. pylori*-uninfected gastric cancer. They were all undifferentiated-type gastric cancer, and 87% of them had lesions with fading[39].
- When a finding that suggests there is no *H. pylori* infection is observed in endoscopy, pay attention to faded mucosa and look for undifferentiated-type gastric cancer. Subsequently, we also found a few cases of gastric adenocarcinoma of fundic gland type with *H. pylori*-uninfected condition.

Side Note Rare accidental symptoms

Around four p.m. as was just finishing up my afternoon endoscopies, I received a phone call from the daughter of a patient on whom I had performed an upper GI endoscopy that same morning. The patient was a female in her 60s. She had come to the hospital on her own. Her endoscopy concluded with a finding of chronic gastritis only. No biopsy was required. After paying the fee, she went home by bus and train. According to her daughter, however, the patient claimed to be unable to remember what she had done that day. When sedation is used, it is pretty common for patients not to notice when their endoscopy has finished. However, I didn't use sedation on this patient. The daughter sounded quite bewildered on the phone, so I advised her to come to the hospital with her mother.

When she returned with her daughter, the patient looked confused and said she couldn't remember anything since she got up that morning. She seemed to possess a normal level of awareness and was able to give her date of birth, address, and phone number without any problem. No abnormal psychiatric findings were observed. Yet even after I explained to her that she had undergone an endoscopy at the hospital, she would soon resume asking why she was there. The daughter meanwhile was watching us all with a dubious expression. Fortunately, I had experienced a similar episode during the first year of my internship — which enabled me to immediately diagnose it as transient global amnesia and explain it appropriately to the patient and her daughter.

In transient global amnesia, retrograde and anterograde amnesia are produced by stress. It is considered a temporary disorder of the hippocampus where short-term memories are formed. In many cases, patients recover within 24 hours. Although there is no impact on conscious awareness, patients become confused because they are unable to understand what condition they are in because they are unable to form any short-term memories. There has been a report on transient global amnesia triggered by endoscopy[a], and I have personally experienced 3 cases of it thus far.

You may be unsure what to do if you are unaware that such accidental phenomena can occur. So I want you to be aware of it.

a) Tsukada K, et al. [Three cases of transient global amnesia after upper endoscopic examination.] Gastroenterol Endosc. 2006; 48: 1215–1220. (In Japanese.)

Answer The gastric cancer is imaged in ① .

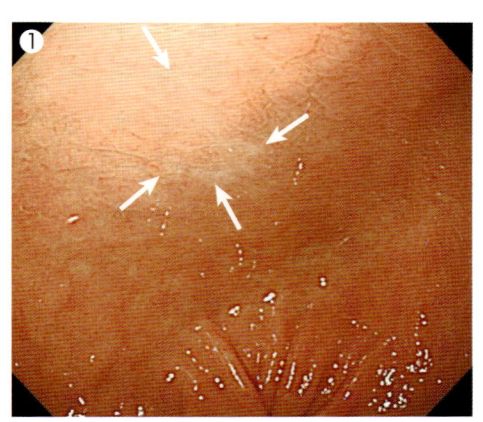

▶ Although the background mucosa is glossy and smooth, it is slightly edematous and RAC appears to be unclear. However, there is no sign of either atrophy or intestinal metaplasia. It is one of those cases that make you hesitant to diagnose *H. pylori* infection.

▶ Slightly faded mucosa (indicated by the arrows) can be seen in the lesser curvature of the antrum. This lesion is very difficult to detect. Because it occurs in a single location and a faded area is observed despite there being no atrophy in the surrounding area, it is suspected to be signet ring cell carcinoma.

Non-magnifying NBI image

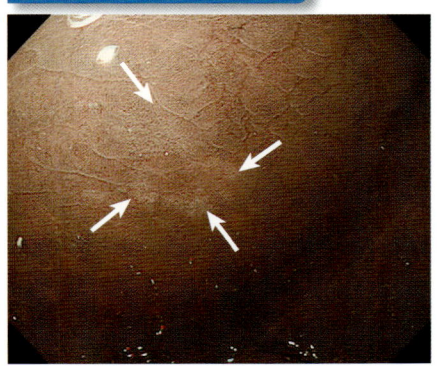

Indigo carmine sprayed image

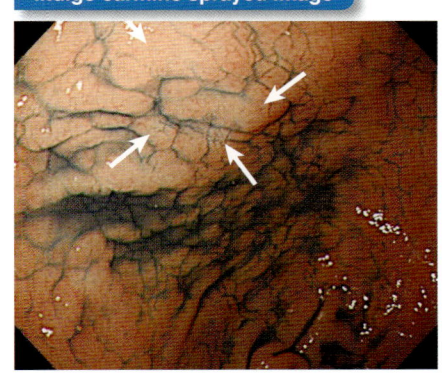

▶ In non-magnifying NBI, the lesion is a lighter shade of brown than the surrounding mucosa.

▶ When indigo carmine is sprayed, the change in color tone is less noticeable. A lack of change in the areae gastricae pattern also causes the visibility of the lesion to deteriorate. When no change is apparent in the mucosal surface as seen here, cancer is not usually exposed on the mucosal surface. As a matter of fact, in this case, signet ring cell carcinoma was present only in the middle layer of the mucosa.

Diagnosis Lesser curvature of the antrum, 0–IIb, 6 mm, sig, T1a (M), UL (–)

Tips

- The presence of cobblestone mucosa makes it difficult to diagnose *H. pylori* infection.
- Look for scanty fading with *H. pylori*-uninfected cases.

Endoscopic image from 1 year previously

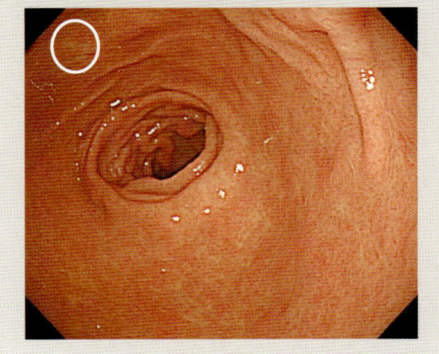

- The faded mucosa is present in the same region (shown in the circle), and looks almost unchanged since then.

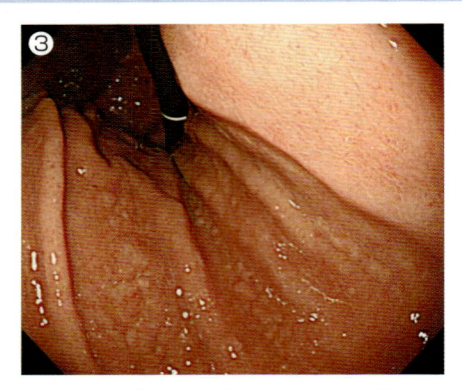

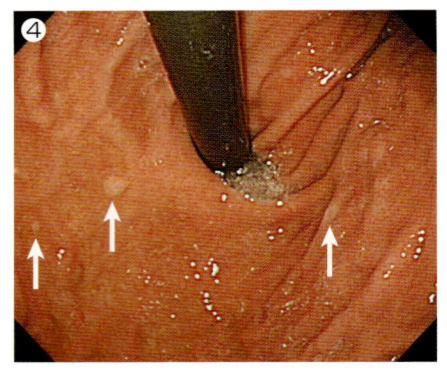

- The mucosa is slightly edematous overall, and multiple hemispherical elevations of various sizes are present between the folds. The color tone is not different from the surrounding mucosa. This is a finding called cobblestone mucosa. Since the mucosa thickens in the elevated parts, RAC is not clear. There had been no *H. pylori* infection in this case, but the cobblestone mucosa made it difficult to evaluate.

- Multiple whitish flat elevated lesions are also present in the fornix (Haruma-Kawaguch lesions).These are different from cobblestone mucosa.

Additional Info Cobblestone mucosa

- A mucosal finding — in which the mucosa in the body becomes edematous, elevated granular mucosa is found in countless numbers, and the surface looks as if it were a stone-paved road —is called cobblestone mucosa. Elevations are often recognized between the folds. Reportedly, this occurs frequently in *H. pylori*-uninfected cases with long-term PPI medication. The elevation is believed to be caused by hyperplastic changes in the parietal cells or by transformation of the parietal cells as a result of long-term treatment with PPIs[40].

- The photos below are of another *H. pylori*-uninfected case and has been treated for 10 years with rabeprazole sodium.

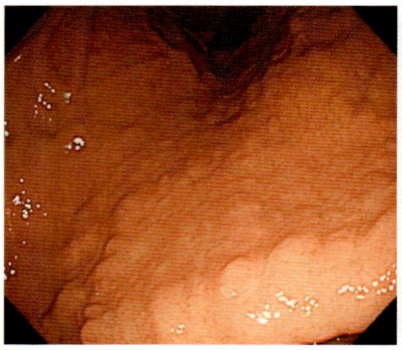

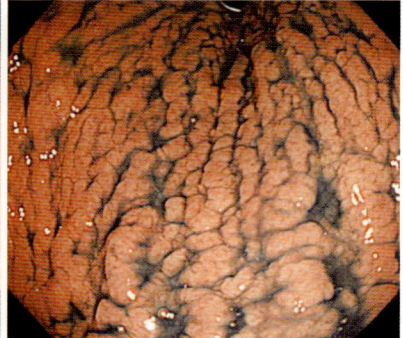

Screening endoscopy at the cancer screening center ⑤

〔*H. pylori*-uninfected gastric cancer〕

Answer   The gastric cancer is imaged in ① .

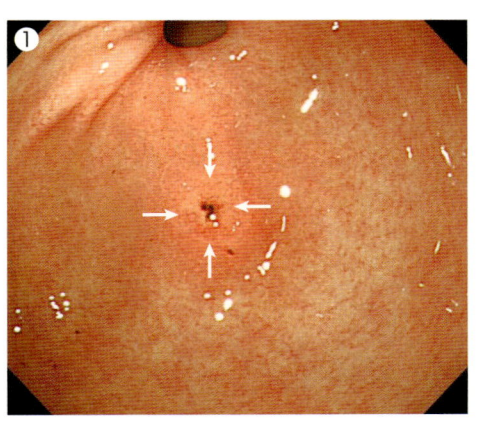

▶ The background mucosa is glossy and uniformly orange-red. It is RAC-positive. Fundic gland polyps are also recognized. It is an *H. pylori*-uninfected case.

▶ Erosion with hematin attached is observed in a single location (indicated by the arrows) in the greater curvature of the prepyloric region. At this point, it is too early to suspect cancer, but the single occurrence makes it worrisome.

Indigo carmine sprayed image

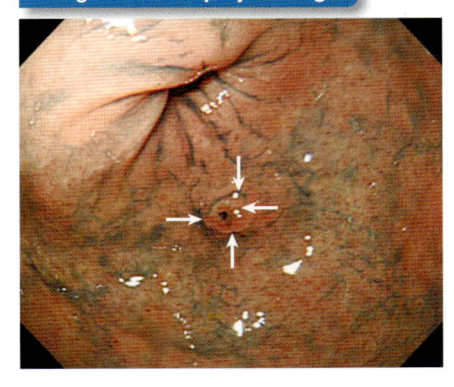

▶ When indigo carmine is sprayed, a depressed surface with clear margins can be recognized. Even though it is a shallow depression, the difference in level makes it look as if it were cut with a knife. This finding alone makes it difficult to diagnose it as cancer. However, since it is a single erosion with clear margins below the level of the surrounding mucosa, cancer should be included in the differential diagnosis and a biopsy should be performed.

▶ It should be noted that benign erosions do not have such clear margins because the transition to the edges is more gradual.

Diagnosis   Greater curvature of the prepyloric region, 0–IIc, 4 mm, sig, T1a (M), UL (−)

Tips

- With a single erosion, include cancer in differential diagnosis.
- Spray indigo carmine to detect findings that suggest cancer.

Answer   The gastric cancer is imaged in ⑥ .

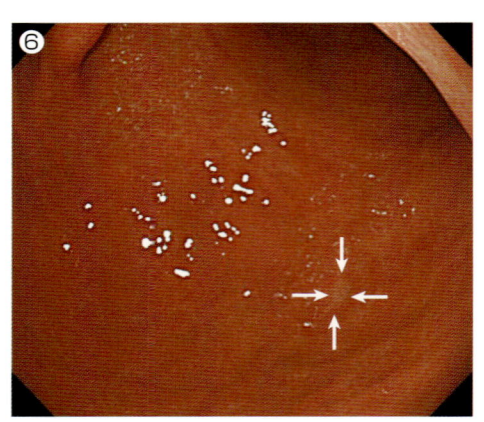

▶ There is C–2 atrophy in the background mucosa. The body exhibits pale diffuse redness. This finding indicates an active *H. pylori* infection.

▶ Faded patches can be seen on the greater curvature of the lower body. Nothing similar is observed in the surrounding area.

Close-up image

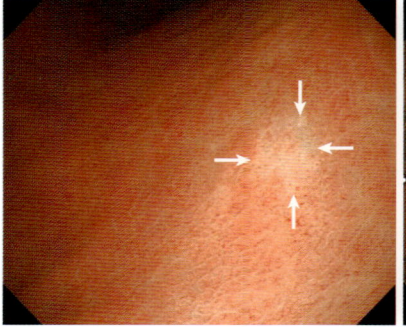

Indigo carmine sprayed images

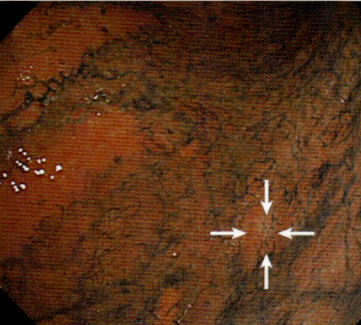 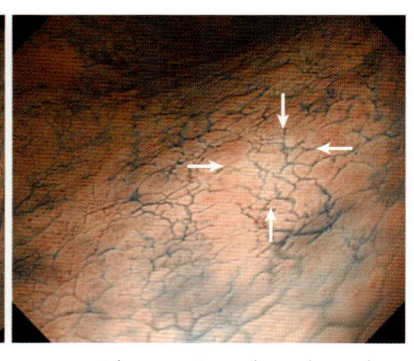

▶ When the endoscope is moved up close, clear margins can be seen around the faded patches.

▶ When indigo carmine is sprayed, areae gastricae patterns in various sizes become visible in the surrounding mucosa. This is a further indication of *H. pylori* infection. The areae gastricae in the faded patches show a similar pattern to the areae gastricae in the surrounding mucosa without surface irregularities, suggesting IIb signet ring cell carcinoma.

Diagnosis   Anterior wall of the lower body, 0–IIc, 6 mm, sig, T1a (M), UL (−)

Tips

• Try to distinguish between faded patches caused by atrophy and those produced by undifferentiated-type gastric cancer.

👓   What's imaged in the other pictures?

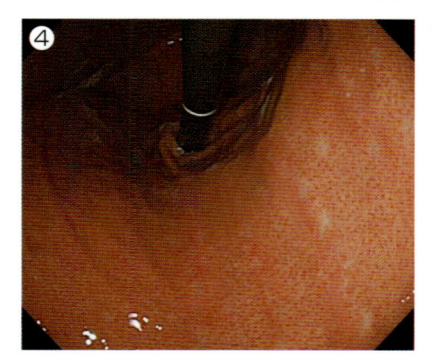

• Multiple faded patches are also present in the lesser curvature of the body. Since they tend to run in a more or less longitudinal direction and are present in multiple locations, we believe they were caused by localized atrophy present in a non-atrophic area.

Answer   The gastric cancer is imaged in ③ and ⑥ .

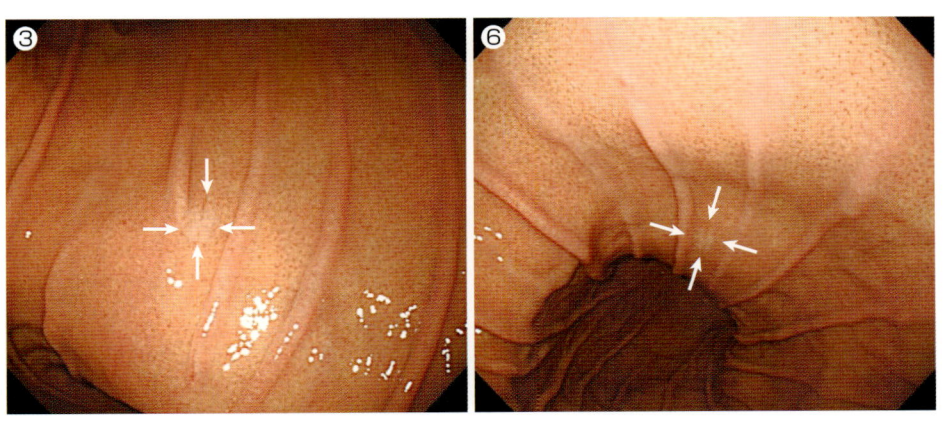

▶ This is a RAC-positive case. The background mucosa is free of atrophy and not infected with *H. pylori*.
▶ Pale faded mucosa is observed in the lesser curvature of the lower body.

Indigo carmine sprayed image

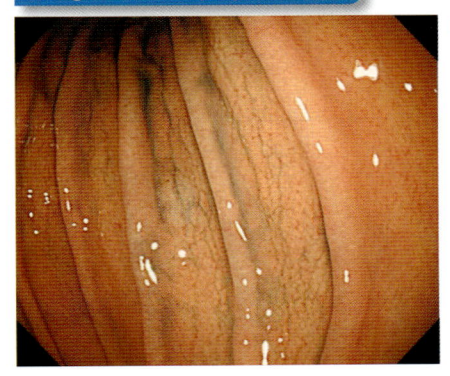

▶ When indigo carmine is sprayed, the lesion appears to be 0–IIb without surface irregularities. As this case presents faded mucosa in the fundic gland region without atrophy, it is suspected to be signet ring cell carcinoma.

Diagnosis   Lesser curvature of the lower body,0–IIc, 4 mm, sig, T1a (M), UL (−)

Tips

• Look for fading when examining an *H. pylori*-uninfected case.

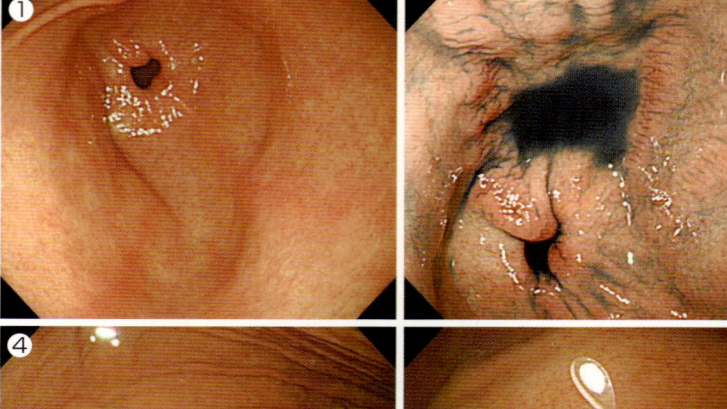

- This is a finding referred to as red streaks where longitudinal red strips of can be seen in the antrum. This finding is often seen on *H. pylori*-un-infected mucosa without gastritis.

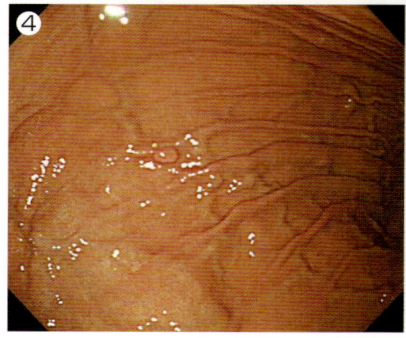
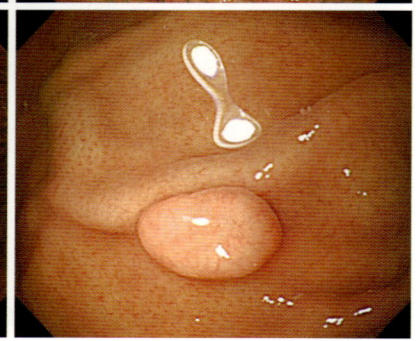

- A Yamada type II polyp can be seen in the greater curvature of the upper body. It is a fundic gland polyp. When observed up close, a slight constriction and circumferential margin can be seen, making it possible to differentiate it from an SMT.

Side Note 📝 What is the color of gastric cancer?

When you look it up in a textbook, it says that the color tone of gastric cancer is red, white, faded, and so on. None of these colors are necessarily the primary color. Rather, it means that the tumor is slightly redder or whiter than the surrounding area, so it is described as reddish or whitish. It is important to capture any subtle differences in color tone from the surrounding background mucosa. Also, although textbooks don't mention this very often, gastric cancer sometimes appears to be yellow. Of course, it's not the primary color yellow; it's just a little more yellowish than the surrounding area. If you can spot this subtle yellow color, your gastric cancer detection rate will improve.

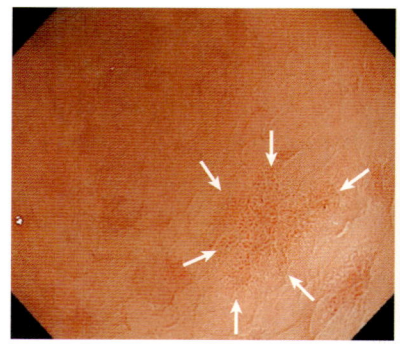
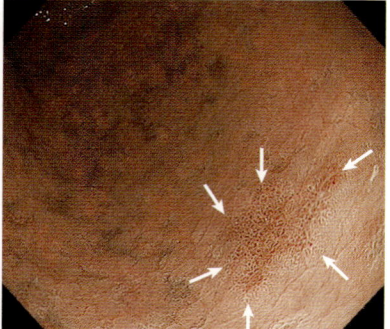

In the background mucosa where intestinal metaplasia and post-eradication reddish depression are present in multiple locations, mucosa that's slightly more yellowish than the surrounding area can be recognized. It exhibits a brownish color in an NBI image (right), making the margins clearer. The margins can also be recognized from the difference in the mucosal patterns. Noting any region that's slightly more yellowish than the surrounding area is important for diagnosis of gastric cancer.

▶ Greater curvature of the lower body, 0–IIb, 5 mm, tub1, T1a (M), UL (–)

Answer The gastric cancer is imaged in ④ and ⑤ .

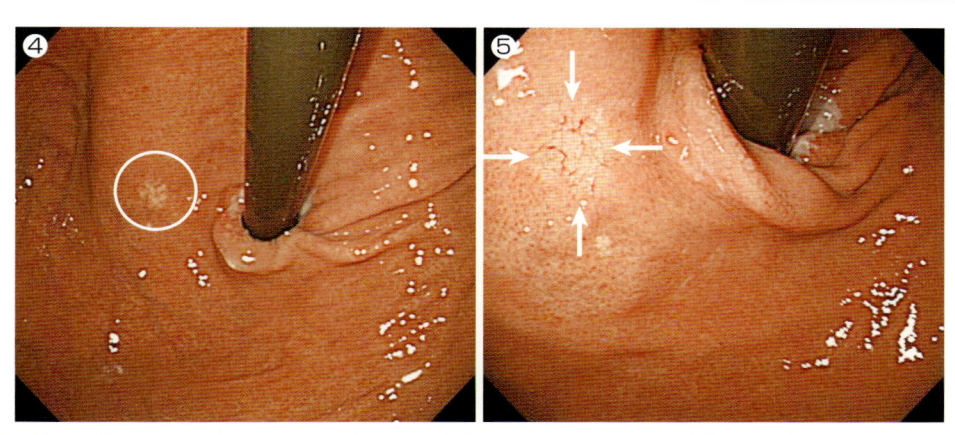

▶ This is a RAC-positive case. The background mucosa is free of atrophy and not infected with *H. pylori*.

▶ Faded mucosa with clear margins (circled) can be seen on the posterior wall of the fornix. The mucosal surface is smooth and glossy. Dilated, tortuous vessels are visible in the superficial layer (indicated by the arrows).

Indigo carmine sprayed images

Non-magnifying NBI image

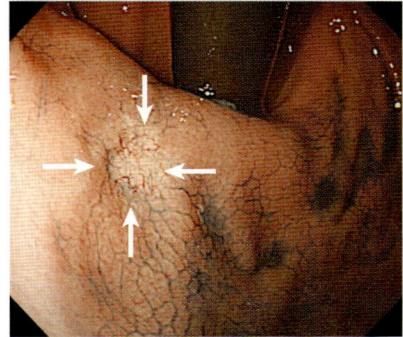
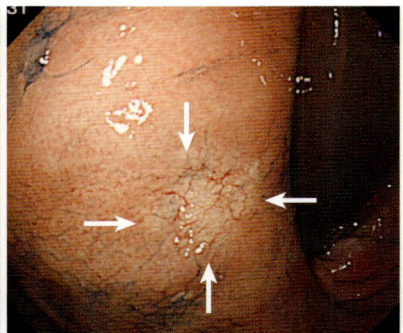
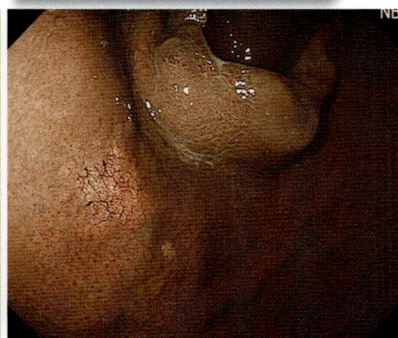

▶ When indigo carmine is sprayed, the surface of the lesion appears to be smooth with no distinctive surface irregularities.

▶ Under non-magnifying NBI observation, the lesion is a lighter shade of brown than the surrounding mucosa and the margins are somewhat unclear.

Histological images of ESD-resected specimen

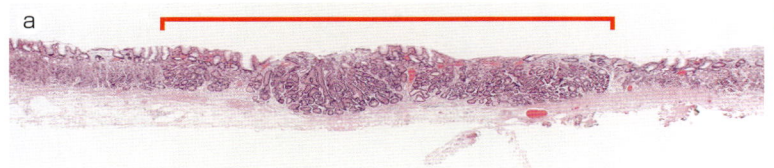
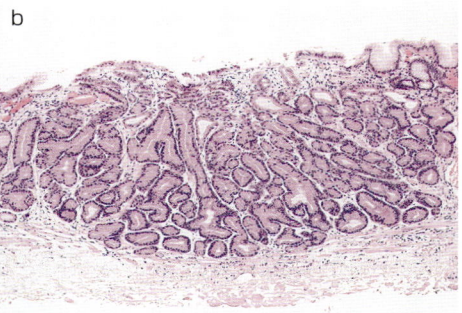
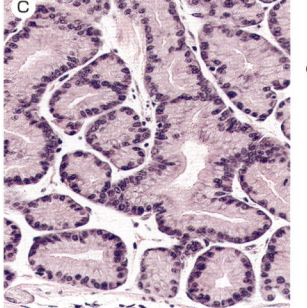

a : HE-stained, low-magnification image. The extent of the tumor is shown under the red line. The background is fundic gland mucosa with inconspicuous atrophy.

b : HE-stained, middle-magnification image of the center of the tumor. Small-sized glands with occasionally branching proliferate in the middle to deep layers of the mucosa.

c : HE-stained, high-magnification image of the tumor. The nuclei are almost round and arrayed on the basal membrane side. The cell bodies appear pale and basophilic and resemble chief cells. The lesion resembled chief cells and corresponded with what is referred to as gastric adenocarcinoma of the fundic gland type (chief cell predominant type), while remaining within the mucosa.

▶ In immunostaining, pepsinogen-I and MUC6 were widely positive and H^+/K^+-ATPase was only partially positive.

Tips

- In *H. pylori*-uninfected cases, also keep an eye out for gastric adenocarcinoma of the fundic gland type.
- Gastric adenocarcinoma of the fundic gland type is a flat, faded lesion, with dilated, tortuous vessels on the surface.
- MALT lymphoma and carcinoid tumor should be included in differential diagnosis of gastric adenocarcinoma of the fundic gland type.

Additional Info   Gastric adenocarcinoma of the fundic gland type

- Gastric adenocarcinoma of the fundic gland type is a relatively new histological subtype of gastric cancer first proposed by Ueyama et al. [41] in 2010. Since it is generated from the fundic glands deep in the mucosa, the superficial layer is covered with non-cancerous mucosa, while cancerous cells — which show similar differentiation to chief cells, mucousus neck cells, and parietal cells — proliferate in the deep portion of mucosa. In immunostaining, pepsinogen-I (specific to chief cells), H^+/K^+-ATPase (specific to parietal cells), and MUC6 (a marker for accessory cells) all show as positive.
- This type of cancer frequently occurs in the upper body of elderly patients, who, in many cases, do not have an *H. pylori* infection. Even small lesions of this type often invade the submucosa, but cell proliferation activity and vascular invasiveness are extremely low. Hence, malignancy is believed to be low and prognosis is favorable [42].
- A typical endoscopic finding is an SMT-like flat elevation. The color is faded, and it is often accompanied by dilated tree-like vessels on the surface [43].

Endoscopic image from 7 years previously

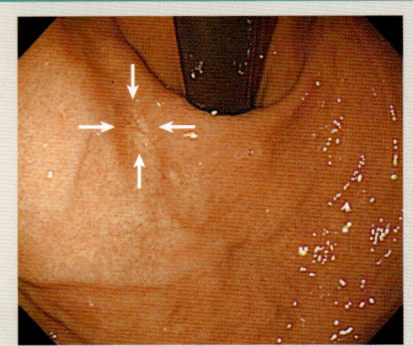

- The image from 7 years earlier shows a similar finding. This indicates that gastric adenocarcinoma of the fundic gland type spreads slowly.

Different case ① : Gastric adenocarcinoma of the fundic gland type

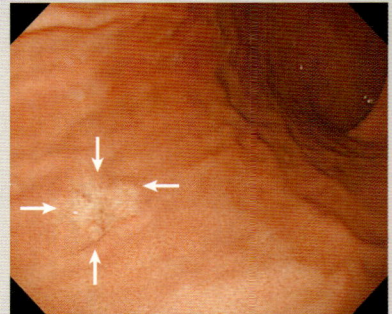 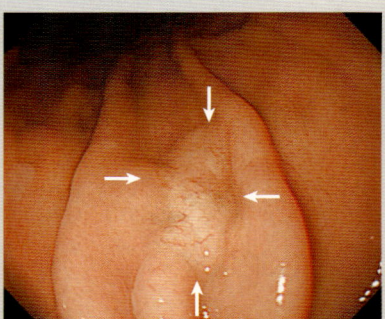 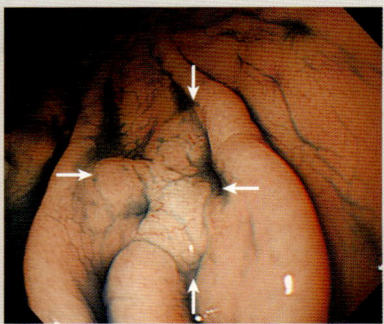

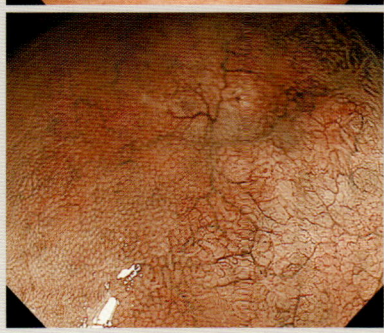

- *H. pylori*-uninfected case. The mucosa is faded and slightly thick. The mucosal surface is smooth and glossy. The margins are slightly unclear, and dilated, tortuous vessels are visible on the surface. Under conventional endoscopy, the diagnosis was MALT lymphoma or gastric adenocarcinoma of the fundic gland type.
- In magnifying NBI (bottom), an abnormal vascular pattern that looks like branches spreading out from the trunk of a tree is recognized. This is a finding similar to the tree-like appearance [44] characteristic of MALT lymphoma. As seen here, MALT lymphoma and gastric adenocarcinoma of the fundic gland type may exhibit similar findings.
- Diagnosis: Greater curvature of the middle body, 0–IIb, 15 mm, gastric adenocarcinoma of the fundic gland type, T1b (SM1, 400 μm), UL (−).

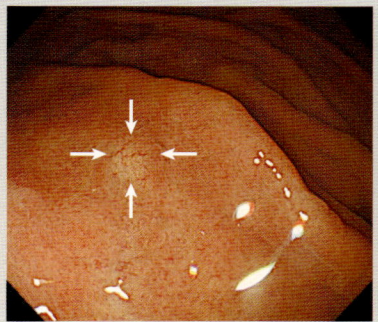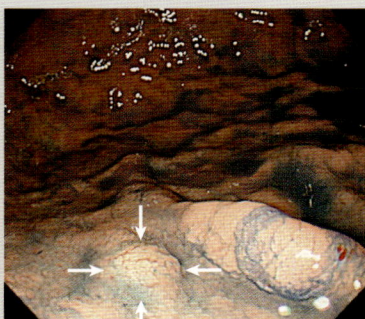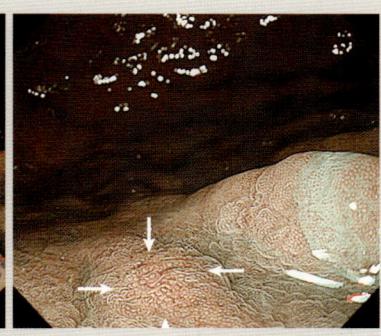

- This is a case of minute gastric adenocarcinoma of the fundic gland type after *H. pylori* eradication. The background mucosa is a fundic gland region without atrophy. An SMT-like elevation with a diameter of 2 mm and a color tone that ranges between yellowish and faded can be seen in the greater curvature of the upper body. It is accompanied by dilated, tortuous vessels on the surface.
- In an NBI medium-magnification image (right), dilated crypt openings can be seen. This finding shows that the crypt openings are extended by a subepithelial tumor.
- As an endoscopic diagnosis, gastric adenocarcinoma of the fundic gland type and carcinoid tumor are both possible, but it is difficult to differentiate them.
- Diagnosis: Greater curvature of the middle body, 0–IIa, 2 mm, gastric adenocarcinoma of the fundic gland type, T1a (M1), UL (–).

Compare! Gastric MALT lymphoma (different case)

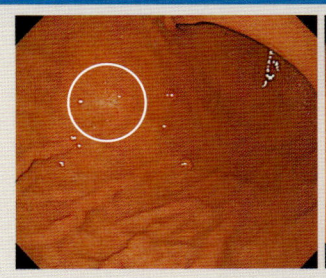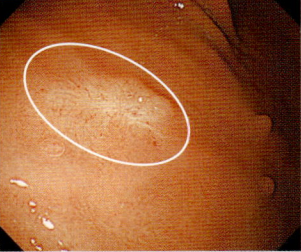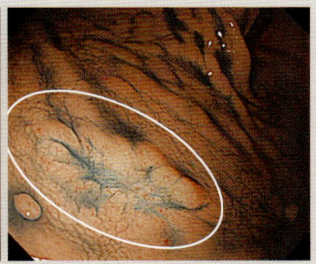

- This is an *H. pylori*-uninfected MALT lymphoma case. As with gastric adenocarcinoma of the fundic gland type, the mucosa is glossy and faded, and there are dilated, tortuous vessels in the superficial layer. Although MALT lymphoma does not have clear margins, occurs in multiple locations, and exhibits various findings, you may also experience cases that are difficult to differentiate from gastric adenocarcinoma of the fundic gland type. The important thing is that you provide the pathologist with any clinical information that makes you suspect gastric adenocarcinoma of the fundic gland type or MALT lymphoma.

Compare! Carcinoid tumors (different case)

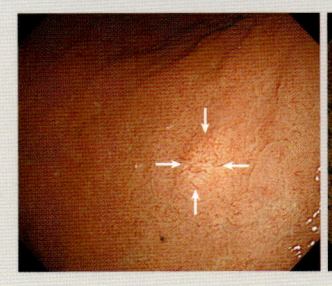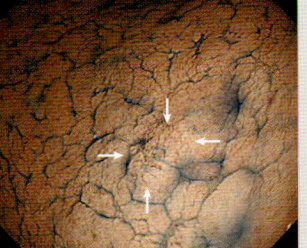

- Multiple carcinoid tumors against a background of Type A gastritis. A yellowish flat elevated lesion is recognized (indicated by the arrows) on the posterior wall of the greater curvature of the middle body. On the surface, dilated, tortuous vessels are visible. It is difficult to differentiate this from gastric adenocarcinoma of the fundic gland type.
- Diagnosis: Posterior wall of the greater curvature of middle body, 0–IIa, 3 mm, carcinoid tumor (neuroendocrine tumor Grade 1), T1a (M1), Type I in Rindi's Classification(See page 165).

👓 What's imaged in the other pictures?

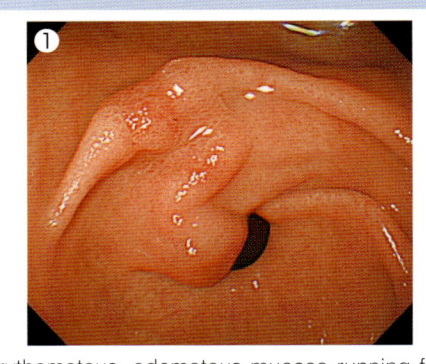

- Erythematous, edematous mucosa running from the pyloric ring to the proximal side can be seen in the lesser curvature of the antrum. Raised erosion is found on the crest of the lesser curvature. This is often seen in the antrum of *H. pylori*-uninfected patients.

Answer The gastric cancer is imaged in ③ .

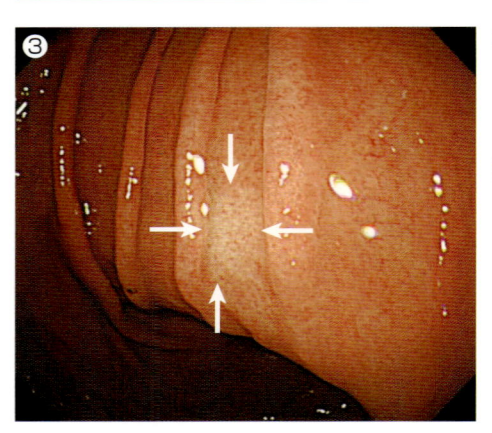

▶ The body has a glossy background mucosa accompanied by RAC. It is determined that there is no *H. pylori* infection. In *H. pylori*-uninfected cases, look for faded mucosa while performing endoscopy.

▶ Mucosa that looks more faded than its surrounding area can be seen in the lesser curvature of the lower body. At this point, signet ring cell carcinoma should be suspected.

Non-magnifying NBI image

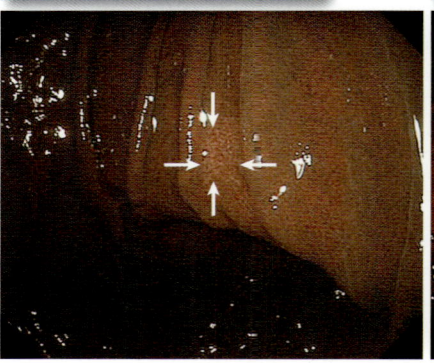

Indigo carmine sprayed image

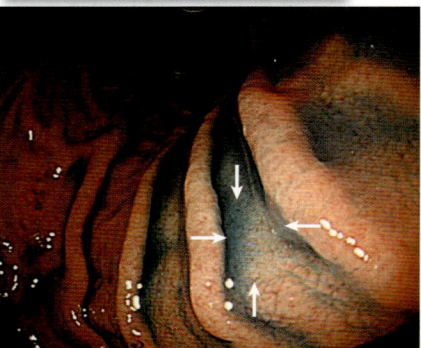

▶ When indigo carmine is sprayed, the lesion becomes harder to see because the mucosal surface has no irregularities.

▶ When signet ring cell carcinoma only exhibits changes in color as seen here, cancer often exists only in the middle layer of the mucosa from a histopathological point of view.

▶ In non-magnifying NBI observation, the lesion is a lighter shade of brown than the surrounding mucosa.

Diagnosis Lesser curvature of lower body, 0–IIb, 5 mm, sig, T1a (M), UL (–)

Tips

Look for fading in *H. pylori*-uninfected cases.

What's imaged in the other pictures?

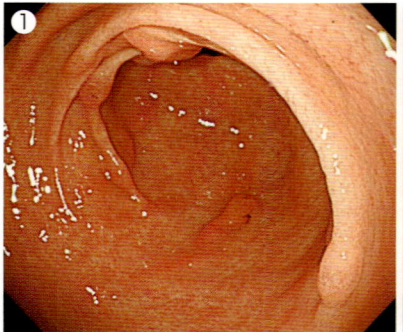

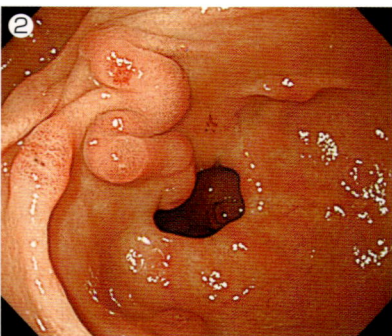

● In the antrum, multiple erosions accompanied by edematous elevations have occurred — some of which are lined up in a row like a string of beads. Edematous changes are not recognized anywhere on the background mucosa, except for the elevations.

● This is a finding referred to as raised erosion in *Kyoto Classification of Gastritis* (See page 30). It is often observed in *H. pylori*-uninfected cases.

Answer　The gastric cancer is imaged in ⑥ .

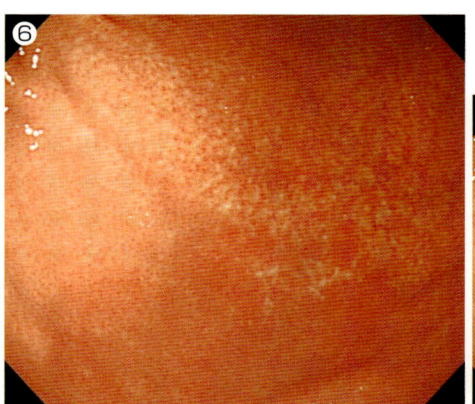

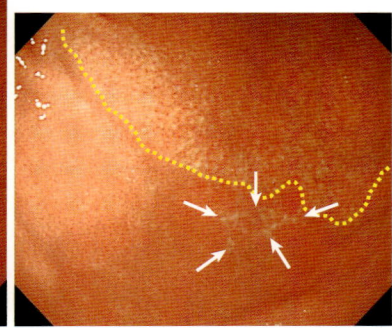

▶ C–2 atrophy can be seen in the background.

▶ The yellow dotted line highlights an atrophic border in the greater curvature of the angulus. On the proximal side is a fundic gland region without atrophy. Triangular faded mucosa (indicated by the arrows) can be seen in the fundic gland region immediately on the proximal side of the atrophic border.

▶ Differential diagnosis of the faded mucosa includes local atrophy, undifferentiated-type gastric cancer, and MALT lymphoma.

Indigo carmine sprayed image

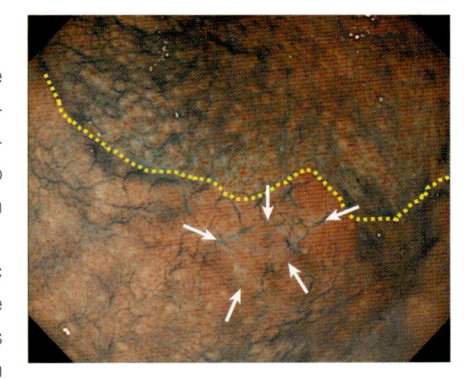

▶ When indigo carmine is sprayed, it becomes clear that the lesion is located on the proximal side of the atrophic border. This makes undifferentiated-type gastric cancer or MALT lymphoma more likely than atrophy. The classifications of undifferentiated-type gastric cancer and MALT lymphoma are shown in **Table**. According to the endoscopic finding of this case, the margins are relatively clear — which makes undifferentiated-type gastric cancer more likely than MALT lymphoma.

▶ Multiple small glandular elevations can be seen on the distal side of the atrophic border. This is a finding referred to as nodular gastritis, and it is considered to be hyperplasia of lymphoid follicles caused by a reaction to *H. pylori* infection. It has been reported that when nodular gastritis is observed, it should be included in the high-risk group of undifferentiated-type gastric cancer in young patients[45].

Table Endoscopic findings of undifferentiated-type gastric cancer and MALT lymphoma

	Undifferentiated-type gastric cancer	MALT lymphoma
No. of lesions	Single	Often multiple
Color tone	Faded	Faded, reddish
Margin	Relatively clear	Unclear
Encroachment	Present (cliff-like)	Absent
Depressed surface	Sometimes accompanied by *insel*	Various findings including erosion and ulcer

Note: MALT lymphoma exhibits various findings and is often difficult to differentiate from undifferentiated-type gastric cancer when the color has faded.

Histological images of ESD-resected specimen

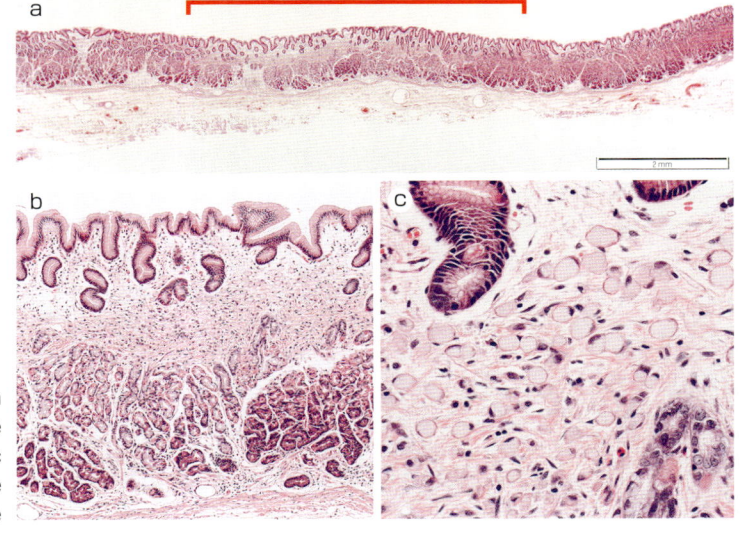

a : HE-stained, low-magnification image. A tumor can be seen extending along the range marked by the red line. The background mucosa is non-atrophic fundic gland mucosa. There is no difference in the thickness of the mucosa on the lesion and on the background.

b : HE-stained, medium-magnification image of the lesion. Centering around the middle layer (glandular neck region) of the mucosa, indistinct strips can be seen in areas where there are foveolar epithelium and fundic glands. Signet-ring cells with pale eosinophilic cytoplasm are distributed throughout this area.

c : HE-stained, high-magnification image of the lesion. Signet-ring cell carcinoma has proliferated in the glandular neck region.

Diagnosis Greater curvature of the angulus, 0–IIb, 10 mm, sig, T1a (M), UL (−)

Tips

- When performing screening endoscopies on young patients, watch for undifferentiated-type gastric cancer.
- Perform observation while being aware of the atrophic border.
- Remember that nodular gastritis is a finding of active *H. pylori* infection.
- Be aware that nodular gastritis poses a high risk for undifferentiated-type gastric cancer.

Compare! Different cases

① Nodular gastritis (See page 28.)
- Small nodular elevations with diameters of 2 to 3 mm are seen mainly in the antrum.
- Spraying indigo carmine clarifies the small elevations and makes it possible to visualize white dots in the centers of the elevations. It has been histopathologically demonstrated that these white dots are lymphoid follicles.

② MALT lymphoma
- Faded mucosa with unclear margins can be seen on the anterior wall of the upper body. Encroachment is not recognized; thus, MALT lymphoma is suspected rather than undifferentiated-type gastric cancer.

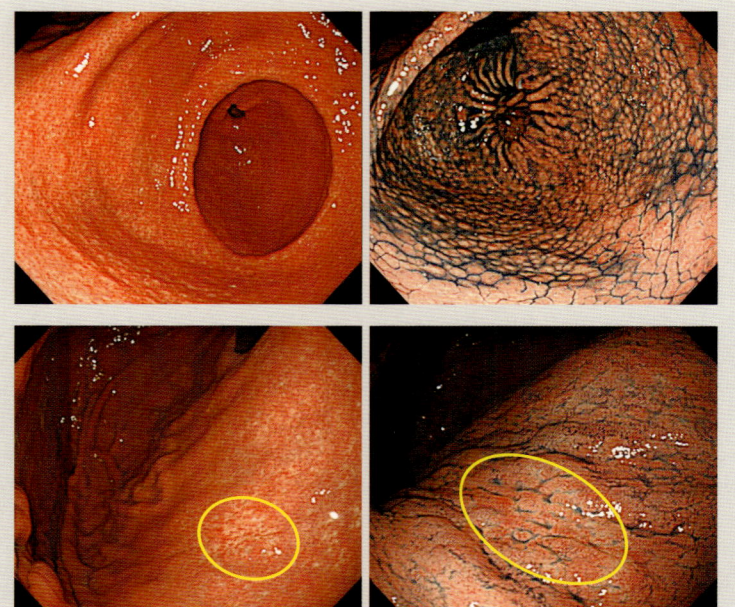

Additional Info Gastric cancer in young patients

- Gastric cancer occurs most frequently in people between the ages of 60 and 70. Gastric cancer in younger patients under the age of 40 is relatively rare — ranging from 4 to 15%. Among the elderly, the gender ratio is about 2:1, whereas among younger patients, the gender ratio is almost 1:1, and the histological type is frequently that of undifferentiated-type gastric cancer[46].
- Gastric cancer in younger patients is often found in an advanced stage, so it is generally considered to have a poor prognosis. However, the popularization of endoscopy now makes it possible to detect gastric cancer in younger patients at a stage where endoscopic treatment is still possible.
- Of the 2,708 cases on which we performed ESD for gastric cancer between 2007 and 2015, patients under the age of 40 numbered just 20 (0.7%) with 9 female patients and 11 male patients. As for the histological type, 16 (80%) were undifferentiated-type gastric cancer and 4 (20%) were differentiated-type gastric cancer (20%). As for color tone, the lesions in 17 cases (85%) exhibited fading.
- Look for fading when performing endoscopy on younger patients.

Answer The gastric cancer is imaged in ④ and ⑤.

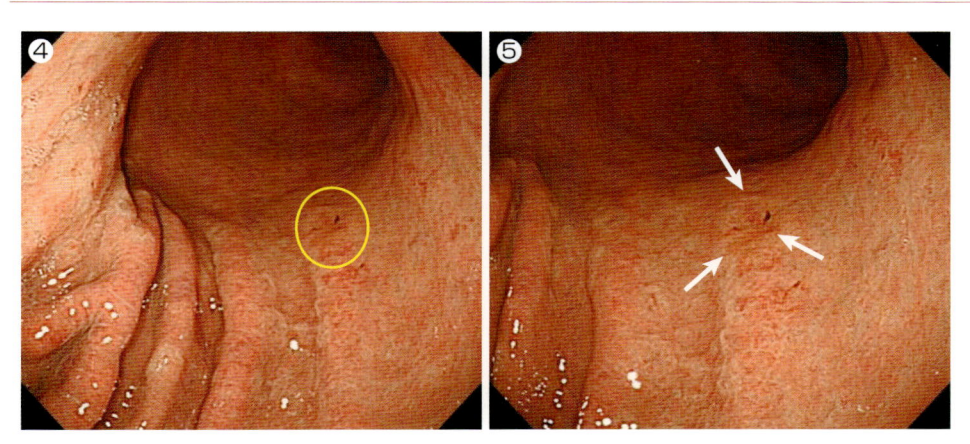

▶ O–3 atrophy and intestinal metaplasia can be seen throughout the background mucosa. Post-eradication map-like redness and erythematous depression appear in multiple locations. With background mucosa like this, it is difficult to find a cancer-caused depression among all the benign erythematous depressions.

▶ In photo ④, a slightly larger and more conspicuous depression than the erythematous depressions surrounding it can be seen on the posterior wall of the greater curvature of the middle body.

▶ When the endoscope is brought up close as in ⑤, a depressed lesion (indicated by the arrows) can be seen. It looks a little more yellowish than the surrounding erythematous depressions. At this point, cancer should be suspected, and detailed observation should be performed.

Indigo carmine sprayed image

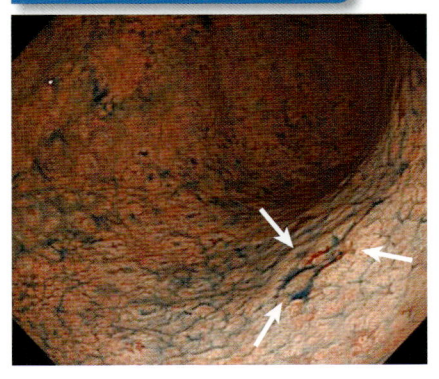

▶ When indigo carmine is sprayed, the depressed surface becomes clearer. Now, it can be seen that it is larger and more irregular than the surrounding erythematous depressions and that its color tone is somewhat yellowish.

▶ All these photos of cancer were taken in antegrade view. However, this makes it difficult to observe the posterior wall of the body because observation is only possible in a tangential direction. It is important to retroflex the endoscope so you can view the site from directly above.

Diagnosis Posterior wall of the greater curvature of the middle body, 0–IIc, 10 mm, tub1, T1a (M), UL (–)

Tips

● In a case where post-*H. pylori* eradication erythematous depressions are present in multiple locations, look for a depression that is larger and more irregular than the surrounding erythematous depressions.

● Spraying indigo carmine facilitates differentiation between benign and malign erythematous depressions.

Answer ❶   The first lesion is imaged in ③ and ④ .

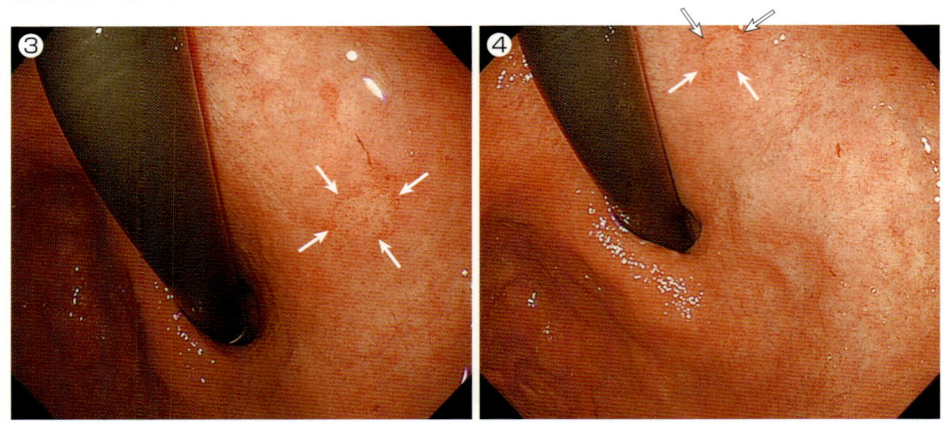

▶ Atrophy and intestinal metaplasia can be seen in the background. The mucosa is a colorful mix of whitish and reddish areas. Scattered attachment of hematin is present as a result of *H. pylori* eradication. A round mucosal area (indicated by the arrows) with a slightly more yellowish-white color tone than the surrounding area can be seen in the lesser curvature of the upper body.

▶ Once you have observed many lesions, you will be able to pick up such subtle alterations in color.

Close-up image

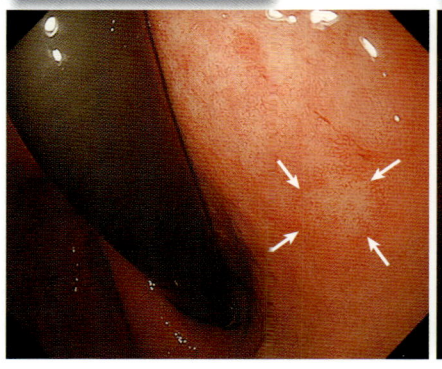

Indigo carmine sprayed image

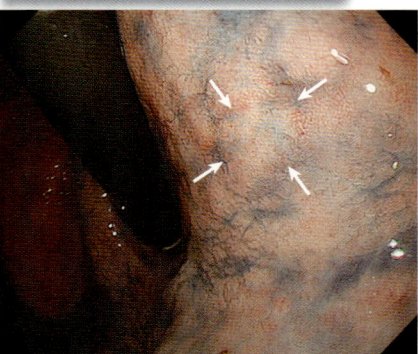

▶ When indigo carmine is sprayed, the visibility of the lesion deteriorates.

▶ When a lesion does not have surface irregularities and shows no noticeable changes on the mucosal surface as in this picture, spraying it with indigo carmine may make it even more difficult to discern.

▶ When the endoscope is brought up close, it becomes clear that the lesion is not accompanied by any changes in surface irregularities, and that there is only a change in color tone.

▶ The margins are relatively clear.

Non-magnifying NBI image

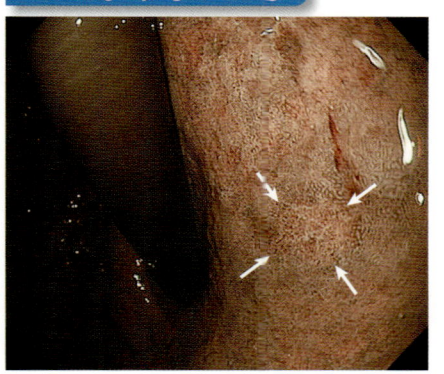

▶ In NBI observation, the lesion is a lighter shade of brown than the surrounding mucosa with clear margins.

Diagnosis ❶   Lesser curvature of the upper body, 0–IIb, 4 mm, tub1, T1a (M), UL (–)

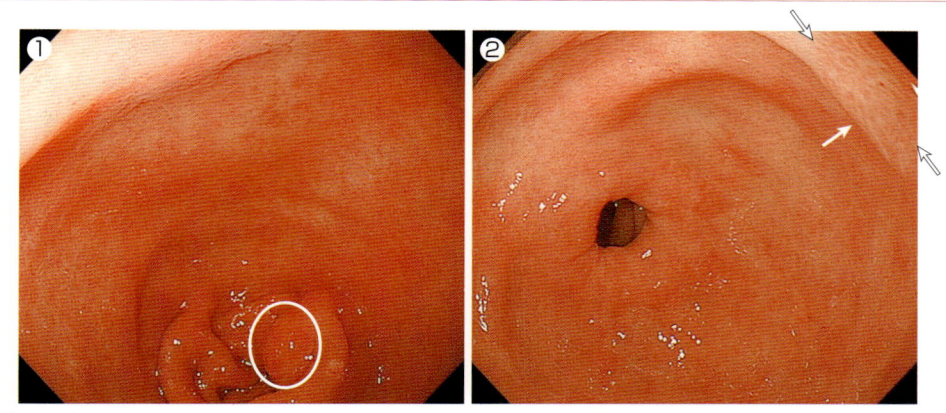

▶ In photo ① , erythematous mucosa is recognized on the posterior wall of the antrum (circled). Since it was viewed from distance and there was peristaltic movement, the details of the lesion are unclear. In close-up photo ② , there is an erythematous depression (indicated by the arrows) at the edge of the view field. This lesion was not noticed during this examination.

▶ Peristalsis is sometimes rapid in the antrum and may cause a lesion to be missed. Peristalsis occurs periodically. It eventually subsides and observation becomes possible. As required, Buscopan® or glucagon should be administered and Minclea® should be sprayed as well.

Endoscopic images 6 months later

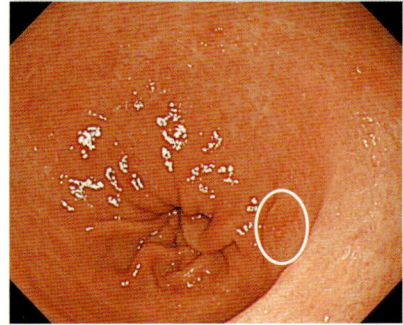 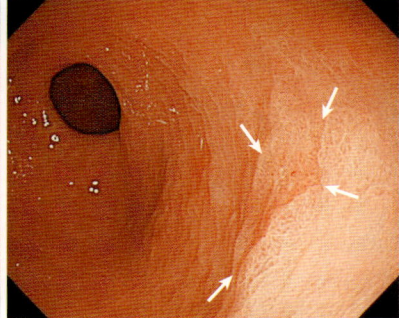

▶ These photos were taken 6 months after the first endoscopy (when the lesion was found). At this time, peristalsis was also rapid. However, once the contractions had subsided, an erythematous depressed lesion (indicated by the arrows) could be recognized. Reactive elevations can be seen in the area around the depression.

Indigo carmine sprayed images

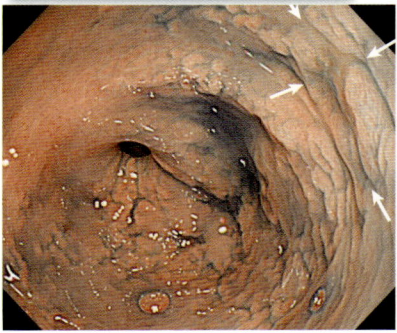 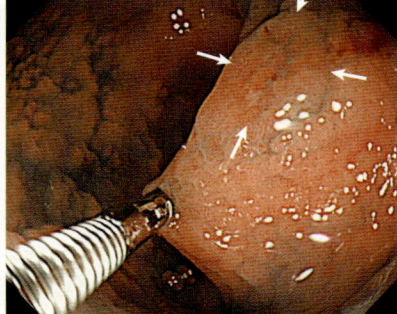

▶ Indigo carmine spraying clarifies the depressed surface.

▶ The posterior wall is in the tangential direction and difficult to observe. When the proximal wall is pulled with forceps, images can be obtained from an angle that is very close to a direct frontal view. A thorn-like encroachment is present, enabling diagnosis of differentiated-type gastric cancer.

Diagnosis ②   Posterior wall of the antrum, 0-IIc, 6 mm, tub1, T1a (M), UL (−)

Tips
- Look for yellowish-white mucosa.
- When the lesion is differentiated only by color, spraying indigo carmine will make it even more difficult to see.
- A lesion in the antrum is likely to go undetected as it may be concealed by peristalsis.

Screening endoscopy of chronic gastritis ③ 〔Gastric adenoma with active *H. pylori* infection〕

Answer The gastric cancer is imaged in ⑥ .

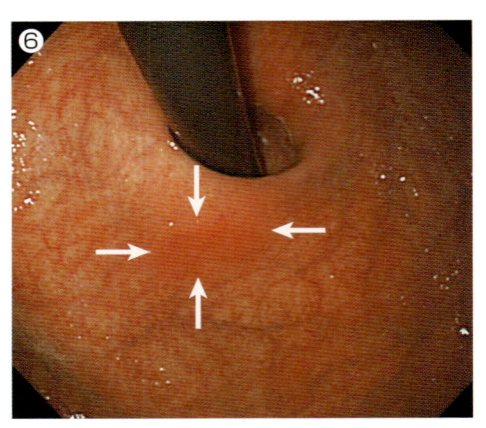

▶ O–2 atrophy is recognized in the background mucosa, and a vascular pattern in the submucosa is visible.

▶ An area that is redder than the surrounding area and where the vascular pattern has disappeared (indicated by the arrows) can be seen on the posterior wall of the cardia.

▶ It cannot be diagnosed as cancer at this point. More detailed observation will be necessary and the possibility of cancer should be kept in mind.

Close-up image

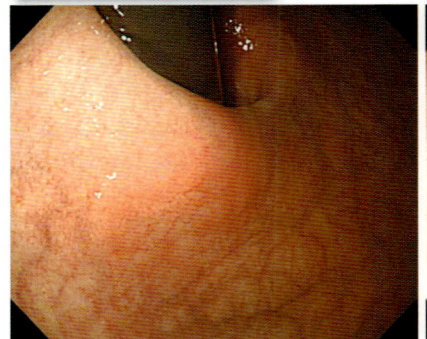

▶ Even when the site is observed from close up, a frontal view does not make it possible to elucidate the details of the lesion.

Changing the angle — in a tangential direction

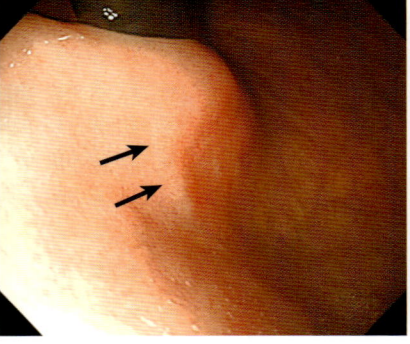

▶ When the site is observed tangentially and air is slightly suctioned, the rising parts of the lesion's edges can be recognized, making it possible to determine that it is an elevated lesion.

Indigo carmine sprayed image

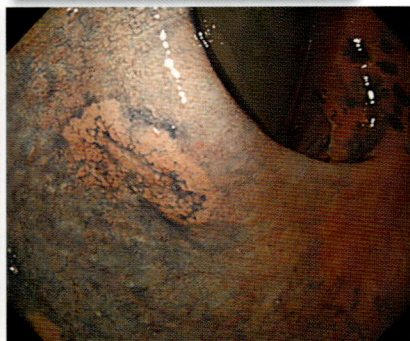

▶ When indigo carmine is sprayed, the lesion's margins can be clearly recognized. The center of the lesion is depressed.

Histological image of ESD-resected specimen

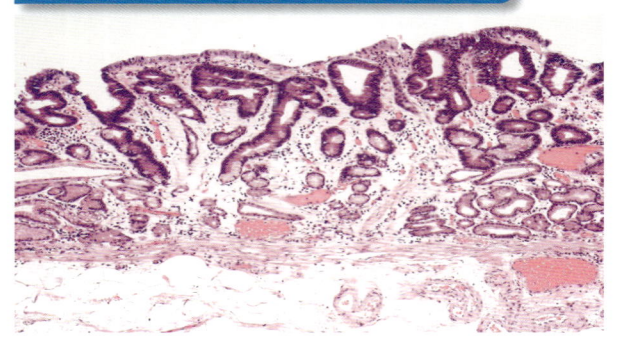

▶ HE-stained, medium-magnification image of the lesion. Tubular adenoma with moderate to severe atypia can be seen on the mucosal surface.

Diagnosis Posterior wall of the cardia, 0–IIa + IIc-like lesion, 16 mm, tubular adenoma with moderate to severe atypia

Tips

- Look for slight redness and disappearance of vascular patterns.
- Whenever the site seems suspicious, observe it from a close distance while changing the angle and adjusting the air amount.
- Surface irregularities are easier to see when observed tangentially.
- Surface irregularities are easier to see when the air amount is decreased.
- If the lesion has surface irregularities, spray indigo carmine to clarify the details.

What's imaged in the other pictures?

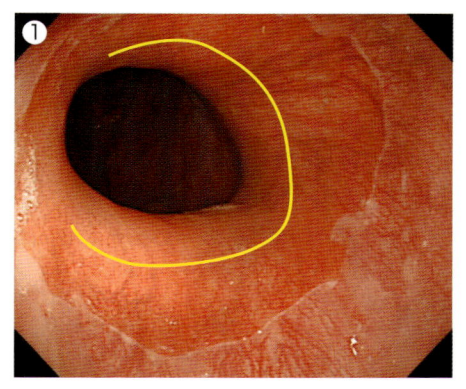

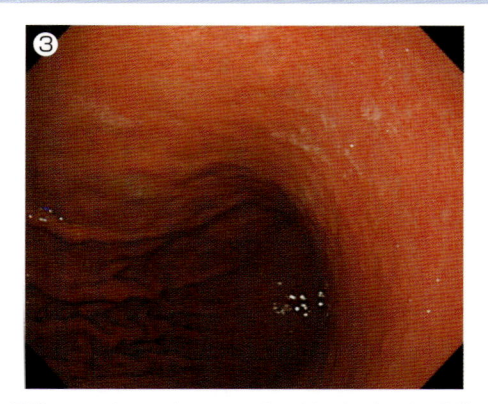

- Evaluate GERD and Barrett's esophagus at the EG junction.
- Because cases of Barrett's esophageal adenocarcinoma have been increasing recently, make sure to perform observation carefully.
- The yellow line — which marks the lower edge of the palisade vessels — shows the EG junction. The columnar epithelium on the proximal side of it is short-segment Barrett's esophagus (SSBE).
- This is Grade M GERD according to the revised Los Angeles Classification.

- Diffuse redness is recognized in the body. Diffuse redness is uniform redness with continuous expansion.
- Sticky mucus is attached.
- These findings indicate active *H. pylori* infection.

Side Note What are the indications of treatment for gastric adenoma?

Indications for gastric adenoma treatment differ from facility to facility. At the Cancer Institute Hospital of JFCR, the following gastric adenoma lesions (diagnosed with biopsy) are considered to be a high risk for cancer[a), b)] and should indicate endoscopic treatment.

  ① 2 cm or more
  ② Remarkable redness
  ③ Depressed type
  ④ Pathologically diagnosed as adenoma with severe atypia
  ⑤ Finding suspected to be cancer in magnifying NBI observation

a) Kasuga A, Yamamoto Y, Fujisaki J, et al. Clinical characterization of gastric lesions initially diagnosed as low-grade adenomas on forceps biopsy. Dig Endosc 2012 ; 24 : 331–338.

b) Tsuji Y, Ohata K, Sekiguchi M, et al. Magnifying endoscopy with narrow-band imaging helps determine the management of gastric adenomas. Gastric Cancer 2012 ; 15 : 414–418.

Answer The gastric cancer is imaged in ② .

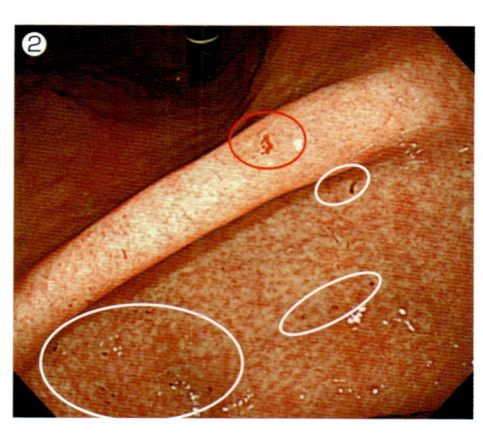

▶ C-2 atrophy is recognized in the background mucosa. Observe an atrophic area while keeping in mind differentiated-type gastric cancer.
▶ Multiple small dark brownish hematin spots (circled in white) are present in the antrum. These are post-eradication changes.
▶ Fresh blood (circled in red) — that is obviously not hematin — is present on the lesser curvature of the angulus. Referred to as spontaneous bleeding, this is one of the findings that suggests a possibility of gastric cancer. The bleeding is induced by stimulation from endoscopic insufflation and irrigation — which happens even though the endoscope is not in direct contact with the site. The reason that bleeding can be so easily stimulated is that the surface of cancerous mucosa is much more delicate than normal mucosa.

During irrigation

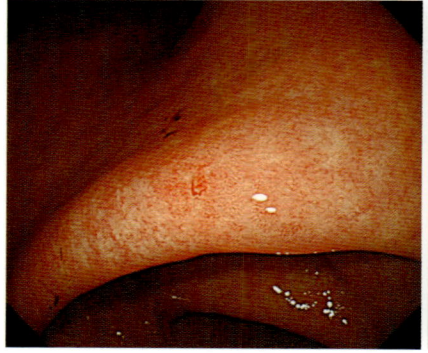

After irrigation

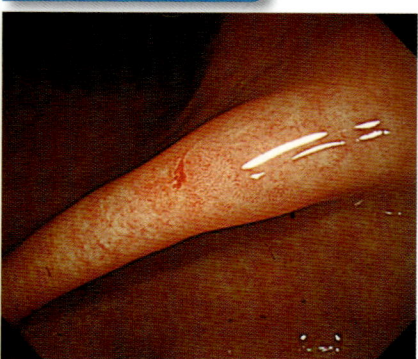

▶ Spontaneous bleeding caused by cancer can be washed away with irrigation, but bleeding will start again immediately.
▶ With hematin that is not related to cancer, bleeding does not restart even when it is washed.

Non-magnifying NBI image

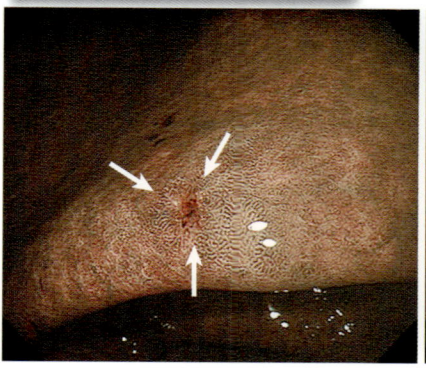

Indigo carmine sprayed image

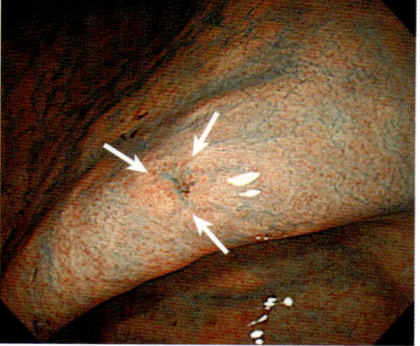

▶ Non-magnifying NBI observation and indigo carmine chromoendoscopy clarifies that the lesion is a small depressed lesion. Small lesions are often not accompanied by typical malignant findings such as encroachment, and in this case, it is also difficult to make a differential diagnosis of benign erosion.
▶ However, spontaneous bleeding was seen, leading to a suspicion of cancer. The site was biopsied and pathologically diagnosed as tub1, so ESD was performed.

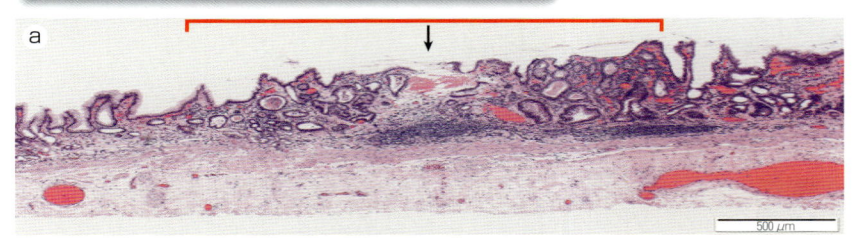

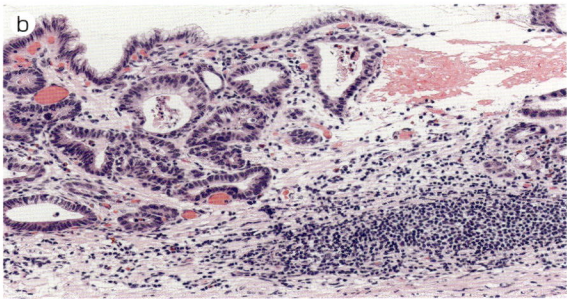

a : HE-stained, low-magnification image of the lesion. A tumor is visible. Its extent is marked by the red line. The diameter of the tumor is 2 mm. A hemorrhagic focus (indicated by the arrow) can be seen in the center of the lesion.

b : HE-stained, medium-magnification image of the lesion. Well-differentiated tubular adenocarcinoma (tub1) showing an irregular tubular structure. On the right of photo b, a bleeding spot can be seen (indicated by the arrow in photo a).

Diagnosis Lesser curvature of the angulus, 0–IIc, 2 mm, tub1, T1a (M), UL (–)

Tips

- Look for differentiated-type gastric cancer in atrophic areas.
- Suspect gastric cancer when you see spontaneous bleeding.
- Note that malignant findings rarely manifest with very small gastric cancers.
- Remember that hematin attachment in multiple locations is a finding that indicates that there is either *H. pylori* uninfection or post-*H. pylori* eradication.

Compare! Different case

Early gastric cancer accompanied by spontaneous bleeding

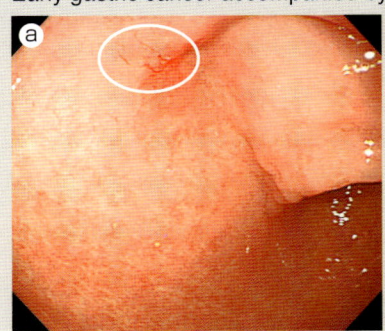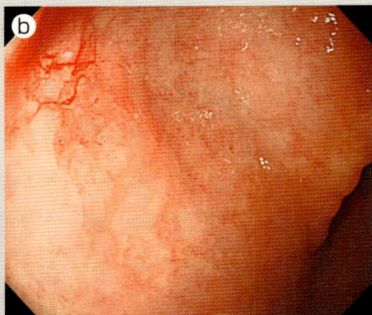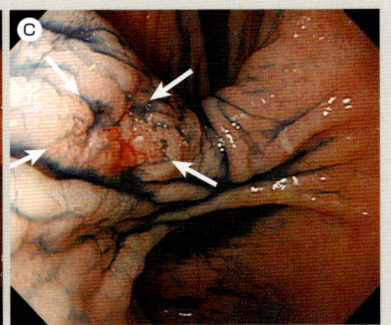

a : Spontaneous bleeding was induced by insufflation on the mucosa of the anterior wall of the lesser curvature of the angulus.

b : When the site is washed and observed from a close distance, it becomes apparent that the erythematous depressed lesion is bleeding.

c : When indigo carmine is sprayed, the margins become clearer. Because the site is accompanied by encroachment, differentiated-type gastric cancer is suspected. The surrounding elevations are reactive elevations, which are hyperplasia of non-cancerous mucosa.

- Pathological diagnosis of the ESD-resected specimen: Anterior wall of the lesser curvature of the angulus, 0–IIc, 10 mm, tub1, T1a (M), UL (–)

Answer   The gastric cancer is imaged in ② .

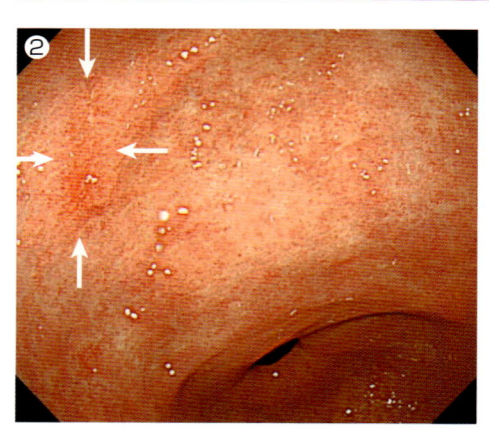

▶ C–3 atrophy is recognized in the background muco-sa. Multiple erythematous patches are present in the antrum.

▶ An erythematous depressed lesion with mild eleva-tions around it is visible in the lesser curvature of the antrum.

Close-up image

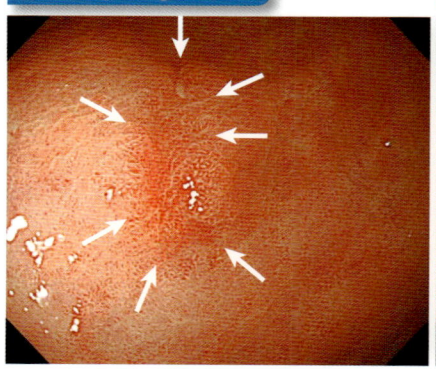

Indigo carmine sprayed image

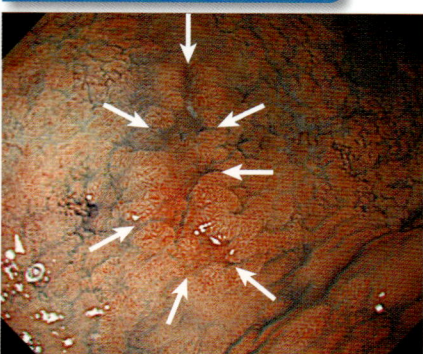

▶ When the endoscope is brought up close, the elevations surrounding the depression can be clearly viewed.

▶ When indigo carmine is sprayed, the depressed surface is easier to see (as indicated by the arrows). A thorn-like encroachment can be seen on the margins. The elevations at the edges of the depression are consid-ered to be reactive elevations, sug-gesting the possibility of differentiat-ed-type gastric cancer.

Diagnosis Lesser curvature of the angulus, 0–IIc, 10 mm, tub1, T1a (M), UL (−)

Tips

- Differentiated-type gastric cancer should be suspected when an erythematous depression surrounded by elevations is seen.
- Spraying indigo carmine makes it possible to see the encroachment.

👓 What's imaged in the other pictures?

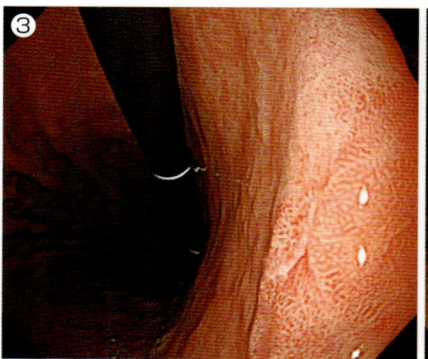

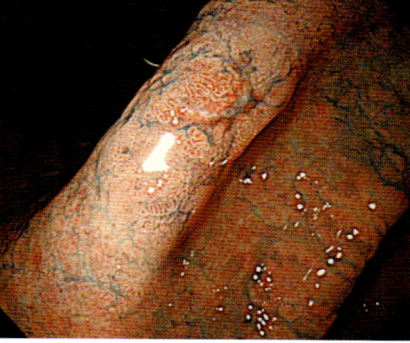

- Irregular erosion is visible in the lesser curvature of the angulus. When indigo carmine is sprayed, the edges of the erosion also re-semble a thorn-like encroachment.
- The biopsy was diagnosed as Group 1. Also because endoscopic diagnosis has limitations, do a bi-opsy for pathological diagnosis whenever you are not sure about lesions.

Answer   The gastric cancer is imaged in ⑥ .

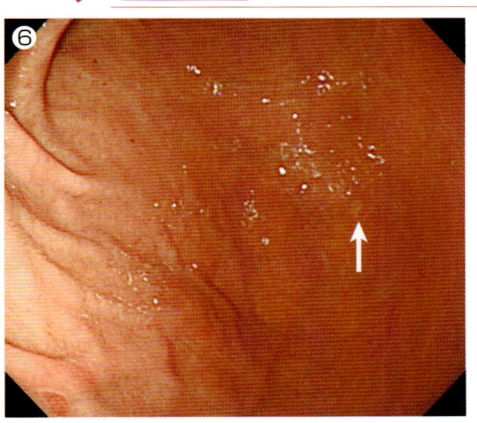

▶ There is no atrophy and RAC is recognized in the background mucosa, which suggests there is no *H. pylori* infection. In cases like this, the possibility of differentiated-type gastric cancer is low, so observation should be performed while keeping in mind the possibility of undifferentiated-type gastric cancer, particularly of signet ring cell carcinoma.

▶ Faded mucosa (indicated by the arrow) that is quite noticeable even from a distance is visible on the greater curvature of the angulus.

Close-up image

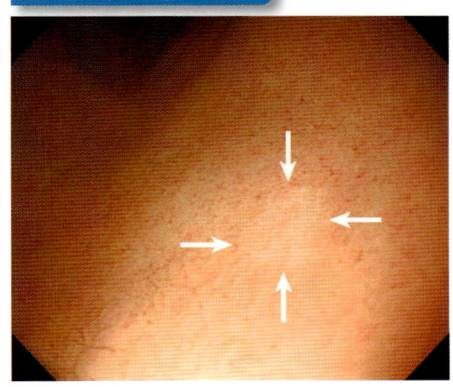

▶ In closed-up view, fading across an area about 3 mm in diameter can be seen. No surface irregularities are evident. There is no finding other than changes in the color of the mucosa.

▶ Because of its location, the lesion is grazed by the endoscope when it is advanced from the antrum to the duodenum. A 0–IIb lesion exhibiting a small faded area is harder to detect when an endoscope comes in contact with it. Such a lesion should be observed and biopsied before the endoscope is advanced to the distal side.

Indigo carmine sprayed images

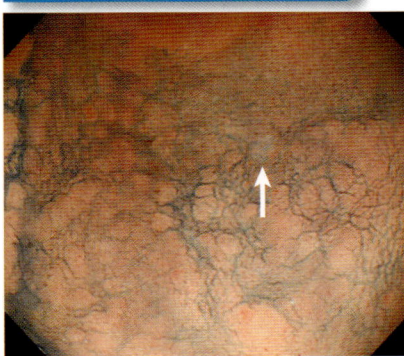
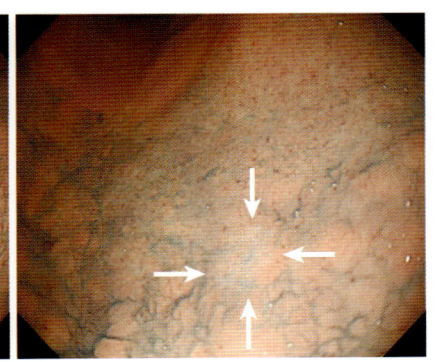

▶ Spraying indigo carmine makes the lesion more difficult to see than in conventional observation.

▶ When a lesion does not have surface irregularities like this, spraying indigo carmine would not be effective.

Diagnosis   Greater curvature of the angulus, 0–IIb, 3 mm, sig, T1a (M), UL (–)

Endoscopic image from 1 year previously

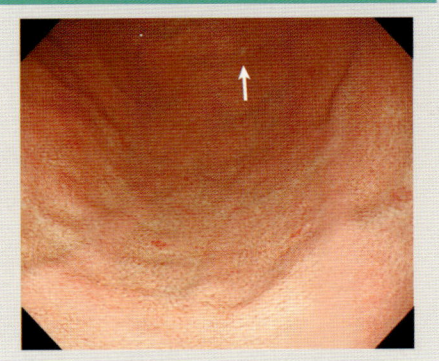

● A small faded area with a diameter of about 2 mm was also recognized in the same site a year earlier. However, it would be difficult to detect it at this point.

Tips

● Look for signet ring cell carcinoma in *H. pylori*-uninfected cases.
● Signet ring cell carcinoma exhibits fading.
● Early signet-ring cell carcinoma is frequently diagnosed as 0–IIb in endoscopy.

Patient complaining of stomach discomfort   〔*H. pylori* -uninfected gastric cancer〕

Answer   The gastric cancer is imaged in ② .

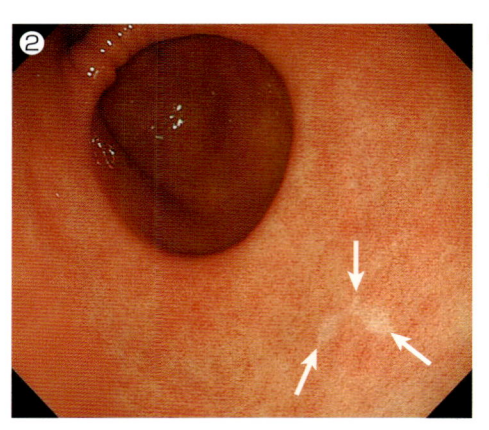

▶ The background mucosa is smooth and uniformly orange-red. RAC can be seen throughout the body, with sporadic occurrence of fundic gland polyps. These are typical findings that indicate there is no *H. pylori* infection.

▶ When *H. pylori* infection is not present, the most common type of gastric cancer found is signet ring cell carcinoma. During observation, if you keep in mind that early signet ring cell carcinoma emerges as a faded 0–IIb lesion, you will notice a single arch-shaped patch on the greater curvature of the antrum. At this point, you should strongly suspect gastric cancer.

Close-up image

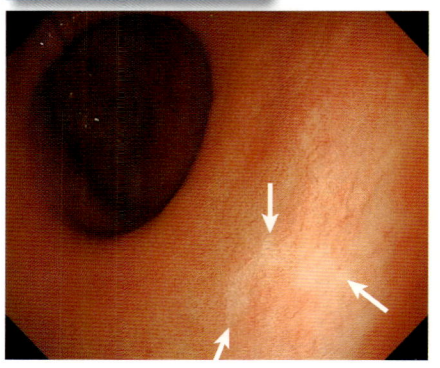

Indigo carmine sprayed image

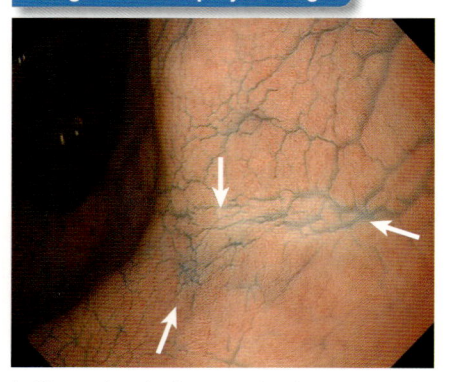

▶ In close-up observation, there is no difference from the surrounding mucosa other than color tones.

▶ Even when indigo carmine is sprayed, the surface irregularities of the lesion and the changes to the areae gastricae pattern remain difficult to see.

Diagnosis   Greater curvature of angulus, 0–IIb, 4 mm, sig, T1a (M), UL (–)

Tips

- Look for undifferentiated-type gastric cancer — especially signet ring cell carcinoma — in *H. pylori*-uninfected cases.
- Undifferentiated-type gastric cancer shows fading.

Answer   The malignant tumor is imaged in ① .

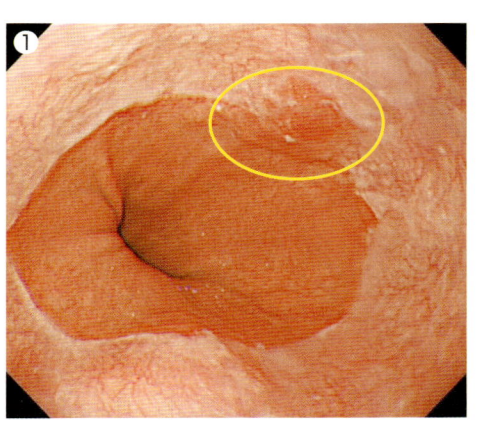

- The gastric mucosa in the background is RAC-positive. It is glossy, smooth and seems to be *H. pylori*-uninfected.
- A reddish flat elevated lesion is recognized at the 2 o'clock position in the esophagogastric junction (EGJ).

- Left : Antegrade view. The palisade vessels can be viewed when observed from a close distance. The distal end of the palisade vessels is marked by the blue dotted line. The proximal side from here is the esophagus. The yellow dotted line shows the squamocolumnar junction (SCJ). At the 2 o'clock position, a reddish flat elevation (indicated by the arrows) can be seen that looks as if it is straddling the SCJ. No palisade vessels can be seen in this area, and the surface is a little coarse. At this point, Barrett's esophageal adenocarcinoma is strongly suspected.
- Right : Retroflex view. The lesion is observed from a close distance after the endoscope has been retroflexed to enter the hernia sac. The margins of the lesion are a little unclear.

Close-up images

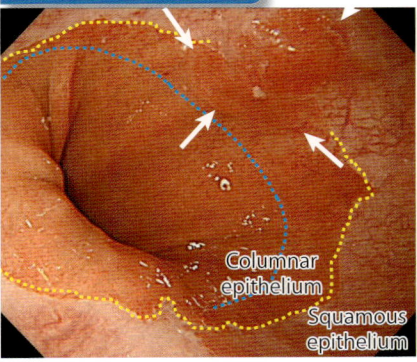

Columnar epithelium
Squamous epithelium

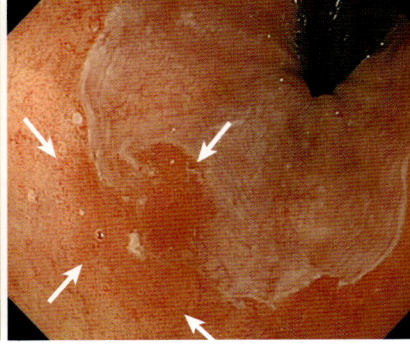

Non-magnifying NBI images

- Left : Antegrade view. Right: Retroflex view.

  The lesion appears to be a darker shade of brown, and the margin looks clearer than in conventional observation.

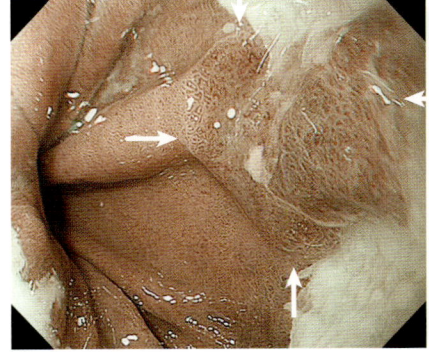

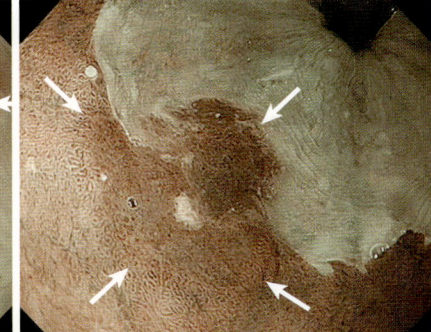

Indigo carmine-sprayed images

- Left : Antegrade view. Right: Retroflex view.

  When indigo carmine is sprayed, the redness of the lesion stands out and the margin becomes distinct.

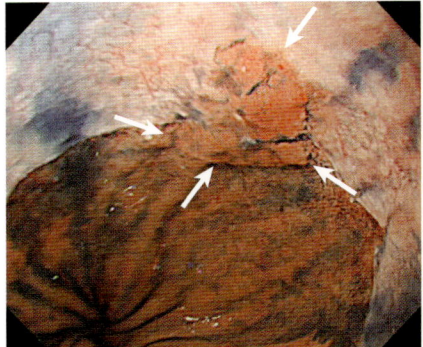

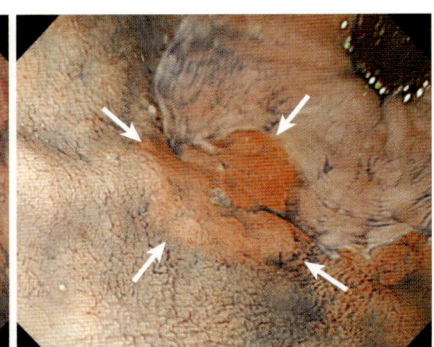

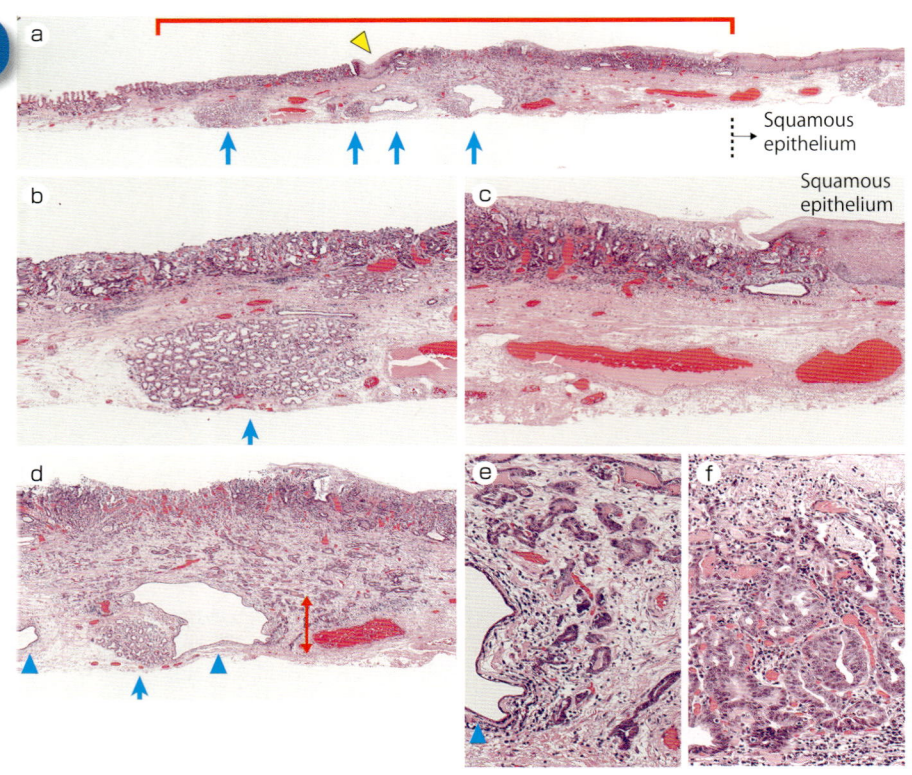

Histological images of ESD-resected specimen

Squamous epithelium

Squamous epithelium

a : HE-stained, low-magnification image. On the right is the esophageal side, and on the left is the gastric side. A tumor can be seen in the region shown under the red line. The end of the esophageal side of the lesion is in contact with the esophageal stratified squamous epithelium (marked with the dotted black line). Within the region of the tumor, a squamous epithelium island (▷) is visible; in addition, esophageal glands proper and their ducts (➙) can be seen in the submucosa. In terms of anatomy, this suggests that the tumor is located in the esophagus. In other words, since most of the lesion seems to be on the esophageal side, there would be no contradiction from a histopathological point of view in diagnosing this case as Barrett's esophageal adenocarcinoma.

b : HE-stained, low-magnification image on the gastric side of the lesion. Moderately differentiated tubular adenocarcinoma extends into the mucosa. Esophageal glands proper can be seen in the submucosa (➙).

c : HE-stained, low-magnification image on the esophageal side of the lesion. Moderately to well differentiated tubular adenocarcinoma is recognized in the mucosa. It has slightly invaded under the squamous epithelium on the proximal side.

d : HE-stained, low-magnification image in the center of the lesion. Moderately differentiated tubular adenocarcinoma that exhibits dense hyperplasia is visible in the mucosa. Adenocarcinoma components showing infiltrative growth associated with fibrosis are recognized in the stratified *muscularis mucosae* and submucosa. In the vicinity of the infiltration, an esophageal gland proper (➙) and dilated ducts (▶) can be seen. The invasion into the submucosa is 500 μm deep (↔) when measured from the lower end of the stratified *muscularis mucosae*. According to the *Japanese Classification of Esophageal Cancer*[47], this corresponds to pT1b-SM2.

e : HE-stained, high-magnification image of the infiltrated areas in the submucosa. Ducts of the esophageal glands proper are visible (▶). These indicate infiltration and expansion of poorly to moderately differentiated adenocarcinoma components that form small ducts and alveolar sacs.

f : HE-stained, high-magnification image of the intramucosal component. Mainly composed of well-differentiated tubular adenocarcinoma.

Diagnosis   Ae, 8 mm, 0–IIa, tub2>tub1>por2 (Barrett's esophageal adenocarcinoma), T1b-SM2 (500 μm)

Tips

- Confirm the distal end of the palisade vessels to identify the EGJ.
- When you see a reddish elevation on the right wall in Barrett's epithelium, you should suspect Barrett's esophageal adenocarcinoma.

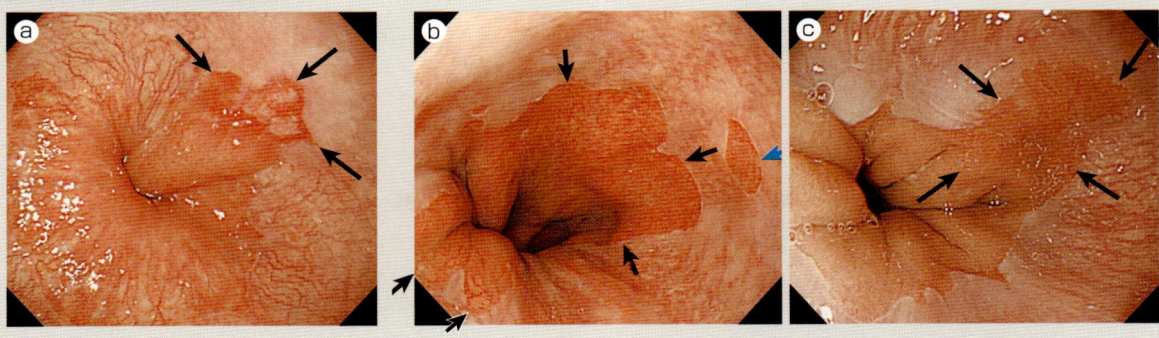

a : **Reflux esophagitis.** The problem with redness on the esophagus side of the EGJ is differentiating between reflux esophagitis and short-segment Barrett's esophagus (SSBE). The morphology of reflux esophagitis consists of triangular and linear shapes and is often associated with opaqueness and fluffiness in the surrounding mucosa. In this case, erythematous mucosa is observed in the 2 o'clock direction (indicated by the black arrows). Since a thin white coat is attached to the center, the surrounding mucosa is opaque, and the margins are accompanied by fluffiness, this case should be diagnosed as reflux esophagitis.

b : **SSBE.** Reddish mucosa is recognized in the 0 to 3 o'clock and 6 to 8 o'clock directions (indicated by the black arrows). On the further proximal side of the 3 o'clock direction, similarly reddish mucosa with a round shape can be seen (indicated by the blue arrow). These mucosal surfaces do not have surface irregularities and are associated with palisade vessels; hence, it is possible to diagnose them as Barrett's epithelium. Furthermore, their less-than-3-cm sizes make it possible to diagnose them also as SSBE.

c : **Barrett's esophageal adenocarcinoma.** Reddish, tongue-shaped mucosa is recognized in the 2 o'clock direction (indicated by the black arrows). The mucosal surface is coarse, and no palisade vessel is recognized. It is not accompanied by fluffiness and erosion on the edges which would lead to a suspicion of reflux esophagitis. Consequently, it is diagnosed as Barrett's esophageal adenocarcinoma.

Additional Info

<What is Barrett's epithelium?>

- To understand Barrett's epithelium, you first have to understand the esophagogastric junction (EGJ) which is an anatomical zone that forms a border between the esophagus and stomach. According to diagnostic criteria defined by the joint working group of the Japanese Gastric Cancer Association and the Japan Esophageal Society, EGJ is determined by the palisade vessels in the lower esophagus. The definition further states that, if the palisade vessels cannot be properly assessed, the EGJ should be regarded as the site at the proximal end of the longitudinal folds of the stomach[29].

- However, we often experience cases in which the identification of the EGJ is difficult. In cases associated with reflux esophagitis, the palisade vessels become unclear. In severe atrophy cases, gastric folds disappear. When the contraction of the lower esophageal sphincter is active, it may not be possible to observe the EGJ. Identifying the EGJ should be done according to the two criteria described above. In principle, however, the first criterion — using the lower end of the palisade vessels — should have priority.

- In normal conditions, the EGJ corresponds with the squamocolumnar junction (SCJ). However, when the esophageal squamous epithelium is replaced by columnar epithelium due to the inflammation caused by reflux esophagitis, the SCJ moves to the proximal side. This area between the EGJ and SCJ is Barrett's epithelium, which is where the carcinogenic tissue associated with Barrett's esophageal adenocarcinoma is generated.

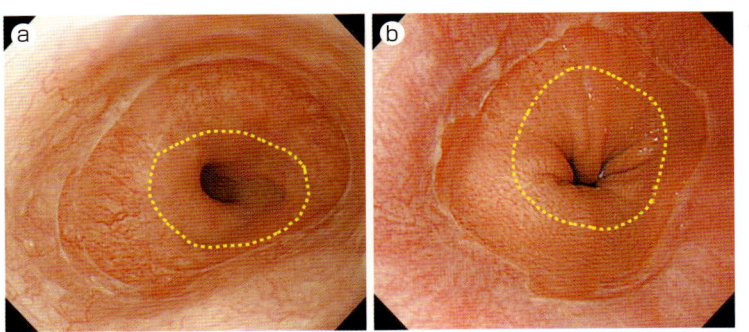

a : The small vessels running longitudinally are the palisade vessels. The dotted line shows the EGJ. The columnar epithelium on the proximal side is Barrett's epithelium.

b : This case has unclear palisade vessels due to reflux esophagitis. The proximal end (shown with the dotted line) of the longitudinal gastric folds should be considered the EGJ.

<Clinical characteristics of Barrett's esophageal adenocarcinoma>

- Barrett's esophagus occurs most frequently in males in their 50s, and it has been reported that most patients are white. Lately, however, Japanese physicians have been learning more about this disease in anticipation of a predicted increase in frequency in Japan. In order to detect Barrett's esophageal adenocarcinoma at an early stage, it is important to be familiar with related endoscopic images. In a study of 23 Barrett's esophageal adenocarcinoma lesions at our hospital, 70% of the macroscopic type showed elevation, 87% exhibited redness, and all cases were located on the right-side wall[48].

- In order to examine the reasons for frequent occurrence of Barrett's esophageal adenocarcinoma on the right side, we used an 8-channel pH monitoring system. Using this 24-hour system, we investigated into the positional relationship between the reflux direction of gastric acid and Barrett's esophageal adenocarcinoma[49]. As a result, we found that the reflux of gastric acid happened most frequently on the right side. The circumferential locations of the cancer and acid reflux corresponded almost exactly. In other words, we were able to prove that acid reflux was deeply involved in the occurrence of Barrett's esophageal adenocarcinoma using pH monitoring.

Answer The gastric cancer is imaged in ② .

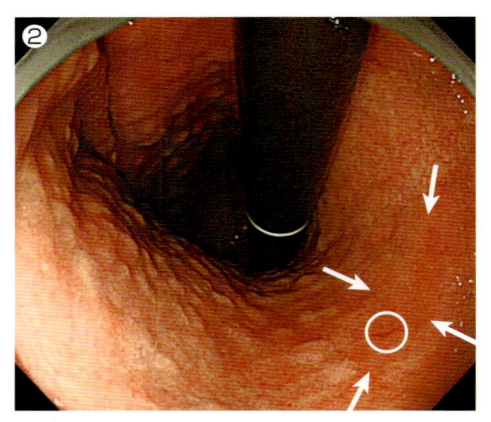

▶ The background mucosa shows O–3 atrophy. Map-like redness, which is a post-eradication change, is visible in the body. Fresh blood (shown in the circle) can be seen on the lesser curvature of the middle body.

▶ The lesion disappears into the surrounding gastritis, which makes it difficult to detect. Such a lesion is referred to as a gastritis-resembling carcinoma.

Indigo carmine sprayed image

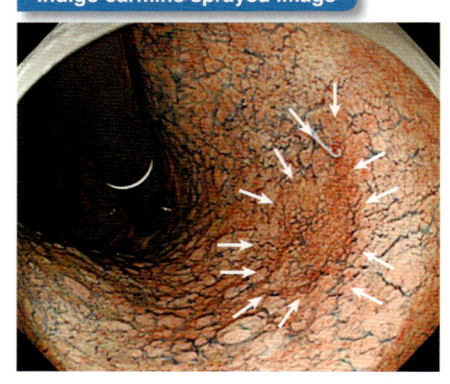

▶ When indigo carmine is sprayed, the redness of the lesion is more noticeable than in conventional endoscopy.

▶ The areae gastricae pattern was also unclear inside the lesion, so we performed detailed diagnosis of the region indicated by the arrows. However, even after indigo carmine was sprayed on the area, it still looked a little unclear.

NBI images Medium magnification High magnification

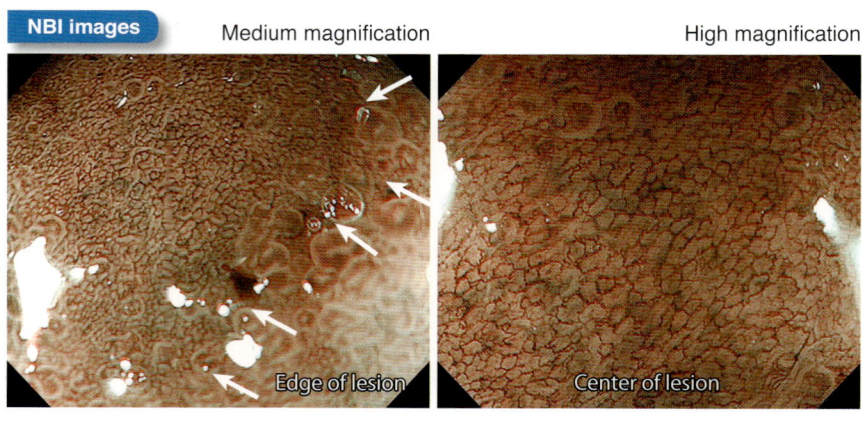

Edge of lesion Center of lesion

▶ In magnifying NBI observation, the inside of the lesion exhibits a reticulated vascular pattern with a clear demarcation line.

Diagnosis Lesser curvature of the middle body, 0–IIc, 19 mm, tub1, T1a (M), UL (−)

Gastric adenoma discovered prior to this examination

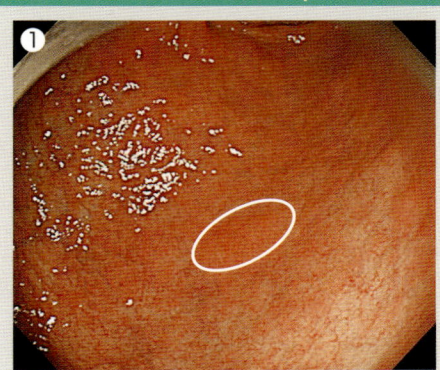

- Slightly yellowish-white mucosa with a vascular pattern that is not as clear as the surrounding area can be seen on the greater curvature of the antrum.

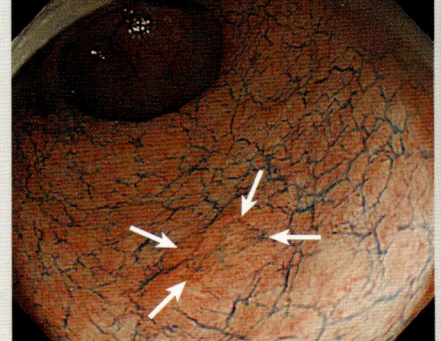

Indigo carmine-sprayed image

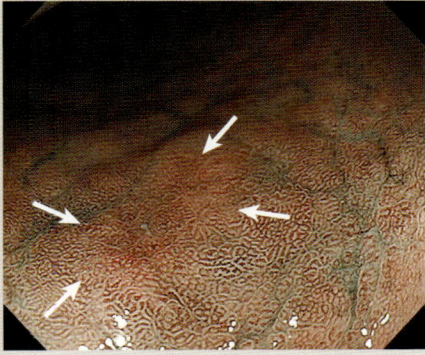

Non-magnifying NBI image

- In indigo carmine sprayed observation, the lesion is the site where the areae gastricae pattern is not as clear as the surrounding area. In non-magnifying NBI observation, that area exhibits a finer ductal structure than the surrounding area.
- Diagnosis: Greater curvature of the antrum, 0–IIb-like lesion equivalent, 5 mm, tubular adenoma with moderate atypia

 Side Note Is an antispasmodic necessary?

Different facilities have different policies as to whether or not an antispasmodic should be used as a routine drug for upper GI screening endoscopy. At the Cancer Institute Hospital of JFCR, we generally do not use Buscopan® or glucagon. When an antispasmodic is used, peristalsis in the antrum is reduced and it is easier to observe accurately. However, even when an antispasmodic is not used, screening endoscopy can be performed with almost no problem as long as you pay close attention during observation. For cases in which observation is hindered because of peristalsis, spraying Minclea®(l-menthol), which acts only locally, would be useful. We do not believe that it is necessary to use Buscopan®, which can cause anticholinergic side effects, or glucagon, which is relatively expensive.

Answer ❶ The gastric cancer is imaged in ⑤ and ⑥ .

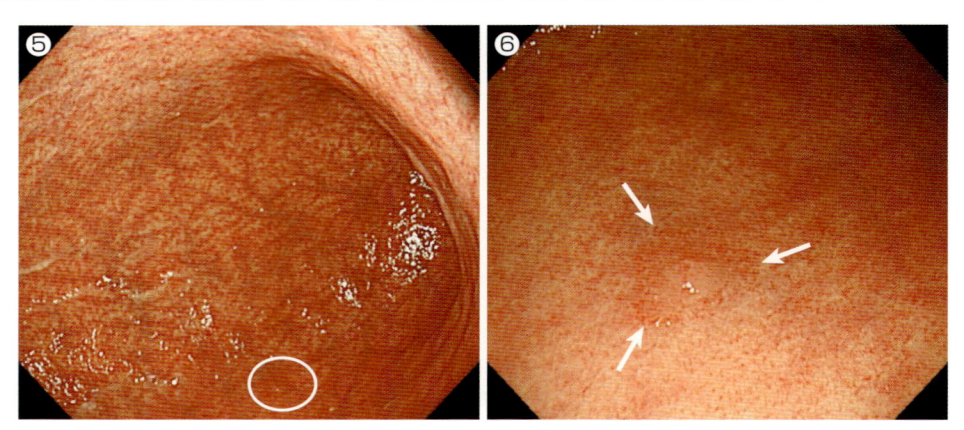

▶ There is O–3 atrophy in the background mucosa, and diffuse redness and attachment of sticky mucus can also be seen. This indicates an active *H. pylori* infection.

▶ A small elevation (shown in the circle) can be seen on the greater curvature of the lower body. When looked at carefully, a reddish surface can be seen spreading around the elevation (indicated by the arrows).

▶ It is difficult to see the lesion from a distance(⑤). However, in close-up observation (⑥) the lesion is visible. Lesions are missed at an unexpectedly high rate in the greater curvature of the body unless observation is conducted from a close distance.

Non-magnifying NBI image

Medium-magnification NBI image

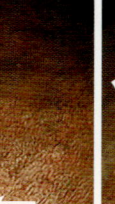
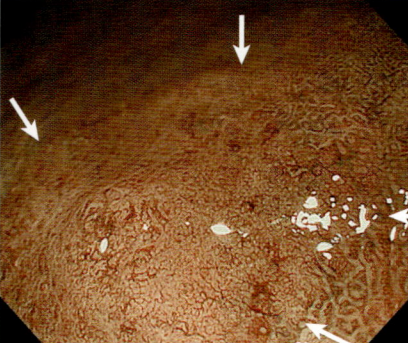

▶ In non-magnifying NBI observation, the lesion is a lighter shade of brown with a clear margin.

▶ In medium-magnification NBI observation, the lesion shows a mesh-patterned vascular structure. This is a finding of differentiated-type gastric cancer.

Indigo carmine sprayed images

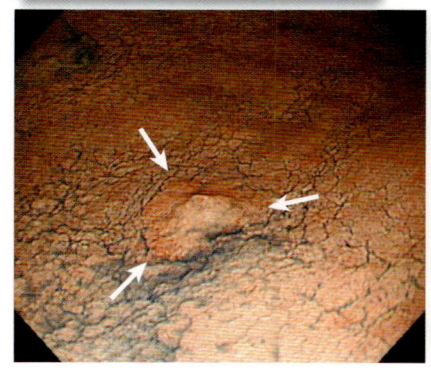
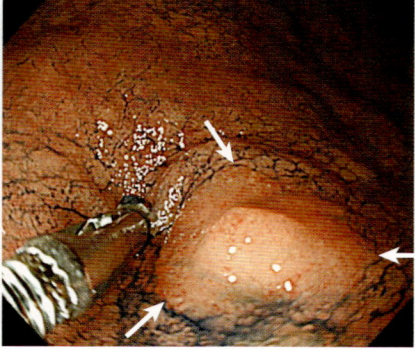

▶ When indigo carmine is sprayed, the areae gastricae pattern observed in the surrounding area is no longer clear inside the lesion. The redness also becomes more noticeable, facilitating recognition of the lesion.

Diagnosis ❶ Greater curvature of the lower body, 0–IIa, 6 mm, tub1, T1a (M), UL (−)

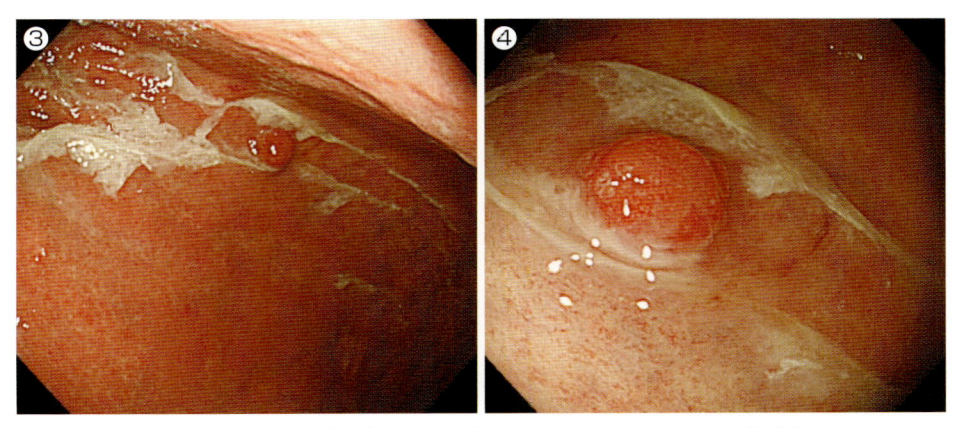

▶ A strongly erythematous polyp-like lesion can be seen near the anterior wall of the greater curvature of the upper body. It is best to take pictures after washing off as much of the sticky mucus as possible. The differential diagnosis at this point was gastric cancer or hyperplastic polyp.

Close-up images (in detailed examination at a subsequent date)

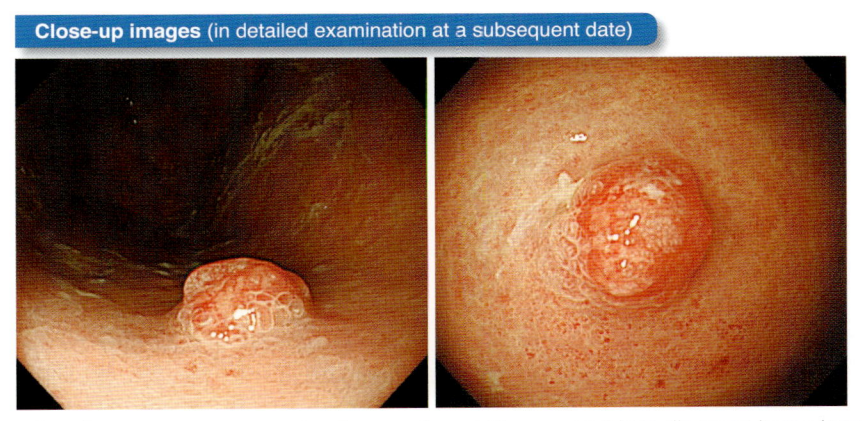

▶ The edge shows a coarse mucosal pattern, so it would be reasonable to diagnose it as a hyperplastic polyp. The top of the lesion is slightly depressed and the mucosal pattern has disappeared.

Magnifying NBI images (in detailed examination at a subsequent date)

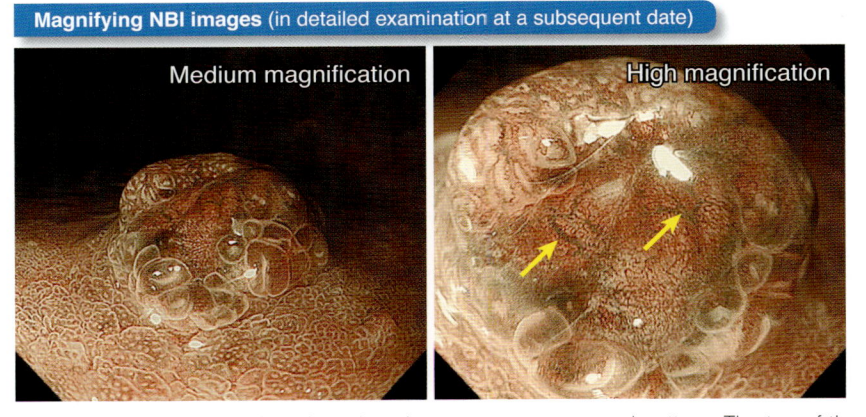

Medium magnification

High magnification

▶ In magnifying NBI observation, the edge shows a coarse mucosal pattern. The top of the lesion is depressed, and the mucosal pattern has disappeared. Also recognized on the top of the polyp are dilated, tortuous vessels (indicated by the yellow arrows).

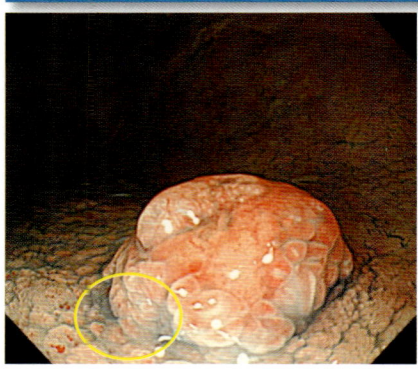 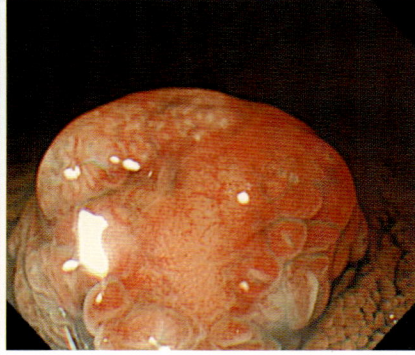

▶ Even when indigo carmine is sprayed, the edge still exhibits a coarse mucosal pattern. On the top of the lesion, the mucosal pattern has disappeared and a slightly yellowish depressed surface accompanied by dilated vessels can be seen.

▶ When the edge (in the yellow circle) is observed carefully, you can see a mucosal pattern that gradually becomes coarser as it approaches the top, while the margin is unclear. In other words, the coarse mucosal pattern is a non-tumorous hyperplastic change. However, the finding on the top of the lesion is not indicative of a hyperplastic polyp. Therefore, an SMT-like tumor accompanied by a central depression is suspected. When the yellowish color tone and dilated vessels are taken into consideration, the differential diagnosis includes a carcinoid tumor. Because a carcinoid tumor is generated from the deep mucosa, it has an SMT-like morphology. However, the mucosa on the top is extended by the tumor and is likely to form a depression.

EUS image

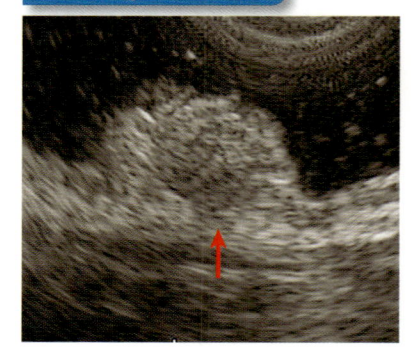

▶ A uniform low echoic mass can be seen in the mucosa. There is a concave finding directing downward to the submucosa as indicated by the arrow, suggesting submucosal invasion.

Diagnosis ❷ Greater curvature of the upper body, 0-I, 6 mm, carcinoid tumor (NET G1), T1b (SM1, 120 μm), Type III in Rindi's Classification*

*See Table 4 on page 165.

Tips

- Observe the greater curvature of the body from a close distance.
- Understand the difference between a hyperplastic polyp, gastric cancer, and carcinoid tumor.

👓 What's imaged in the other pictures?

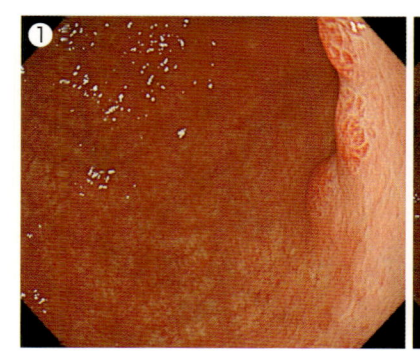 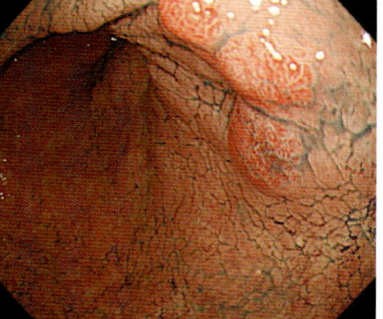

- A long and narrow erythematous polyp is visible on the posterior wall of the angulus. It has a coarse mucosal pattern and is a hyperplastic polyp.

Patient referred to us due to suspected gastric cancer

(Gastric cancer with active *H. pylori* infection)

[1] Is the ulcer on the posterior wall of the middle body benign or malignant?

Answer ❶   Pay attention to ②, ④, and ⑤.

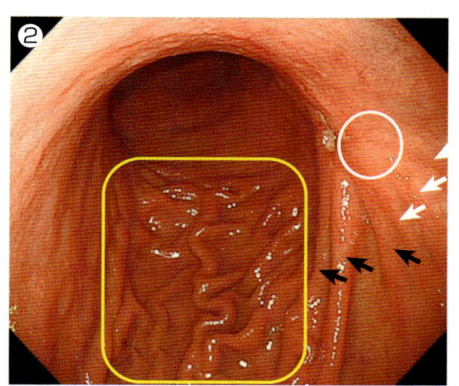

▶ In the gastric mucosa in the background, O–1 atrophy and diffuse redness are observed. The folds in the greater curvature are enlarged (enclosed in the yellow rectangle), which is indicative of an active *H. pylori* infection.

▶ On the posterior wall of the middle body, an ulcer accompanied by converging folds (indicated by the black arrows) can be seen. The folds do not have malignant findings (such as abrupt cutting, clubbing, adhesion and encroachment). They converge smoothly in the center, suggesting benign gastric ulcer.

▶ Converging folds are also present on the proximal side of the ulcer (indicated by the white arrows). An old ulcer scar (enclosed in the white circle) is visible nearby. We believe this a recurring chronic ulcer.

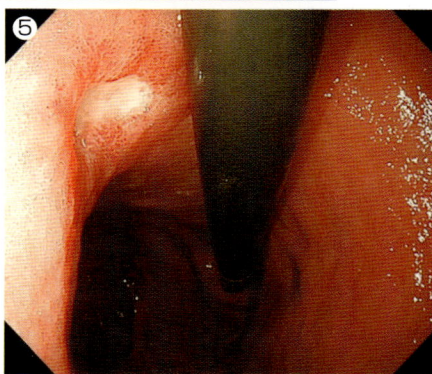
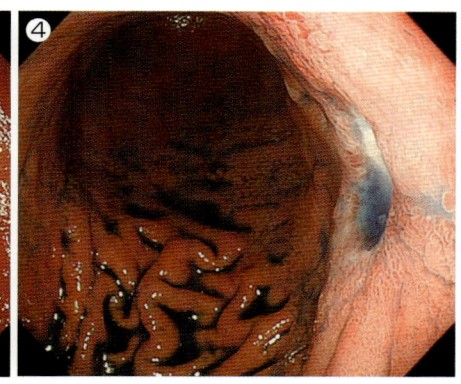

▶ In close-up observation (⑤), the base of the ulcer is uniform, and the edges of the ulcer are clear. Erythematous palisade regenerative epithelium can be seen in the surrounding area, suggesting that the ulcer is benign.

▶ In indigo carmine-sprayed observation (④), no depressed surface suggestive of 0–IIc can be seen in the surrounding area. Two points on the edge were biopsied, and the result of the pathological diagnosis was gastritis.

Diagnosis ❶ Posterior wall of the middle body, benign gastric ulcer

Two months after PPI administration

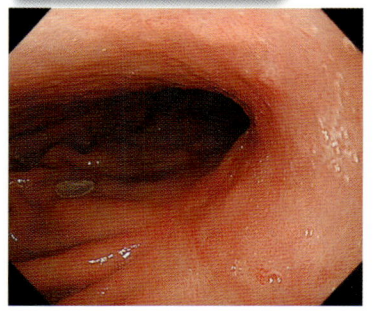

▶ The ulcer has healed into a scar (S1).

Compare! Different case

Malignant ulcer

To differentiate between early gastric cancer and a benign tumor, it is important to look for 0–IIc around the ulcer. Pure 0–III is rare, and in most cases 0–IIc exists concurrently in the surrounding area in combinations such as 0–IIc+III and 0–III+IIc. The finding of 0–IIc is a depressed surface with a margin. Inside the depressed surface, surface irregularities, granular change and mucosal pattern disappearance are present.

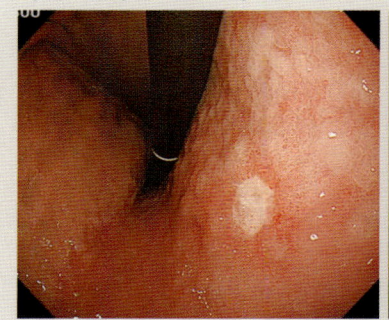
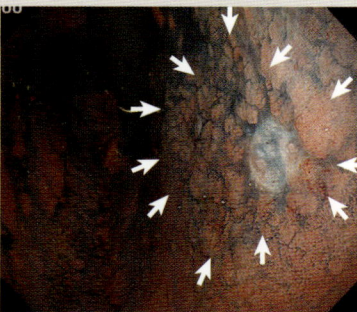

- The base and edge of ulcer are clear, which makes it look benign at first glance. However, when indigo carmine is sprayed, a 0–IIc surface becomes visible in the surrounding area, making it possible to diagnose it as gastric cancer.
- Diagnosis: Posterior wall of middle body, 0–IIc+III, 30 mm por1, T1b (SM2)

Answer ❷ Here is the cancer! It's imaged in ⑪ and ⑫ .

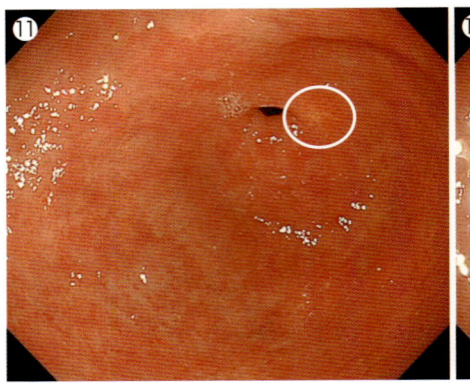 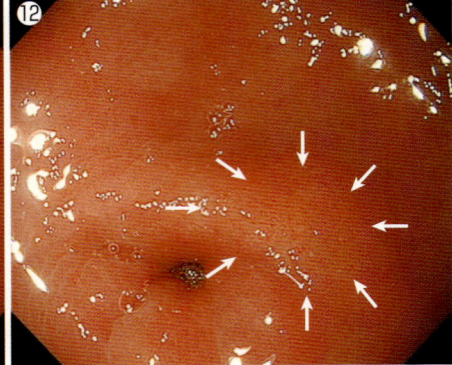

▶ On the posterior wall of the prepyloric region, the mucosa is slightly more yellowish than the surrounding area. When the endoscope is brought up close (⑫), the mucosal surface no longer looks glossy, making us surmise that the surface is coarse. At this point, cancer should be suspected. NBI and indigo carmine spraying would be necessary for detailed observation of the mucosal surface.

Non-magnifying NBI image

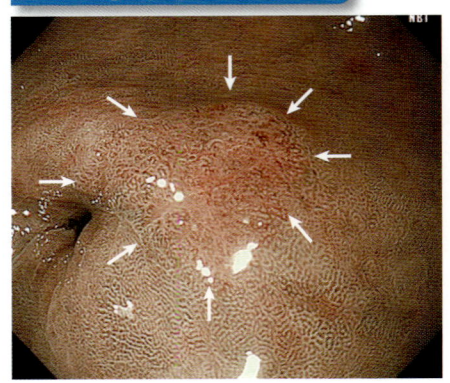

▶ In non-magnifying NBI observation, the lesion is a darker shade of brown than the surrounding mucosa. The mucosal surface of the lesion exhibits a fine granular texture and structural patterns in various sizes. These findings strongly suggest cancer.

Histopathologic image of biopsy specimen

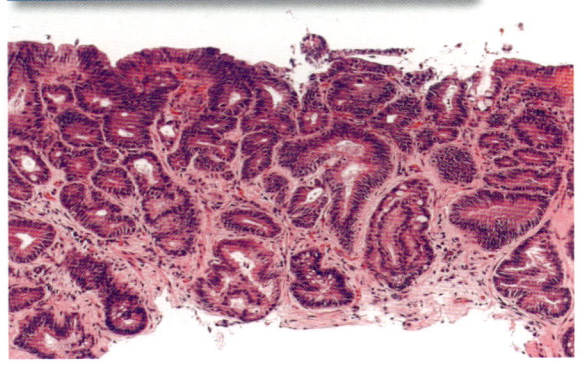

▶ HE-stained, middle-magnification image. The nuclei of the cells that form the ducts are irregular and deeply dyed. An increase in the nuclear-to-cytoplasmic ratio (N/C ratio) is observed (cytologic atypia). The ducts vary in size (structural atypia) and have high density. Hence, the lesion is diagnosed as well-differentiated tubular adenocarcinoma.

Diagnosis ❷ Posterior wall of prepyloric region, 0–IIc, 6 mm, tub1, T1a (M), UL (–)

Tips

- To evaluate whether an ulcer is benign or malignant, observe it while paying attention to : ① properties of the folds, ② properties of the base and margins of the ulcer, and ③ presence of a 0–IIc surface in the surrounding area.
- You should suspect differentiated-type gastric cancer when you see mucosa that is a little more yellowish than the surrounding area.
- Whenever suspecting cancer, bring the endoscope up close and perform indigo carmine-sprayed chromoendoscopy or NBI observation to confirm the changes in the surface structure of the mucosa.

Unacceptable endoscopic picture

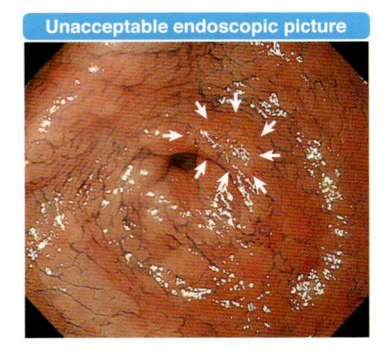

- This was the only picture from indigo carmine-sprayed chromoendoscopy at the time the lesion was discovered. Although spraying indigo carmine can show surface irregularities on the mucosal surface in detail, this picture is too distant view.
- If the endoscope is brought closer to the site, it will be possible to capture changes in the fine surface irregularities on the lesion. Always be sure to also take close-up pictures.

Patient referred to us after being diagnosed with gastric SMT

〔Gastric cancer with active *H. pylori* infection〕

Answer The gastric cancer is imaged in ①, ④, and ⑤.

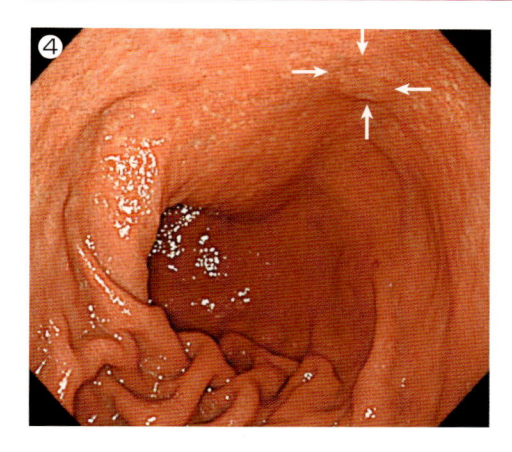

- ▶ In the background mucosa, C-3 atrophy can be seen along the lesser curvature of the body. Because diffuse redness, enlarged folds, and tortuous folds are also visible, this case can be considered active *H. pylori* infection.
- ▶ Although it is difficult to differentiate from the surrounding atrophy, mucosa that is a little more yellowish-white than the surrounding area can be seen in the lesser curvature of the middle body.

Close-up images

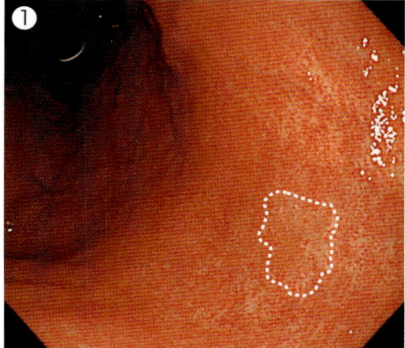
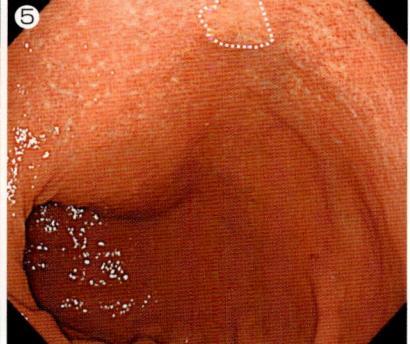

- ▶ Yellowish-white mucosa can also be seen in the distal view.
- ▶ Despite having a similar color tone to the surrounding atrophy, the lesion stands out as a relatively large area of uniformly yellowish-white mucosa, whereas the atrophy features spotty and patchy patterns. A significant change in the mucosa is critical when making a cancer diagnosis.

Non-magnifying NBI image

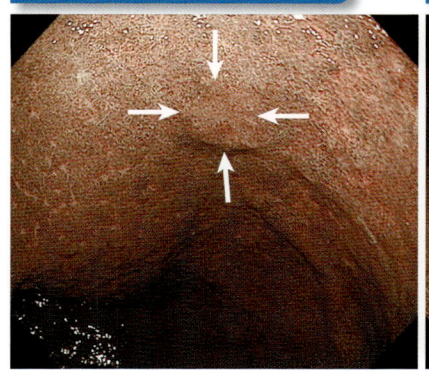

Medium-magnification NBI image

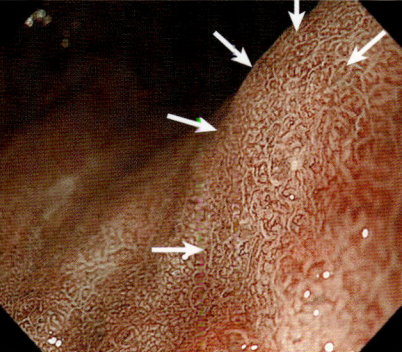

- ▶ In non-magnifying NBI observation, the lesion is a lighter shade of brown than the surrounding gastritis.
- ▶ In magnifying NBI observation, loop-shaped dilated and tortuous vessels of different sizes can be seen in the fine structure of the lesion, suggesting differentiated-type gastric cancer.

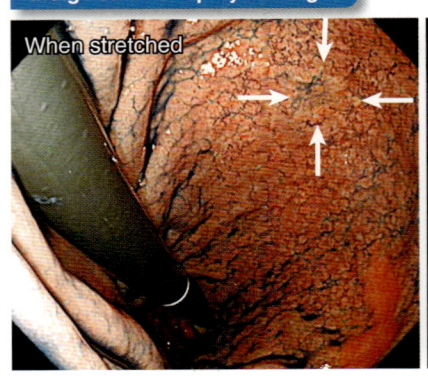

When stretched

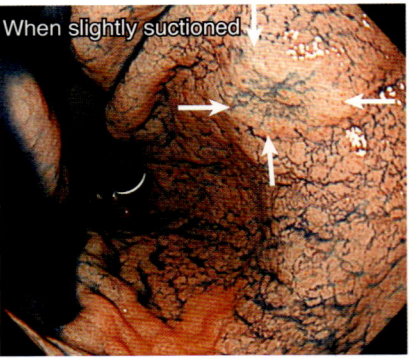

When slightly suctioned

▶ When indigo carmine is sprayed on the lesion, there is no sign of an areae gastricae pattern similar to the patterns in the surrounding mucosa. Instead, irregular narrow grooves can be seen. The change in the color tone is also more apparent.

▶ Visibility of lesions with fewer surface irregularities can be improved by slightly suctioning air rather than by insufflation to stretch the site.

Diagnosis Lesser curvature of the middle body, 0-IIb, 7 mm, tub1, T1a (M), UL (−)

Tips

- Pay attention to changes in color tone over a significant area.
- Indigo carmine sprayed chromoendoscopy and NBI observation improve the visibility of a lesion.

What's imaged in the other pictures?

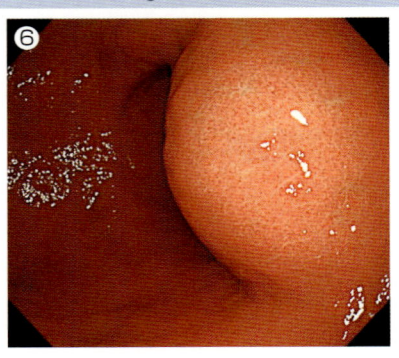

- An SMT with a diameter of about 5 cm can be seen in the region between the angulus and the posterior wall of the lesser curvature of the antrum. After performing ESD on the early gastric cancer, we performed laparoscopy and endoscopy cooperative surgery (LECS) on the SMT, which was later determined to be a gastrointestinal stromal tumor (GIST) in a histopathological examination.

Side Note Laparoscopy and endoscopy cooperative surgery (LECS)

A treatment method that combines laparoscopic surgery with endoscopy, LECS was introduced by Hiki et al.[a] in 2008 as an operation to resect a gastric SMT with minimal invasiveness. Thanks to this technique, intragastric growth-type SMTs that conventionally had to be resected using only a laparoscope can now be resected in minimum necessary ranges, also minimizing postoperative distortion of the gastric wall. It is now possible to avoid proximal gastrectomy and total gastrectomy, especially with lesions in the vicinity of the EG junction. This is a significant benefit[b].

a) Hiki N, Yamamoto Y, Fukunaga T, et al. Laparoscopic and endoscopic cooperative surgery for gastrointestinal stromal tumor dissection. Surg. Endosc. 2008 ; 22 : 1729–1735.
b) Hirasawa T, Hiki N, Yamamoto Y, et al. [Laparoscopy and endoscopy cooperative surgery for gastric submucosal tumor in the cardiac region of the stomach.] Gastroenterol Endosc. 2014; 56 : 2359–2366. (In Japanese with English abstract.)

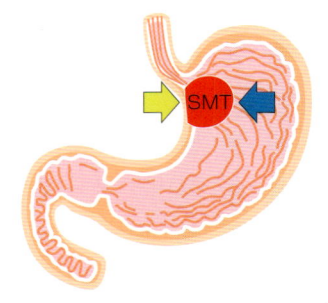

Difference in views between a laparoscope and GI endoscope

Intragastric growth-type SMT lesions cannot be recognized in the laparoscopic approach (⮕), making it necessary to perform a wide-range resection that includes part of the surrounding non-cancerous area. When the lesion is in the cardiac region, it may even be necessary to perform a total gastrectomy. In the GI endoscopic approach (⮕), on the other hand, you can resect the lesion in a minimal range, enabling you to perform local resection while preserving the cardia.

Patient referred to us due to a high CA19-9 level   〔Carcinoid tumor (*H. pylori*-uninfected case)〕

Answer   The malignant tumor is imaged in ③ and ④ .

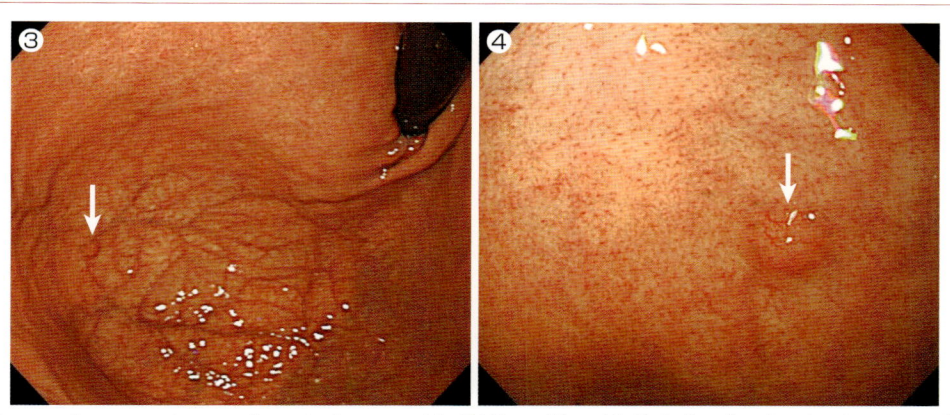

▶ The background mucosa is smooth and glossy and is RAC-positive. Multiple fundic gland polyps are also present. Hence, this is a typical *H. pylori*-uninfected case.

▶ A polyp-like elevation can be seen in the greater curvature of the fornix. At first glance, it looks like a fundic gland polyp. However, when viewed from a close distance, it does not have a margin. As fundic gland polyps typically have a margin, this should be considered an SMT lesion.

Close-up image

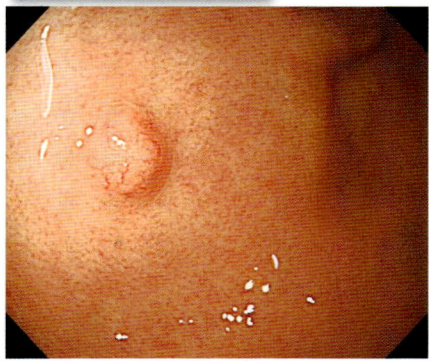

Non-magnifying NBI image

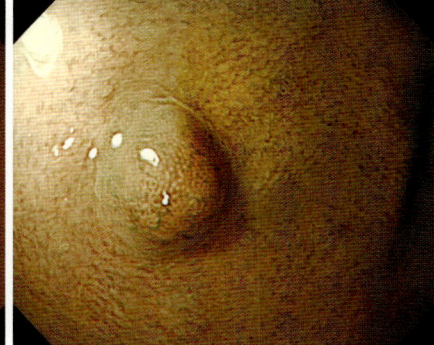

▶ In close-up observation, the lesion exhibits a slightly yellowish SMT-like elevation covered with normal mucosa, accompanied by dilated, tortuous vessels.

▶ In non-magnifying NBI observation, dilated crypt openings are recognized on the upper surface of the lesion. This happens because the submucosal tumor has extended the area where the crypt openings are located.

Indigo carmine sprayed images

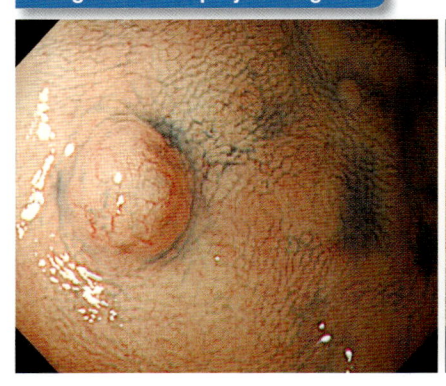 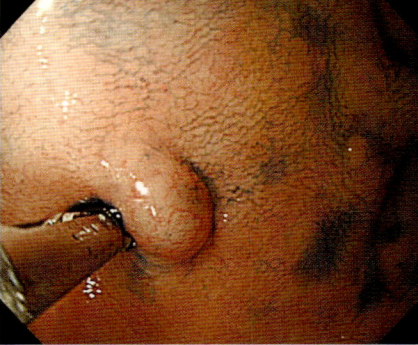

▶ The originating portion of the lesion rises while being covered with normal mucosa. The surface is smooth. Because the top of the lesion is thinned, a yellowish color tone is exhibited, influenced by the color tone of the tumor.

▶ When palpated with forceps, the tumor is discovered to be hard with poor mobility. When an SMT-like elevation has poor mobility, you should suspect a tumor originating in the deep mucosa (carcinoid tumor or fundic gland type gastric cancer).

Diagnosis   Greater curvature of the fornix, SMT, 2 mm, carcinoid tumor (NET G2), T1b (SM1, 250 μm), Type III in Rindi's classification*

*See Table 4.

Tips

- Differentiate between a fundic gland polyp and SMT.
- A carcinoid tumor is a hard SMT-like elevation with poor mobility.
- A carcinoid tumor has a yellowish color tone and is accompanied by dilated, tortuous vessels.

Additional Info   Gastric carcinoid tumor

- A gastric carcinoid tumor originates in endocrine cells present in the deep mucosa. It is a relatively a rare type of gastric cancer and grows slowly. While it has similar findings to an SMT since it is generated from the deep mucosa, it is classified as an epithelial tumor
- One hundred years have passed since a gastrointestinal carcinoid was first reported, and the concept of carcinoid has changed since then (**Table 1**). According to the 2010 WHO Classification of Digestive Neuroendocrine Neoplasms (**Table 2**), pancreatic and gastrointestinal tumors that have endocrine properties and phenotypes are generically called neuroendocrine neoplasms (NENs). NENs are classified into well-differentiated neuroendocrine tumors (NETs) and poorly differentiated neuroendocrine carcinomas (NECs). NETs are further subclassified into Grades 1 and 2 (NET G1 and NET G2) based on the rate of proliferation(mitotic rate or ki-67 index). The *Japanese Classification of Gastric Cancer* (14th edition)[29], meanwhile, divides neuroendocrine tumors into carcinoid tumors (mainly corresponding to the WHO Classification's NET G1 and G2) and endocrine cell carcinomas (mainly corresponding to the WHO Classification's NEC).
- Gastric carcinoid tumors are classified into types I to III in Rindi's classification, and there are differences in their clinical characteristics (**Tables 3 and 4**).

Table 1 Evolution of the concept of carcinoid

1980 WHO Classification	2000 WHO Classification	2010 WHO Classification	*Japanese Classification of Gastric Cancer* (14th ed.)
Carcinoid	Well-differentiated endocrine tumor (WDET)	Neuroendocrine tumor: NET G1	Carcinoid tumor
	Well-differentiated endocrine carcinoma (WDEC)	Neuroendocrine tumor: NET G2	
	Poorly differentiated endocrine carcinoma (PDEC)	Neuroendocrine carcinoma: NEC	Endocrine cell carcinoma

〔Based on various sources[29), 50]〕

Table 2 Grading system(2010 WHO Classification)

2010 WHO Classification	Mitotic rate (/10HPF)	Ki-67 index (%)
NET G1	<2	≤2
NET G2	2 to 20	3 to 20
NEC	>20	>20

- Mitotic rate: At least 50 of the high-magnification fields of view (2 mm^2) are investigated, and the number of mitoses per 10 fields of view is measured.
- Ki-67 index: The precentage of tumor cells that immunolabel positively for the ki-67 antigen.

〔Based on various sources[50]〕

Table 3 Treatment policies for gastric carcinoid tumor according to the guidelines

	Types I, II*	Type III
Japanese guideline (2015)	• Tumor diameter: ≤1 cm; no. of tumors: ≤5; MP invasion absent; lymph node metastasis absent → Follow-up observation or endoscopic resection • Tumor diameter: 1 to 2 cm; no. of tumors: ≤5; MP invasion absent; lymph node metastasis absent → Endoscopic resection or gastrectomy + lymphadenectomy • Tumor diameter: >2 cm; no. of tumors: ≥6; MP invasion present; lymph node metastasis present → Gastrectomy + lymphadenectomy	Gastrectomy + lymphadenectomy
ENETS (2016)	• Tumor diameter: ≤1 cm → Follow-up observation or endoscopic resection • Tumor diameter: ≥1 cm → Endoscopic resection • MP invasion, positive resection stump → Surgical local resection	Gastrectomy + lymphadenectomy
NCCN (2016)	• Follow-up observation and endoscopic resection for conspicuous tumors. • Anterectomy should also be considered when the tumor is enlarged.	• Gastrectomy + lymphadenectomy • Surgical local resection for cases without lymph node metastasis while endoscopic resection is also considered. However, only lesions with ≤1 cm tumor diameter that are NET G1 and have no MP invasion are subject to endoscopic resection.

*With type II, resection of a gastrin-producing tumor should be performed as a rule.

〔Based on various sources[51)-53]〕

Table 4 Rindi's classification

	Type I	Type II	Type III
Endoscopic image	Multiple small submucosal tumor-like elevations	Multiple small submucosal tumor-like elevations	Often singular and large
Occurrence site	Body	Body	Body, antrum
Patient history	Type A gastritis	MEN–1 type	None in particular
Serum gastrin	High	High	Normal
Malignant potential	Low	Low	High

[Based on various sources[54)]]

- Unlike other gastrointestinal carcinoid tumors, gastric carcinoid tumors are classified as types I to III in Rindi's classification. They also differ in biological malignancy.
- With Rindi's types I and II, multiple carcinoids occur in the fundic gland region due to hypergastrinemia.
- With Rindi's type I, severe atrophic gastritis in the body caused by auto-immune gastritis (type A gastritis) causes an increase in the intragastric pH and gastrin is excessively secreted from the G cells of the pyloric region, resulting in hypergastrinemia.
- With Rindi's type II, hypergastrinemia is caused by a gastrin-producing tumor represented by multiple endocrine neoplasia type 1 (MEN1).
- Rindi's type III occurs sporadically and is considered to be highly malignant.

👓 What's imaged in the other pictures?

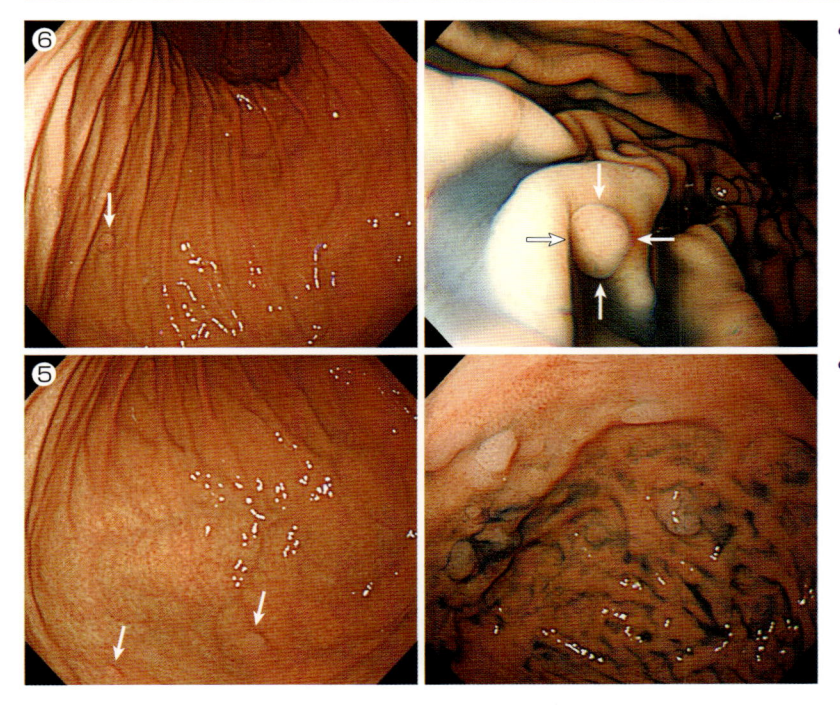

- Multiple fundic gland polyps are present in the body. Both fundic gland polyps and SMTs are elevated lesions. They have smooth surfaces and their color tones correspond with the surrounding area. It is sometimes difficult to differentiate a small SMT from a fundic gland polyp. However, a fundic gland polyp is slightly constricted and possesses a clear circumferential margin, making it possible to differentiate it from an SMT.

- Although it is difficult to recognize in conventional endoscopy, spraying indigo carmine reveals multiple low-height white flat elevations of different sizes in the region between the fornix and the upper body. These are called multiple white flat elevations (Haruma-Kawaguchi lesions). They are hyperplasia of the foveolar epithelium of the fundic glands.

Side Note **Make good use of sedatives!**

To mitigate the patient's anxiety and the discomfort of endoscopy, many facilities use sedatives and analgesics. At the Cancer Institute Hospital of JFCR, we perform more than 20,000 endoscopies a year and administer a sedative (midazolam) or analgesic (pethidine) to 73% of the patients. Being a sedative, midazolam has anti-anxiety and hypnotic properties, but no analgesic property. Pethidine is an opioid and alleviates pain in the pharynx and suppresses reflex. If you administer midazolam alone to suppress the reflex in a patient who has a strong gag reflex, you may end up using too much. When the patient has a strong gag reflex, the use of pethidine can often reduce discomfort and make the examination less difficult.

Synchronous multiple lesions found in detailed preoperative examination ①

[Gastric cancer with active *H. pylori* infection]

Answer The synchronous multiple lesions are imaged in ④.

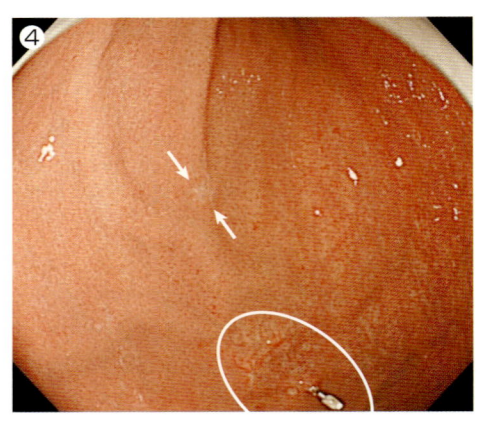

▶ On the proximal side of the lesion (circled) discovered by the previous doctor, a small patch of faded mucosa (indicated by the arrows) is visible. Fading in non-atrophic mucosa stands out even when it covers a small area. A small faded area in non-atrophic mucosa should be suspected to be undifferentiated-type gastric cancer.

▶ In preoperative endoscopies, synchronous multiple lesions are often found. Surgical procedures and resection ranges are subject to change depending on preoperative endoscopic findings. It is important to be aware of the possibility synchronous multiple lesions when performing endoscopic observation.

Indigo carmine sprayed image

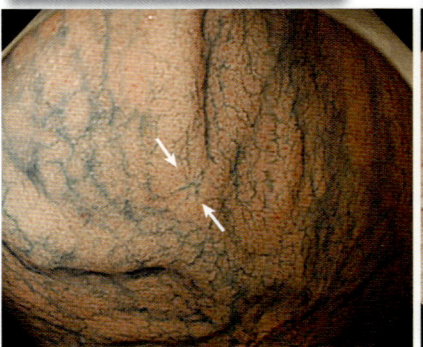

Magnifying NBI image

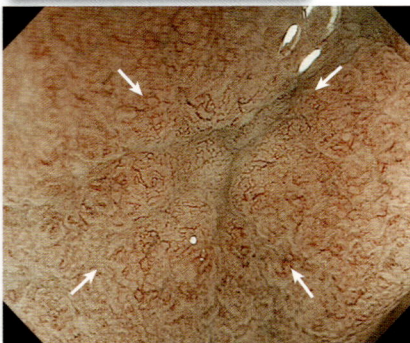

▶ When indigo carmine is sprayed, the fading is less noticeable and the visibility of the lesion deteriorates. It can be seen, however, that the lesion is slightly depressed.

▶ In magnifying NBI observation, dilated and tortuous vessels are visible inside the fine structure that is about to disappear. This makes it possible to diagnose it as cancer.

Diagnosis Anterior wall of the lesser curvature of the middle body, 0–IIc, 3 mm, sig, T1a (M), UL (–)

Tips
- There can always be more than one lesion.
- Suspect undifferentiated-type gastric cancer when you see fading in non-atrophic mucosa.

Gastric cancer found by the previous doctor

Shown in ②.

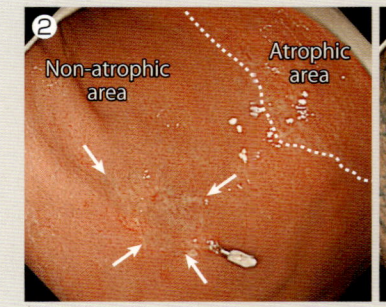

Non-atrophic area

Atrophic area

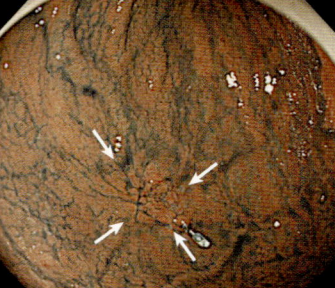

- The background mucosa is accompanied by diffuse redness and attachment of sticky mucus, which leads to a diagnosis of active *H. pylori* infection. C–3 atrophy is visible in the lesser curvature of the body, but has not expanded into either the anterior or posterior walls, or the greater curvature of the body. A depression with mixture of fading and redness is visible in the non-atrophic mucosa. A clip is attached to the distal side of the lesion. This was attached by the previous doctor to stop bleeding after biopsy. When indigo carmine was sprayed, the depressed surface became a little clearer.
- Diagnosis: Anterior wall near the lesser curvature of the middle body, 0–IIc, 20 mm, por>sig>tub2, T1a (M) UL (+)

Synchronous multiple lesions found in detailed preoperative examination ②

〔Gastric cancer with active *H. pylori* infection〕

case 25

Answer The gastric cancer is imaged in ⑤ and ⑥ .

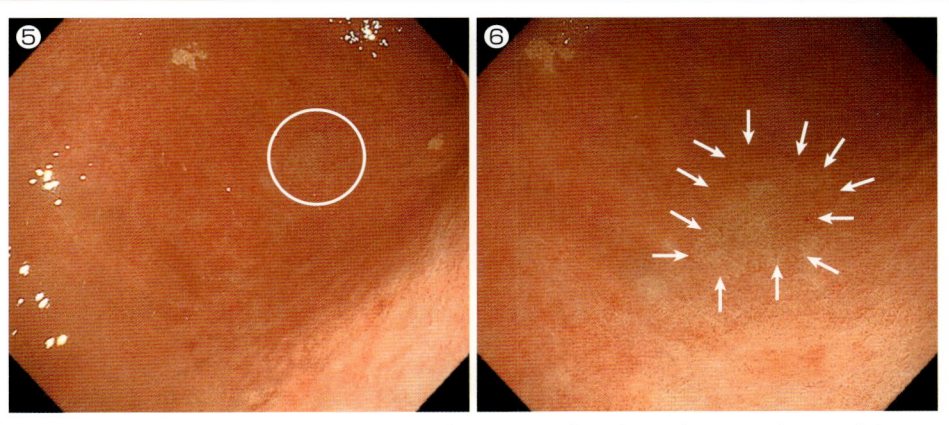

▶ O–3 atrophy can be seen in the background mucosa and xanthoma is present here and there.
▶ Diffuse redness is exhibited, suggesting an active *H. pylori* infection.
▶ When viewed from a distance (⑤), mucosa that is slightly more yellowish-white than the surrounding mucosa can be seen in the greater curvature of the lower body.
▶ In close-up observation (⑥), the proximal side of the lesion is yellowish-white. There is some redness on the distal side of the lesion that is almost the same color tone as the surrounding mucosa. The margin on the distal side is somewhat unclear in conventional endoscopy.

Non-magnifying NBI image

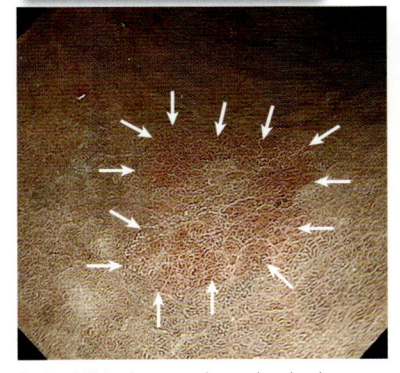

Indigo carmine sprayed image

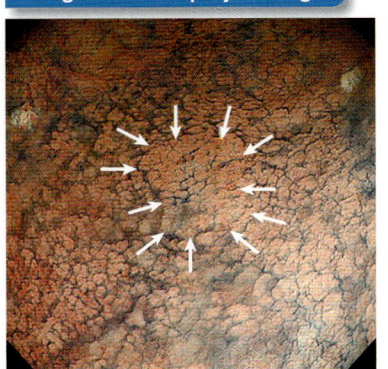

▶ When indigo carmine is sprayed, there seems to be almost no difference between the height of the lesion and that of its surroundings. Nor is there any clear difference between the areae gastricae patterns inside and outside of the lesion. As a result, the lesion is not as conspicuous as it is in NBI observation.
▶ However, indigo carmine does not adhere to the lesion as tenaciously as it does to the surrounding area, which makes it easier to see the margin (indicated by the arrows).

▶ In NBI observation, the lesion exhibits a brownish color with clear margins.

Diagnosis Greater curvature of the lower body, 0–IIb, 14 mm, tub1, T1a (M), UL (−)

Tips

- Watch for multiple lesions.
- Watch for any change in color tone that is more yellowish-white than the surroundings.
- Remember that a 0–IIb is easy to miss.
- Note that NBI may be useful for detection of a 0–IIb lesion.

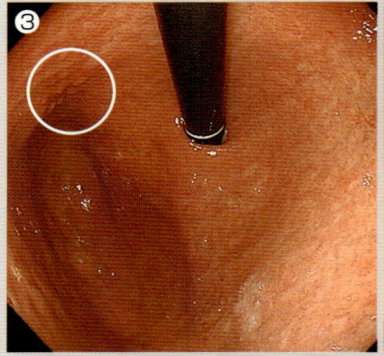
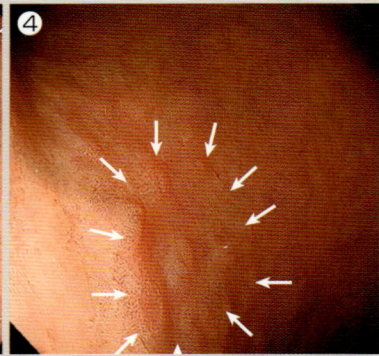

- In observation with the endoscope retroflexed (③), a reddish depressed lesion with conspicuous surface irregularities can be seen on the posterior wall of the upper body.
- In close-up observation with antegrade view (④), it can be seen that the lesion is depressed with a slightly unclear margin.

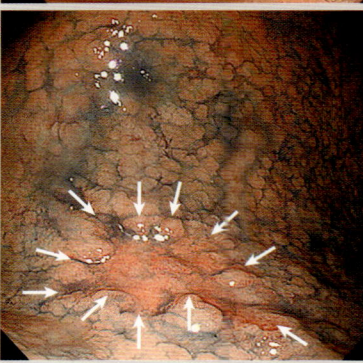

- When indigo carmine is sprayed, the surface irregularities become clear and the lesion's redness stands out, facilitating recognition of the margin. It is a reddish depressed lesion accompanied by a thorn-like encroachment. The surrounding area features reactive elevations. For these reasons, it can be diagnosed as differentiated-type gastric cancer.
- Diagnosis: Posterior wall of the upper body, 0–IIc, 31 mm, tub1>pap, T1a (M), UL (–)

Side Note What is the appropriate number of photos to take?

How many endoscopic pictures should we take during an upper GI endoscopy? According to the guidelines of the European Society of Gastrointestinal Endoscopy (ESGE)[a], the recommended number of images to be recorded during an upper GI endoscopy is 8. Of those, only 4 should be of the stomach. Of course, in Japan, where the rate of chronic gastritis and gastric cancer is much higher, European-style guidelines are not suitable. In Japan, the standard number of pictures recommended is 30 to 40 between the esophagus and the duodenum. When a lesion is found, detailed observation is necessary, so naturally the number of pictures taken should be increased. Recently, I've noticed that young doctors these days often take more than 100 pictures, needlessly shooting similar images because today's digital filing systems have virtually no limit on the number of storable images. But you won't make good progress in endoscopy if you think you should take as many pictures as possible. I don't believe that we should take any pictures without good reason.

a) Rey JF, Lambert R. ESGE recommendations for quality control in gastrointestinal endoscopy: guidelines for image documentation in upper and lower GI endoscopy. Endoscopy. 2001; 33: 901–903.

Synchronous multiple lesions found in detailed preoperative examination ③
〔Gastric cancer with active *H. pylori* infection〕

Answer ❶ The first lesion is imaged in ② and ④ .

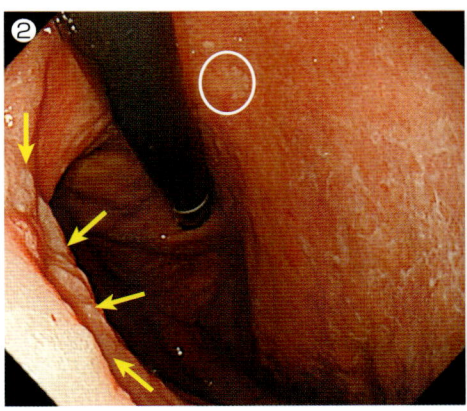
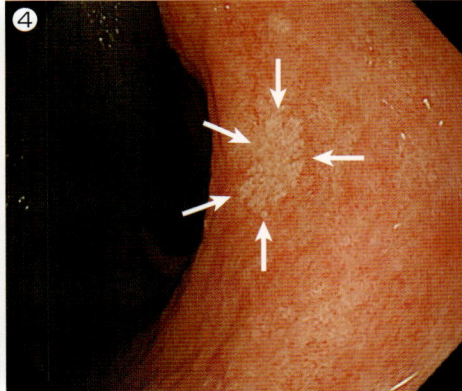

▶ Severe O–2 atrophy is recognized in the background mucosa, while the non-atrophic mucosa exhibits diffuse redness. This is a finding of active *H. pylori* infection.

▶ White mucosa with a clear margin (enclosed in the white circle) can be seen in the lesser curvature of the upper body. This is change in color tone (indicated by the white arrows). As it covers a relatively substantial area, it needs to be examined in detail as it suggests the possibility of adenoma or cancer. Additionally, the lesion on the posterior wall of the upper body (indicated by the yellow arrows) is already-known early cancer.

Non-magnifying NBI image   **Medium-magnification NBI image**   **Indigo carmine sprayed image**

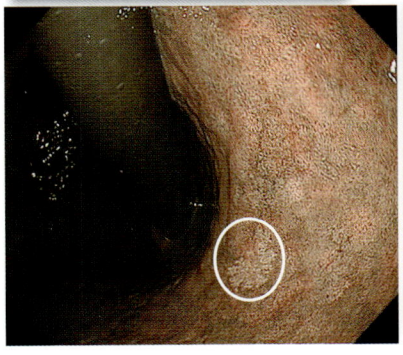
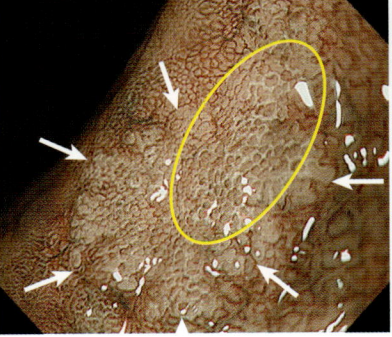
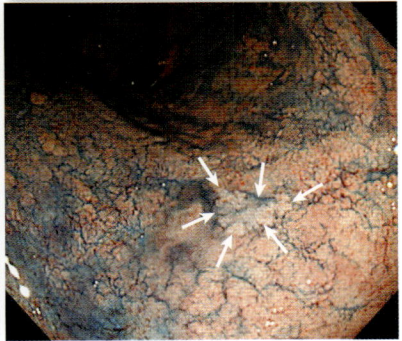

▶ In non-magnifying NBI observation, the lesion is a lighter shade of brown than the surrounding mucosa while the margin is clear. Under medium magnification, mesh-like vessels are visible. There is also a white opaque substance (WOS) partially attached in a mesh-like pattern (enclosed in the yellow circle).

▶ When indigo carmine is sprayed, it becomes apparent that the lesion is a 0–IIb lesion with no surface irregularities compared to the surrounding area. The margin is clear due to the difference in color tone.

Diagnosis ❶ Lesser curvature of the middle body, 0–IIa-like lesion, 5 mm, tubular adenoma with moderate atypia

Answer ❷ The second lesion is imaged in ③.

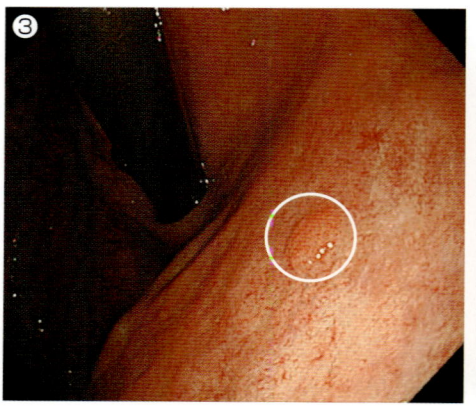

▶ A small reddish flat elevation can be seen on the anterior wall of the middle body.

Close-up image

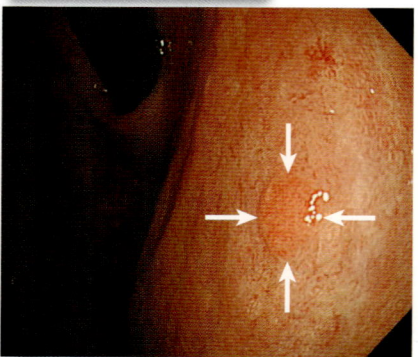

▶ Among reddish polyps inside atrophic mucosa, hyperplastic polyps have one of the highest occurrence rates.

▶ However, the coarse mucosal pattern characteristic of hyperplastic polyps is not present here, and the redness looks a little dark and dull. This suggests that cancer should be considered.

Non-magnifying NBI image

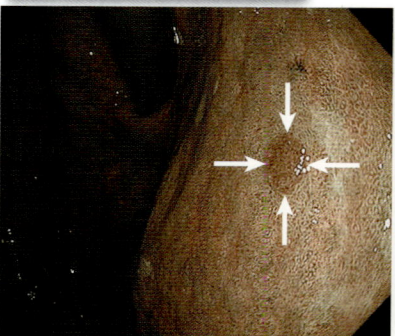

Medium-magnification NBI image

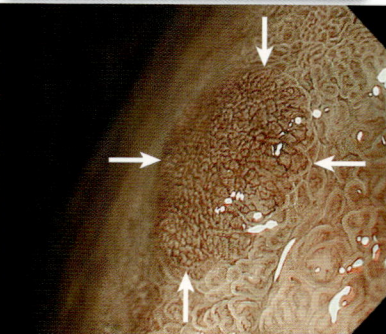

Indigo carmine sprayed image

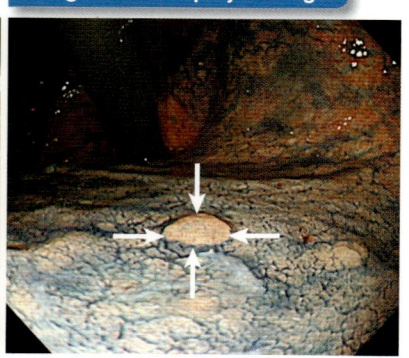

▶ In non-magnifying NBI observation, the lesion is a darker shade of brown than the surrounding mucosa while the margin is clear. When magnified, clear mesh-like vessels can be seen, leading to a diagnosis of cancer.

▶ Even when indigo carmine is sprayed, the coarse mucosal pattern characteristic of hyperplastic polyps is not recognized.

▶ The background mucosa appears bluish due to the indigo carmine, but the dye does not adhere as well to the lesion, making the redness stand out.

Diagnosis ❷ Anterior wall of the middle body, 0–IIa, 3 mm, tub1, T1a (M), UL (−)

Additional Info White opaque substance (WOS)

● WOS was first reported by Yao et al. It is a white opaque substance that exists in the superficial mucosal layer of gastric epithelial tumors[55]. Since WOS does not transmit light from an endoscope, it obstructs observation of microvascular patterns in the area where it is present. It is not a permanent finding; it may, over the course of follow-up observation, disappear or newly emerge. The main component of WOS is considered to be lipid droplets deposited in the intraepithelial cells of a tumor[56].

● WOS is frequently observed in adenoma cases but also observed in differentiated-type gastric cancer cases. It takes on different shapes in adenoma and cancer — in the former it exhibits regular patterns such as mesh-like and labyrinth-like, while in the latter it has low density, no regular shape, and exhibits irregular, asymmetrical distribution[55].

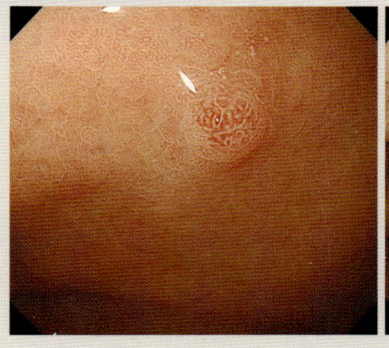 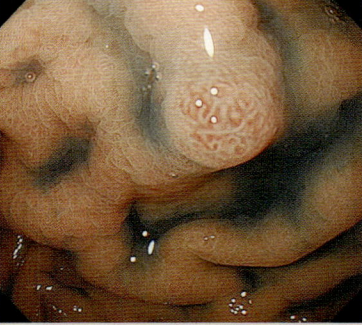

- Hyperplastic polyps and reddish 0–IIa lesions resemble each other at first glance when they are small. However, a hyperplastic polyp exhibits its characteristic coarse mucosal pattern, making it possible to differentiate it without having to perform a biopsy.

Lesion discovered by the previous doctor

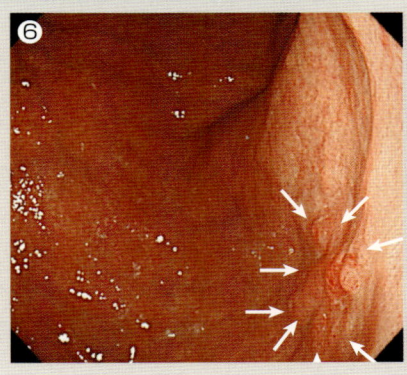 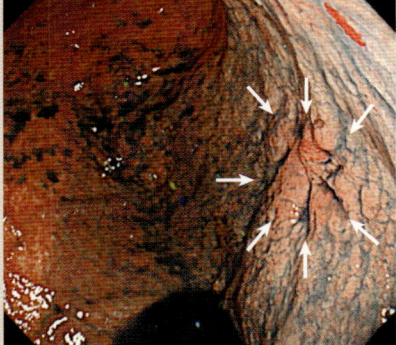

- A reddish depressed lesion accompanied by convergence of folds (indicated by the arrows) can be seen on the posterior wall of the middle body. Most of it is elevated, including the depressed portion. Due to conspicuous surface irregularities, the preoperative diagnosis was T1b (SM2). However, the postoperative diagnosis was T1a (M), UL (+). When this type of lesion is accompanied by an ulcer scar, invasion depth diagnosis can be difficult.
- Diagnosis: Posterior wall of the middle body, 0–IIc, 30 mm, tub1>tub2>por, T1a (M), UL (+)

Tips

- When you've found one lesion, look for a second and third one.
- Look for a reddish or whitish flat elevation on atrophic mucosa.
- Note that invasion depth diagnosis is difficult with gastric cancer accompanied by an ulcer scar.

Synchronous multiple lesions found in detailed preoperative examination ④

〔Gastric cancer detected after *H. pylori* eradication〕

Answer The gastric cancer is imaged in ① .

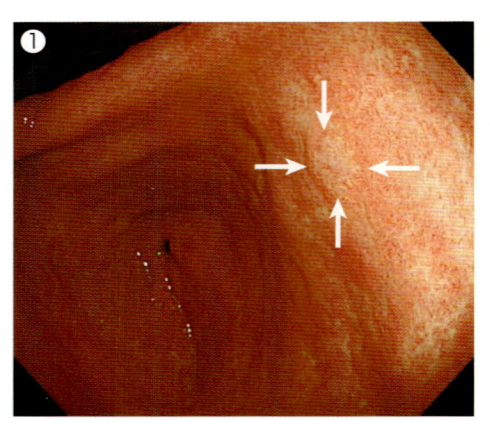

▶ The background mucosa exhibits C–3 atrophy. In atrophic areas, keep an eye out for differentiated-type gastric cancer.

▶ Yellowish-white mucosa that is a little more conspicuous than the surrounding atrophy is seen on the posterior wall of the antrum.

Close-up image

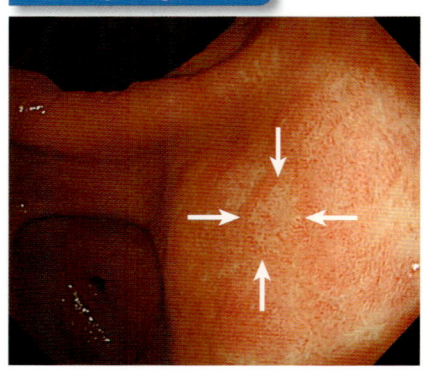

Indigo carmine-sprayed image

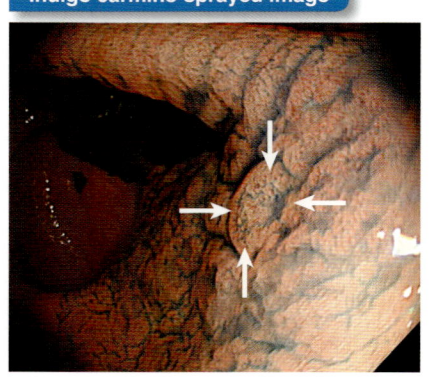

▶ It is difficult to distinguish this lesion from the surrounding atrophy. However, while the atrophy shows patchy fading, the lesion appears as an area of patchy yellowish-white flat mucosa with clear margins. Perform detailed observation while considering the possibility of cancer.

▶ When indigo carmine is sprayed, it becomes apparent that the lesion has both a coarse texture and a fine mucosal pattern. However, it cannot be diagnosed as cancer at this time.

Non-magnifying NBI image

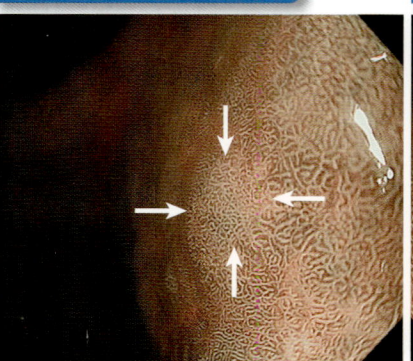

Medium-magnification NBI image

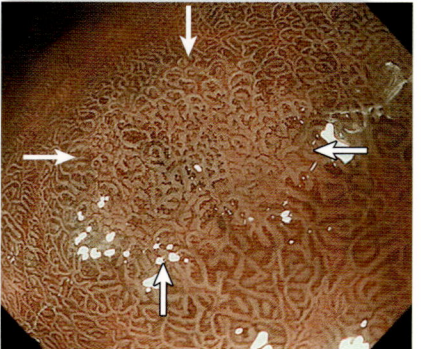

▶ A finer surface microstructure than present in the surrounding gastritis is visible in NBI observation. Because looped dilated and tortuous vessels can be seen when magnified, this should be diagnosed as differentiated-type gastric cancer.

Diagnosis   Posterior wall of the antrum, 0–IIb, 3 mm, tub1, T1a (M), UL (–)

Tips

- In an atrophic area: Look for differentiated-type gastric cancer.
- In a non-atrophic area: Look for undifferentiated-type gastric cancer.

Lesion discovered by the previous doctor

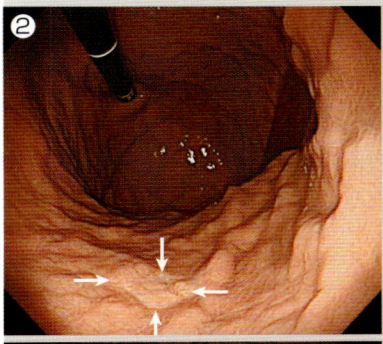 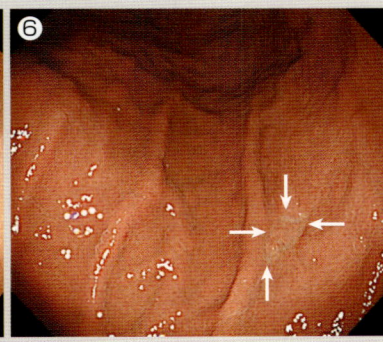

- A faded depressed lesion with a clear margin can be seen near the posterior wall of the greater curvature of the middle body. The background mucosa is a fundic gland region with no atrophy, suggesting undifferentiated-type gastric cancer.

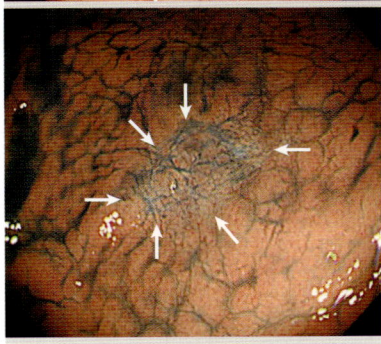

- When indigo carmine is sprayed, the areae gastricae on the depressed surface seem less clear than in the surrounding area.
- Diagnosis: Greater curvature of the middle body, 0–IIc, 15 mm, sig, T1a (M), UL (–)

Side Note Synchronous multiple lesions

Synchronous multiple lesions are often defined as cancer discovered within one year after the first endoscopic treatment. It has been reported that their occurrence frequency is 9.2 to 19.2%[a), b)]. Synchronous multiple lesions are often seen in the elderly. It is reasonable to assume that if you don't find synchronous multiple lesions at least once in every ten times in preoperative gastric cancer endoscopies, then you are probably missing some cases of gastric cancer. Don't let yourself be distracted by a single lesion. You have to perform observation very carefully to see if there are any other hidden cancerous lesions.

a) Nakajima T, Oda I, Gotoda T, et al. Metachronous gastric cancers after endoscopic resection: how effective is annual endoscopic surveillance? Gastric Cancer. 2006; 9: 93–98.
b) Kobayashi M, Narisawa R, Sato Y, et al. [Self-limiting risk of metachronous gastric cancers after endoscopic resection.] Gastroenterol Endosc. 2012; 54: 1498–1505. (In Japanese with English abstract.)

case
28

Synchronous multiple lesions found in detailed preoperative examination ⑤

〔Gastric cancer with active *H. pylori* infection〕

Answer The gastric cancer is imaged in ② and ⑥ .

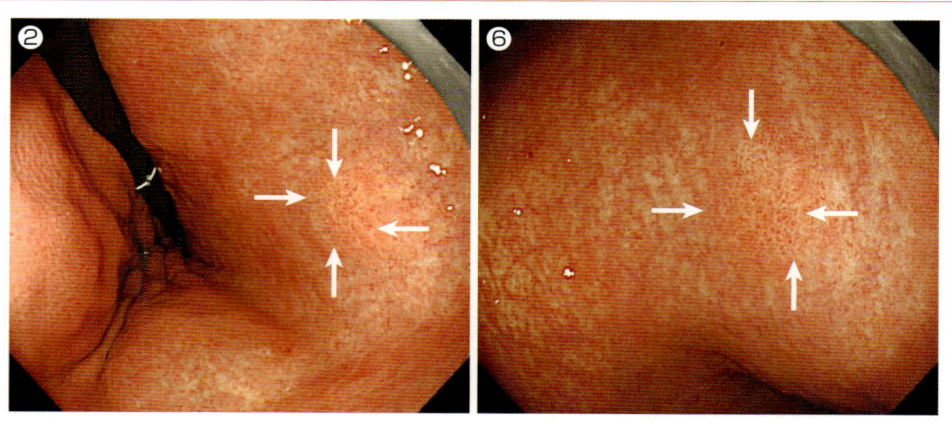

▶ O-3 atrophy is present in the background mucosa. Non-atrophic mucosa in the greater curvature of the body exhibits diffuse redness. This indicates an active *H. pylori* infection.

▶ An area that contains a mix of redness and yellowish-white mucosa can be seen in the lesser curvature of the lower body. It is difficult to be differentiate from the surrounding mucosa. However, even though the fading of the atrophy s patchy, there is a certain degree of regularity to the mix of color tones in the lesion. This makes it possible to detect the lesion.

Close-up image

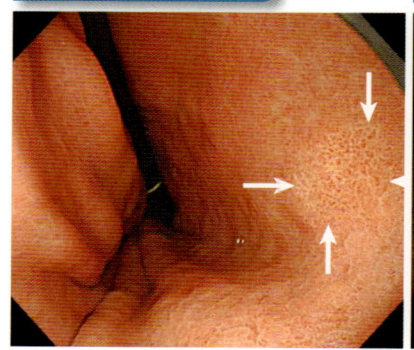

Non-magnifying NBI image

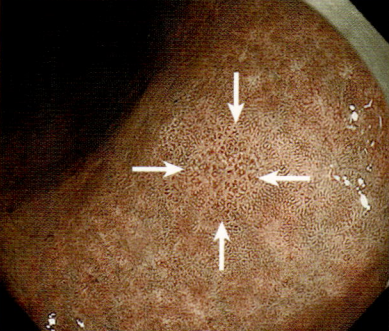

Magnifying NBI image

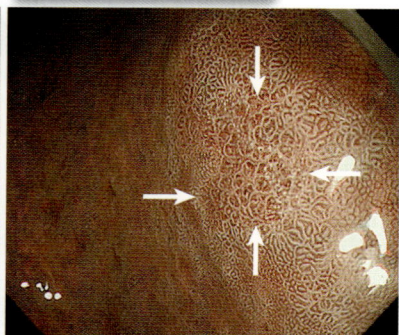

▶ In close-up observation, multiple small areas of redness can be seen in the mucosa that is more yellowish-white than the surrounding area.

▶ In NBI observation, a fine granular surface microstructure is visible on the lesion.

Indigo carmine sprayed image

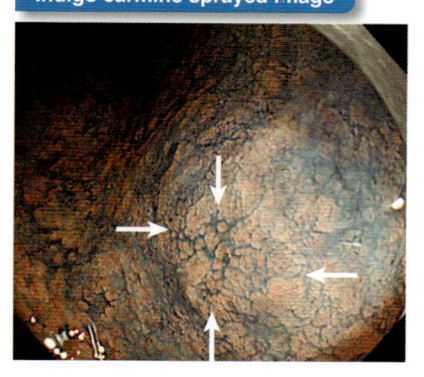

▶ When indigo carmine is sprayed, a fine granular mucosal pattern becomes clear.

Tips

- Perform endoscopy while keeping an eye out for synchronous multiple lesions.
- Pay attention to subtle differences in color tone of atrophy and cancer.

Lesion discovered by the previous doctor

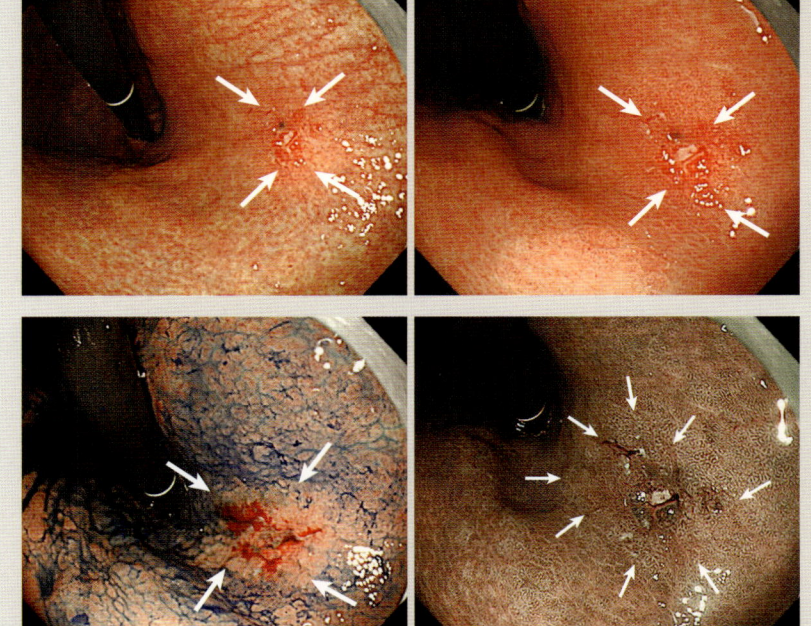

- A reddish depressed lesion can be seen in the lesser curvature of the upper body. Erosion and regenerative epithelium in the lesion have occurred as a consequence of multiple biopsies performed by the previous doctor. When numerous biopsies are performed, the removal of a significant amount of tissue can change the properties of the lesion.

- It is a hemorrhagic lesion. The bleeding makes it harder to visualize.
- Diagnosis: Lesser curvature of the upper body, 0–IIc, 22 mm, tub1, T1b (SM1, 450 µm), UL (–)

 Side Note   Eyes can only see what the brain knows

Whenever I am standing behind one of our residents watching while they perform an endoscopy, various thoughts pop into my head like, "What about that depression? Aren't you going to spray indigo carmine?" and "Hey, what about that redness there? Why not look at it in close up?" It's hard for me not to comment when the resident tries to wrap up the procedure without covering the points I'm not comfortable with. But I was like that once, and the truth is you can't recognize cancer even when you see a finding of cancer unless you have actually seen cancer with your own eyes. A pioneer of ESD for gastric cancer, Dr. Gotoda once said, "Eyes can only see what the brain knows," referring to endoscopic diagnosis of gastric cancer[a]. I think it's a marvelous way of putting it.

a) Gotoda T, Uedo N, Yoshinaga S, et al. Basic principles and practice of gastric cancer screening using high-definition white-light gastroscopy: Eyes can only see what the brain knows. Dig Endosc. 2016; 28(Suppl 1): 2–15.

Synchronous multiple lesions found in detailed preoperative examination ⑥

Answer The gastric cancer is imaged in ② , ③ and ⑥ .

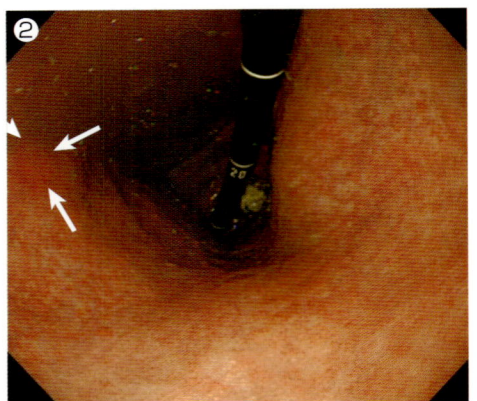

▶ Due to the presence of severe O–3 atrophy in the background mucosa, the examination was performed with the assumption that there was a high risk of differentiated-type gastric cancer.
▶ Reddish mucosa can be seen on the anterior wall of the middle body. It is a distant view and the details are unclear.

Retroflex view

Antegrade view

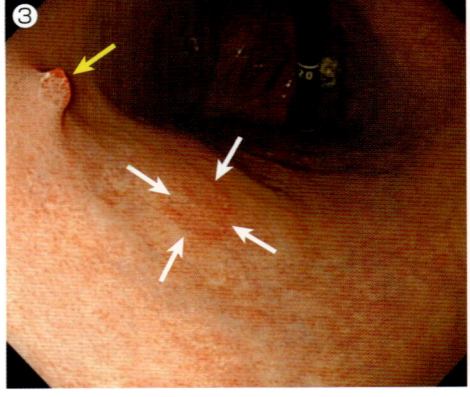 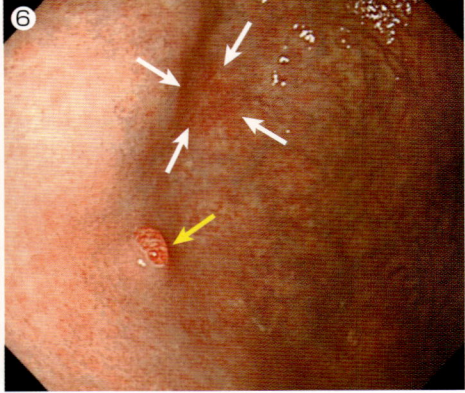

▶ In close up, the lesion is recognized as a reddish surface with no vascular pattern. The only thing noticeable is the difference in color tone. The surface irregularities are unclear.
▶ A reddish polyp that exhibits a coarse mucosal pattern is observed nearby. This is a typical hyperplastic polyp (indicated by the yellow arrow).

Indigo carmine sprayed image

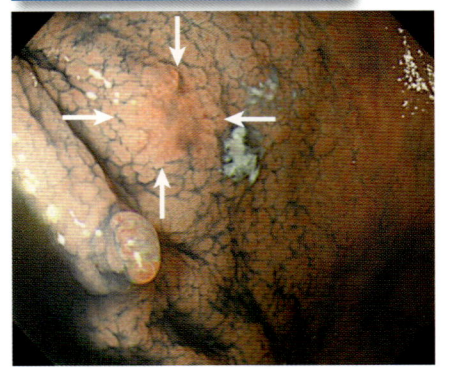

▶ When indigo carmine is sprayed, the difference in color tone becomes more apparent. The areae gastricae pattern visible in the surrounding area is less clear on the lesion, making it easier to see.
▶ This lesion was not detected in conventional endoscopy and was only discovered when indigo carmine was sprayed on the entire gastric mucosa at the end of the examination. Gastric cancer is often found when indigo carmine is sprayed.

Histological images of ESD-resected specimen

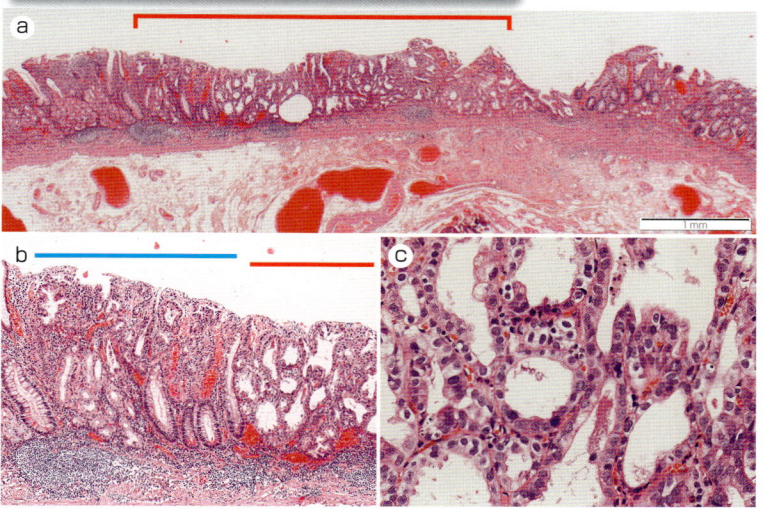

a : HE-stained, low-magnification image. A tumor can be seen in the area shown under the red line. In the background, there is body fundic gland mucosa that shows inflammatory cell infiltration accompanied by intestinal metaplasia and lymphoid follicles. The lesion is slightly depressed.

b : HE-stained, medium-magnification image of the edge of the lesion. A dense growth of tubular structures can be seen in all mucosal layers at the center of the lesion (shown under the red line) and in the main portion of the surface layer of the mucosa at the edge (shown under the blue line).

c : HE-stained, high-magnification image of the lesion. A dense growth of glands comprised of cells with enlarged oval nuclei can be seen. It is diagnosed as well-differentiated tubular adenocarcinoma (tub 1).

Diagnosis   Anterior wall of the middle body, 0–IIc, 7 mm, tub1, T1a (M), UL (–)

Tips

- Multiple lesions tend to occur in gastric cancer.
- There is a high risk of differentiated-type gastric cancer with severe atrophic gastritis.
- Gastric cancer is often found when indigo carmine is sprayed.

What's imaged in the other pictures?

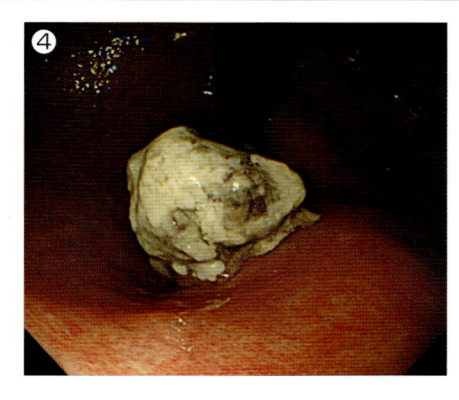

- An elevated lesion with a diameter of about 30 mm can be seen in the lesser curvature of the cardia. The lesion is covered with necrotic tissue. It is the early cancer pointed out by the previous doctor.
- After ESD had been performed on the lesion on the anterior wall of the middle body, proximal gastrectomy was performed on this lesion.
- Diagnosis: Lesser curvature of the cardia, 0–I, 30 mm, tub1>tub2, T1b (SM2)

case

30

Answer ❶ The gastric cancer discovered by the previous doctor is imaged in ⑥ .

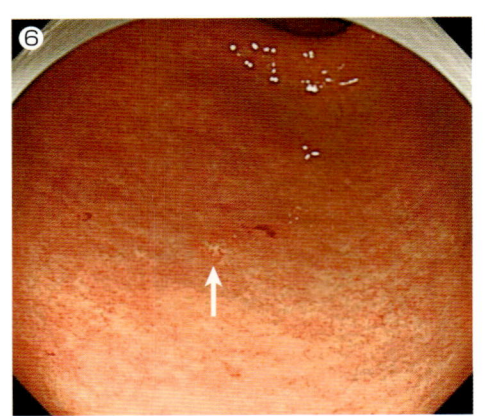

⑥

▶ Diffuse redness, minor mucosal swelling, and enlarged folds can be seen, suggesting an active *H. pylori* infection.

▶ O–2 atrophy is recognized in the background mucosa.

▶ A biopsy scar (indicated by the arrow) can be seen in the greater curvature of the antrum. The periphery is slightly reddish, and fresh blood is attached. However, it is too early to suspect cancer.

Indigo carmine sprayed image

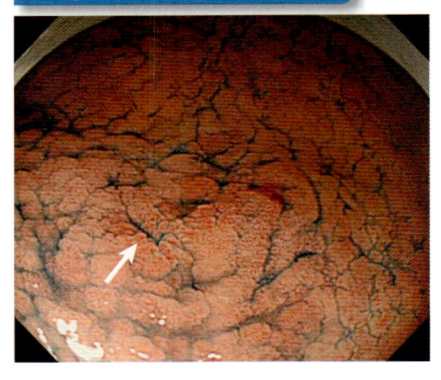

▶ When the site is observed up close after spraying indigo carmine, a biopsy scar (indicated by the arrow) can be seen on the proximal side. However, the surface irregularities are inconspicuous, and there is no clear finding of cancer.

▶ With a small lesion, the effects of a biopsy often make a finding of cancer hard to see.

Non-magnifying NBI image

High-magnification NBI image

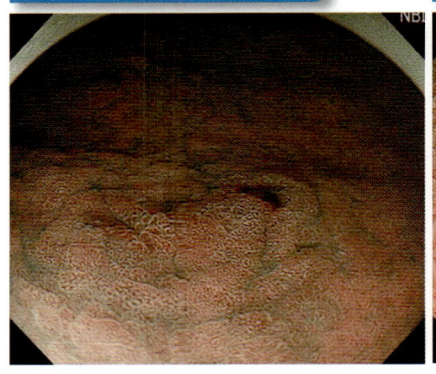

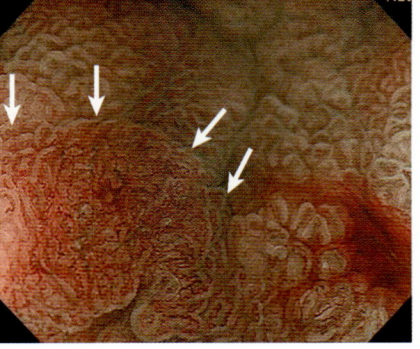

▶ In non-magnifying NBI observation, the lesion is recognized as a brownish area. When magnified, the demarcation line (indicated by the arrows) can be clearly recognized and dilated, tortuous abnormal vessels can be seen in the lesion, making it possible diagnose this lesion as cancer.

Diagnosis ❶ Greater curvature of the antrum, 0–IIc, 12 mm, tub1, T1a (M), UL (–)

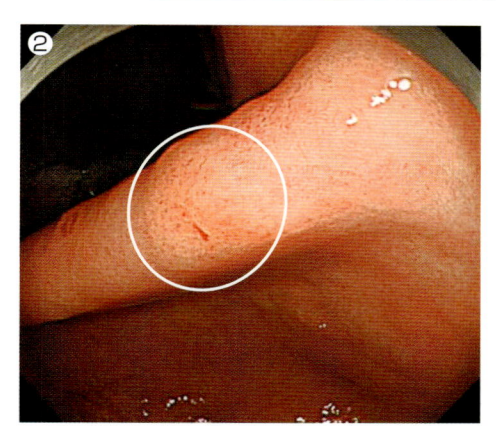

▶ On the anterior wall of the lesser curvature of the angulus, a flat elevated lesion can be seen that is a little more yellowish than the surrounding area.

▶ The lesion is accompanied by spontaneous bleeding, posing the possibility that it is a neoplastic lesion.

Indigo carmine sprayed image

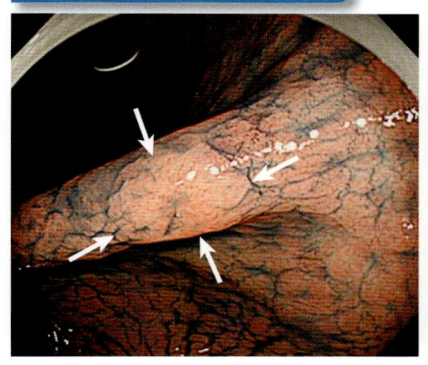

Non-magnifying NBI image

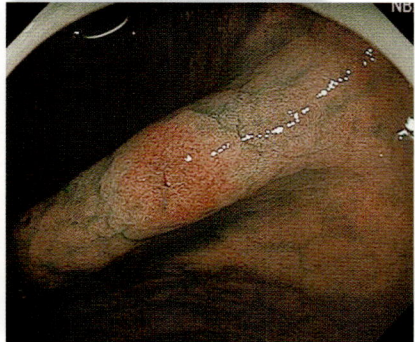

Low-magnification NBI image

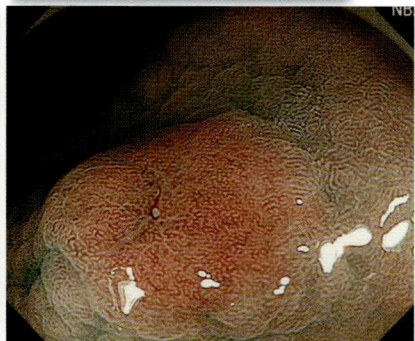

▶ When indigo carmine is sprayed, the areae gastricae in the lesion are no longer visible and the redness stands out from the surroundings.

▶ In non-magnifying NBI observation, the lesion is clearly imaged as a brownish area.

▶ When magnified, both the structure and vessels look more irregular, suggesting an adenoma rather than cancer.

Diagnosis ② Posterior wall of the lesser curvature of the angulus, 0–IIa-like lesion, 6 mm, tubular adenoma with moderate atypia

Tips

- Watch for synchronous multiple lesions.
- Spontaneous bleeding is a sign of a tumor.
- Watch for subtle differences in color tone.
- Non-magnifying NBI observation is sometimes useful for detection of lesions.

case 31

Answer   The gastric tumor is imaged in ① and ② .

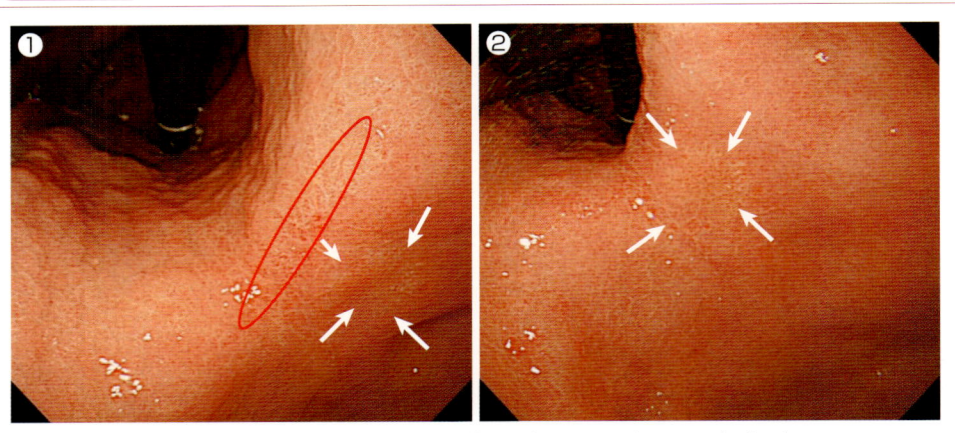

▶ O-2 atrophy is present in the background mucosa. Map-like redness can be seen in the lesser curvature of the body. This is a post-eradication change. A linear ulcer scar (in the red elliptical circle) is visible in the lesser curvature of the angulus, extending across the anterior and posterior walls. Linear ulcer scars like this frequently occur in the angulus.

▶ Reddish regenerative epithelium is visible in the middle of the view field. None of the mucosa appears to have a depressed surface or surface irregularities, so this can be judged as benign ulcer scar.

▶ Slightly to the distal side of the ulcer scar, the mucosa (indicated by the arrows) appears to be slightly more yellowish white than the surrounding mucosa. There is almost no difference in surface irregularities; only differences in color tones can be seen.

Indigo carmine-sprayed image

Non-magnifying NBI image

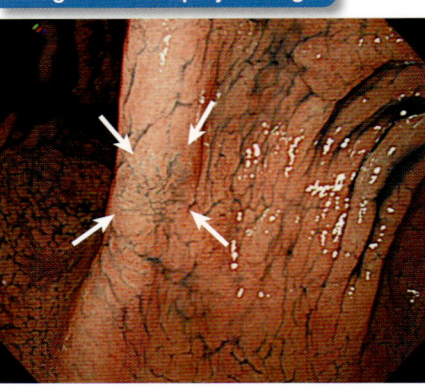 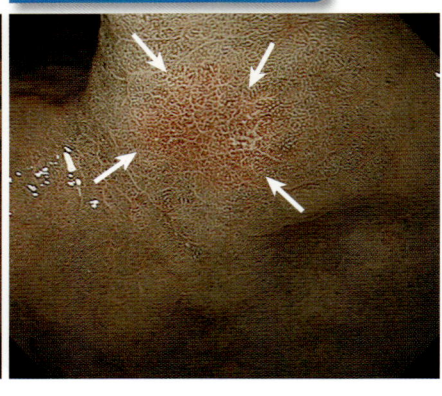

▶ When indigo carmine is sprayed, the lesion is revealed to be a flat 0-IIb type.

▶ The indigo carmine pools in the narrow grooves inside the lesion, which do not resemble the areae gastricae pattern in the surrounding mucosa.

▶ NBI offers the best visibility in this case. The lesion shows as brownish mucosa, and its extent is clear even in non-magnifying NBI observation.

Histological image of biopsied specimen

100 μm

▶ HE-stained, medium-magnification image. A tubular adenoma with moderate atypia can be seen in the superficial side of the mucosa, while in the deep mucosa the non-neoplastic glands are dilated in cyst-like forms.

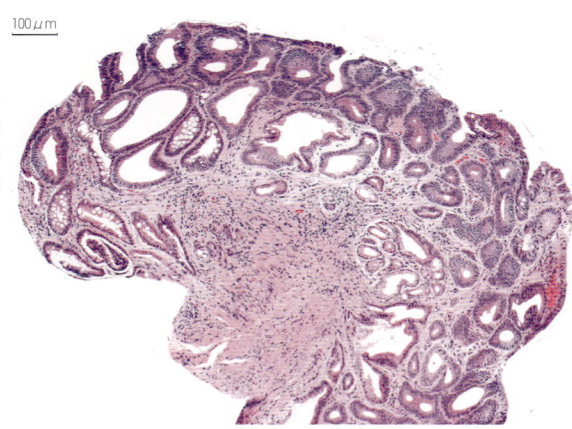

Tips

- Look for differentiated-type gastric cancer and gastric adenoma in stomachs with severe atrophy and intestinal metaplasia.
- Typical gastric adenoma should manifest as a whitish flat elevated lesion. However, many other flat lesions appear after *H. pylori* eradication.
- Gastric adenoma and differentiated-type gastric cancer may exhibit a color tone that is a little yellower than the surrounding area.
- Gastric adenoma and differentiated-type gastric cancer lesions can be observed clearly in non-magnifying NBI observation.

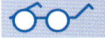 What's imaged in the other pictures?

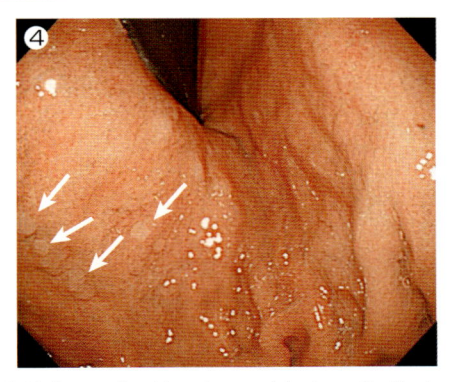

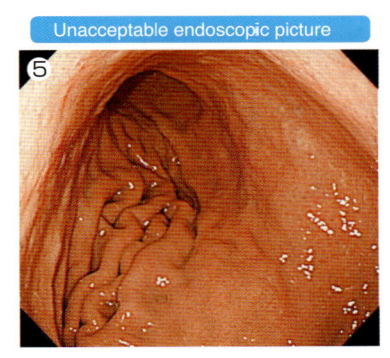

Unacceptable endoscopic picture

- Multiple small white elevated lesions (indicated by the arrows) are present in the region from the cardia to the fornix.
- Since the background mucosa is atrophic, these white flat elevated lesions can be identified as intestinal metaplasia.

- The areas between the folds in the greater curvature of the body are not extended, so this picture is not very useful.
- If cancer is hidden between the folds, it will not be found. In antegrade view, it is important that you perform sufficient insufflation to make it possible to observe the areas between the folds.

Compare! Different case

Typical gastric adenoma

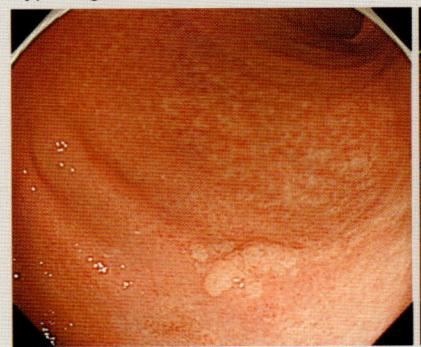
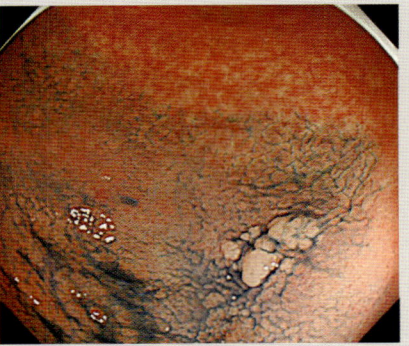

- This is a whitish flat elevated lesion with low height.
- The surface and margins are smooth. The surface of an adenoma is often nodular.
- The margins are clear.

Screening endoscopy after chemotherapy for gastric malignant lymphoma
[Gastric cancer detected after *H. pylori* eradication]

Answer The gastric cancer is imaged in ② .

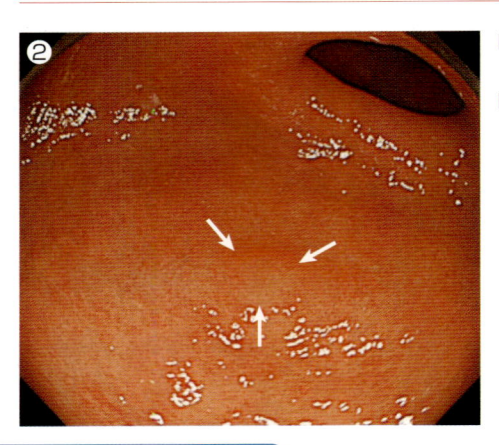

▶ O-3 atrophy can be seen in the background mucosa.

▶ The mucosa in the greater curvature of the prepyloric region (indicated by the arrows) looks slightly more yellowish-white than the surrounding mucosa. If you are not able to spot slight changes in color tone, you will not be able to find minute gastric cancers.

Indigo carmine-sprayed images

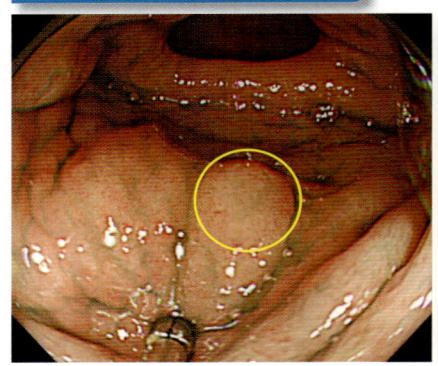
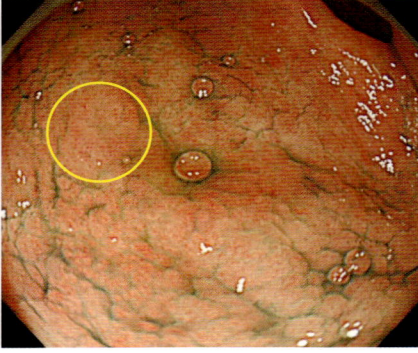

▶ When indigo carmine is sprayed, it is possible to see that the mucosal surface is slightly depressed.

Diagnosis Greater curvature of the prepyloric region, 0-IIc, 3 mm, tub1, T1a (M), UL (−)

Tips
- Watch for subtle changes in color tone.
- Keep in mind that when a lesion has a yellowish-white color tone, it is more likely to be a differentiated-type gastric cancer.
- Whenever you have the slightest suspicion about a lesion, spray it with indigo carmine and move the endoscope in close for detailed examination.

What's imaged in the other pictures?

▶ Many scars (enclosed in the elliptical circle) are visible. These are the result of chemotherapy for gastric malignant lymphoma.

▶ A biopsy was later performed on the coarse mucosa indicated by the arrow. The histopathological diagnosis was intestinal metaplasia.

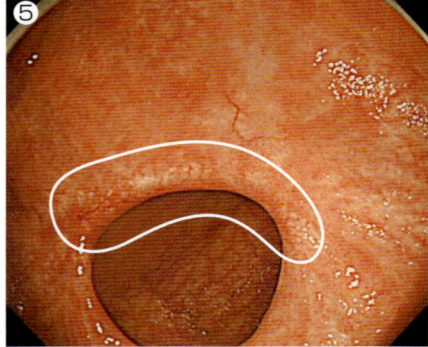
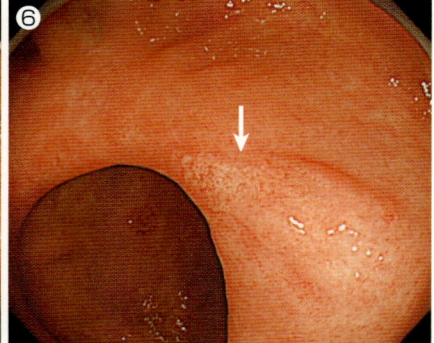

case 33 Patient referred to us after uncurative ESD for gastric cancer

[Gastric cancer with active *H. pylori* infection]

Answer The gastric cancer is imaged in ③ and ④ .

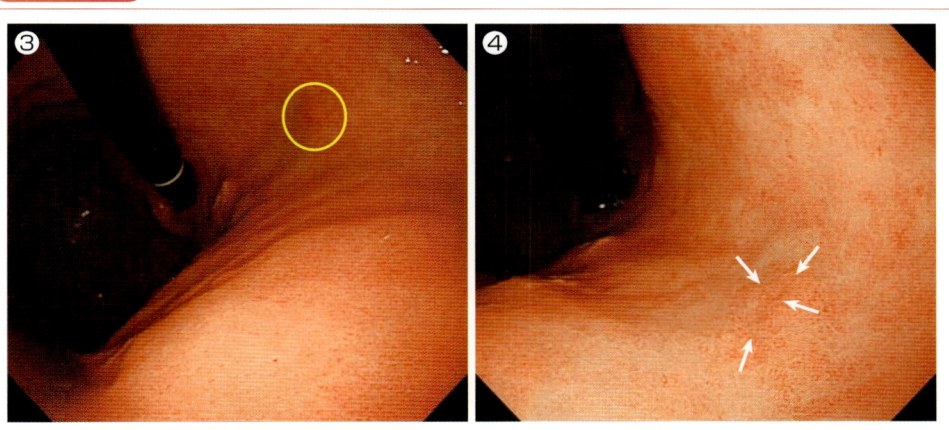

▶ C-3 atrophy and diffuse redness are present in the background mucosa, indicating an active *H. pylori* infection.
▶ Atrophy and intestinal metaplasia are conspicuous in the lesser curvature of the body. When the background mucosa is in this condition, keep an eye out for differentiated-type gastric cancer.
▶ In photo ③ , a reddish depressed lesion (circled) can be seen in the lesser curvature of the middle body. There seem to be elevations in the surrounding area as well.
▶ In close-up photo ④ , conspicuous surface irregularities are visible, which are obviously different from the surrounding mucosa. If you look at it carefully, you can see that the lesion is depressed as indicated by the arrows. It is not possible, however, to obtain a detailed finding using conventional endoscopy alone.

Indigo carmine sprayed images

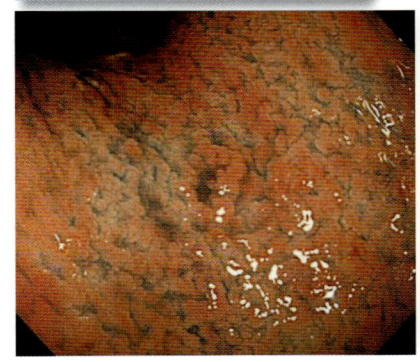 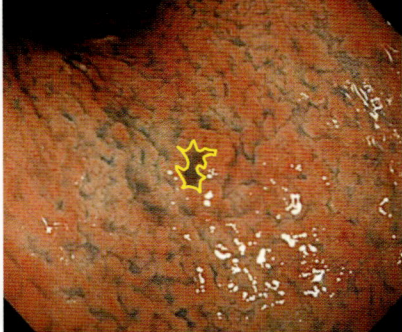 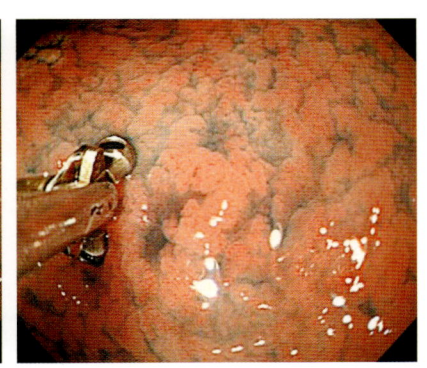

▶ When indigo carmine is sprayed, an encroachment (thorn-like intrusion into the surrounding area) can be seen. At this point, you can be certain that it is cancer.
▶ There are some minor elevations around the lesion. These are reactive elevations and are often seen with differentiated-type gastric cancer.

▶ The size of the lesion is equivalent to that of the fully opened jaws of the forceps, which tells you that it is a 6-mm lesion. Taking pictures like this makes it possible to better evaluate the lesion later.

Diagnosis Lesser curvature of the middle body, 0–IIc, 6 mm, tub1, T1a (M), UL (–)

Tips

- Note that atrophic gastritis and intestinal metaplasia suggest a high risk of differentiated-type gastric cancer.
- Closely observe regions with conspicuous surface irregularities after spraying indigo carmine.
- Remember that a thorn-like intrusion into the surrounding area is a sign of gastric cancer.

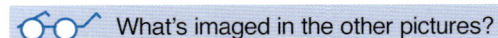 **What's imaged in the other pictures?**

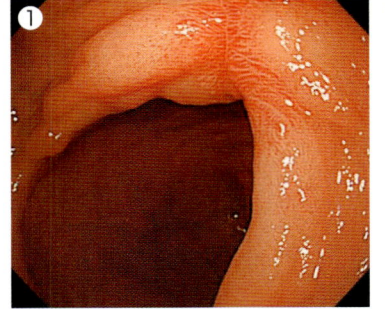

- This is an ESD scar from a procedure performed 1 month previously. As seen in this photo, benign ulcer scars are accompanied by a reddish regenerative epithelium with a palisade-like structure as seen in this photo.

183

Answer ① The first lesion is imaged in ④.

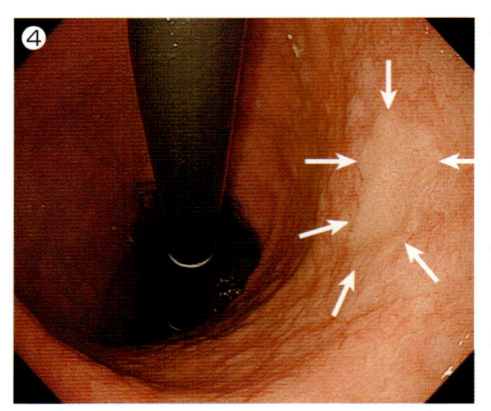

▶ O–3 atrophy is present in the background mucosa. Multiple white flat elevations can also be seen. These are signs of intestinal metaplasia.
▶ Post-ESD scars can be seen on the anterior walls of the antrum and middle body.
▶ On the posterior wall of the lower body, a flat elevation can be seen. It is slightly yellowish compared to the white color of the surrounding mucosa.
▶ To find this lesion, you need to be able to spot the subtle difference in color tone. Also note that it is noticeably larger than the flat elevations in the surrounding area.
▶ The posterior wall of the lower body is an easy-to-miss site. You will not see it in the field of view in retroflexed observation unless you deliberately push in the endoscope.

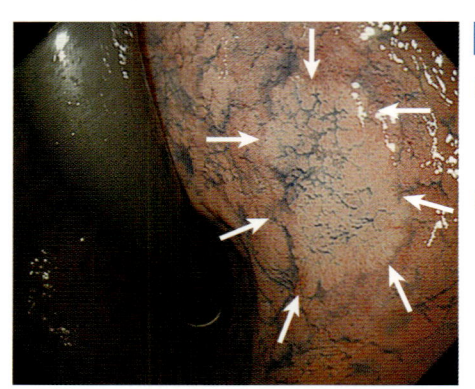

Indigo carmine sprayed image

▶ When indigo carmine is sprayed, the surface grooves in the lesion become much clearer than the grooves in the atrophic gastritis and intestinal metaplasia around it.
▶ The margin is also clearer after spraying indigo carmine. To get a direct frontal view of a lesion on the posterior wall of the body, twist the endoscope counterclockwise first, and then angulate it all the way to the left and suction a little air.

Diagnosis ① Posterior wall of the lower body, 0–IIa-like lesion, 20 mm, tubular adenoma with moderate atypia

---

 Side Note Metachronous gastric cancer

Metachronous gastric cancer occuring after curative endoscopic resection of ealy gastric cancer is not rare. According to some studies, the incidence rate ranges from 8.2 to 15%[a)–c)]. On an annual basis, this means that new gastric cancer is found at a rate of 2 to 3% per year. This is by no means insignificant. The occurrence of metachronous gastric cancer is high especially among males, as well as among patients who have a history of severe atrophic gastritis and multiple cancers[a)]. One prospective study has reported that incidence of metachronous gastric cancer can be reduced to one third with the intervention of *H. pylori* eradication[d)]. This suggests that *H. pylori* eradication and annual endoscopy are indispensable after endoscopic treatment. When examining such patients after endoscopic treatment, always keep in mind that hidden gastric cancer is very likely to be present.

a) Mori G, Nakajima T, Asada K, et al. Incidence of and risk factors for metachronous gastric cancer after endoscopic resection and successful Helicobacter pylori eradication: results of a large-scale, multicenter cohort study in Japan. Gastric Cancer. 2016; 19: 911–918.
b) Nakajima T, Oda I, Gotoda T, et al. Metachronous gastric cancers after endoscopic resection: how effective is annual endoscopic surveillance? Gastric Cancer. 2006; 9: 93–98.
c) Kobayashi M, Narisawa R, Sato Y, et al. [Self-limiting risk of metachronous gastric cancers after endoscopic resection.] Gastroenterol Endosc. 2012; 54: 1498–1505. (In Japanese with English abstract.)
d) Fukase K, Kato M, Kikuchi S, et al. Effect of eradication of Helicobacter pylori on incidence of metachronous gastric carcinoma after endoscopic resection of early gastric cancer: an o -label, randomized controlled trial. Lancet. 2008; 372: 392–397.

Answer ❷   The second lesion is imaged in ⑤.

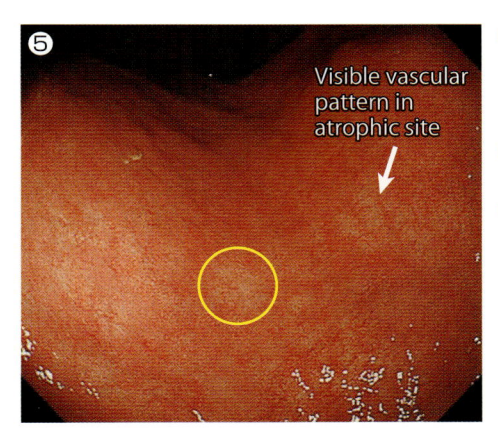

Visible vascular pattern in atrophic site

▶ The color of the mucosa near the anterior wall of the lesser curvature of the middle body is slightly more yellowish-white (circled) than in surrounding intestinal metaplasia.

▶ Vascular patterns are not as conspicuous as they are with atrophy.

▶ Detailed observation is necessary as cancer is suggested by the subtle difference from the surrounding mucosa.

Indigo carmine-sprayed image

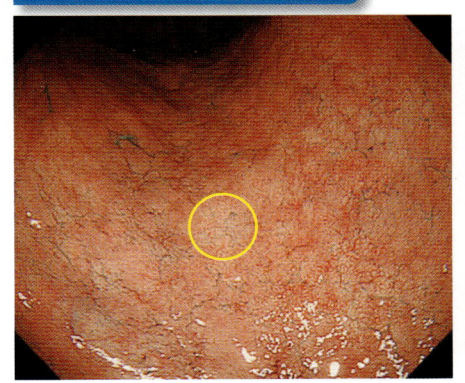

Non-magnifying NBI image

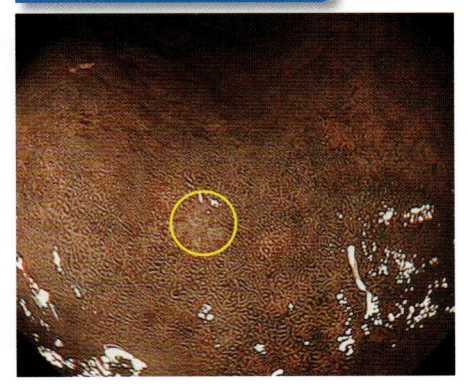

▶ When indigo carmine is sprayed, the mucosa looks coarser than the chronic gastritis in the background.

▶ Even without magnification, NBI allows you to see that the lesion has a finer structure than the surroundings mucosa.

Diagnosis ❷   Anterior wall of the lesser curvature of the middle body, 0–IIb, 3 mm, tub1, T1a (M), UL (–)

Tips

- Watch for metachronous multiple occurrences and synchronous multiple occurrences of gastric cancer.
- Make sure you observe the posterior wall of the lower body carefully since this a region where it is very likely that a lesion will be missed.
- Try to detect any subtle differences between the atrophic area and the intestinal metaplasia in the background.
- When you see a whitish flat elevation, include intestinal metaplasia and adenoma in the differential diagnosis.

Screening endoscopy after ESD for gastric cancer ②
[Gastric cancer detected after *H. pylori* eradication]

Answer The gastric cancer is imaged in ① .

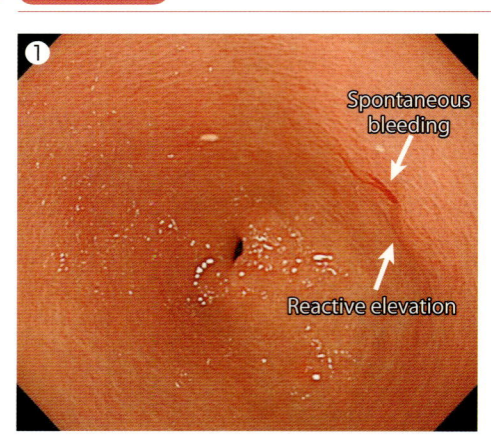

Spontaneous bleeding

Reactive elevation

▶ O–1 atrophy is present in the background mucosa. Intestinal metaplasia is conspicuous and xanthoma is scattered around. This is a case with a high risk of differentiated-type gastric cancer.

▶ The first thing to notice is the bleeding on the posterior wall of the antrum. The area around the hemorrhage is elevated. At this point, spontaneous bleeding from the cancer is suspected. The elevation around the lesion is believed to be a reactive elevation of a 0–IIc lesion.

After irrigation

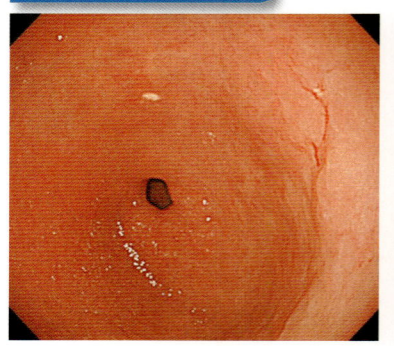

Indigo carmine-sprayed images

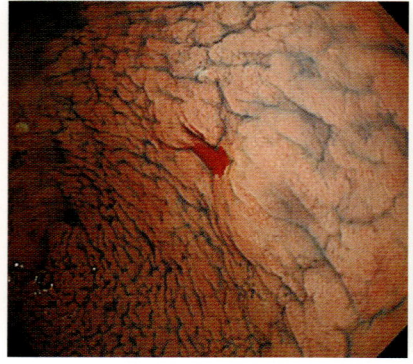
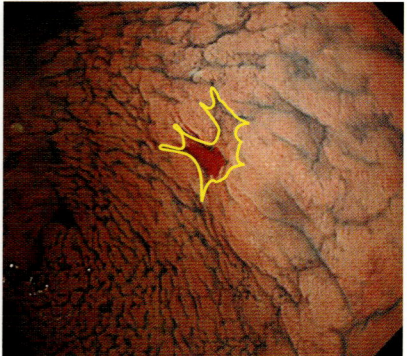

▶ After the blood has been rinsed away, more blood starts oozing from the site. In cases like this, there is a very good chance that the bleeding is from a cancerous lesion as the cancerous tissue on the surface is very delicate.

▶ When indigo carmine is sprayed, it is possible to see a thorn-like intrusion spreading into the surrounding mucosa. Reactive elevations can also be seen, suggesting differentiated-type gastric cancer.

Tips
- Look for synchronous multiple lesions after ESD for gastric cancer.
- Remember that spontaneous bleeding is a sign of gastric cancer.
- Note that a thorn-like intrusion into the surrounding mucosa and reactive elevations are findings of differentiated-type gastric cancer.

Diagnosis Posterior wall of the antrum, 0–IIc, 4 mm, tub1, T1a (M), UL (–)

What's imaged in the other pictures?

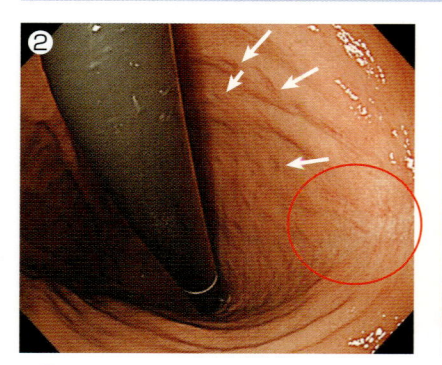
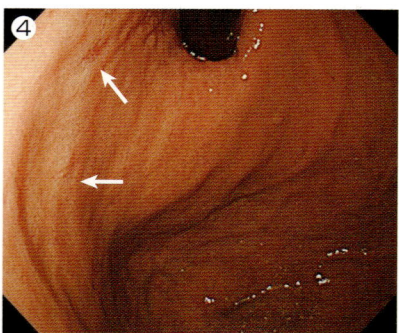

- An ESD scar (enclosed in the red circle) can be seen in the lesser curvature of the lower body. The folds converge smoothly at the scar. There is no sign of any malignancy.
- Multiple reddish depressions (indicated by the arrows) have occurred in the body. These are changes that took place after *H. pylori* eradication. A single reddish depression would suggest gastric cancer. Multiple depressions, on the other hand, indicate a strong possibility of post-eradication alteration.

Answer The gastric cancer is imaged in ② and ③ .

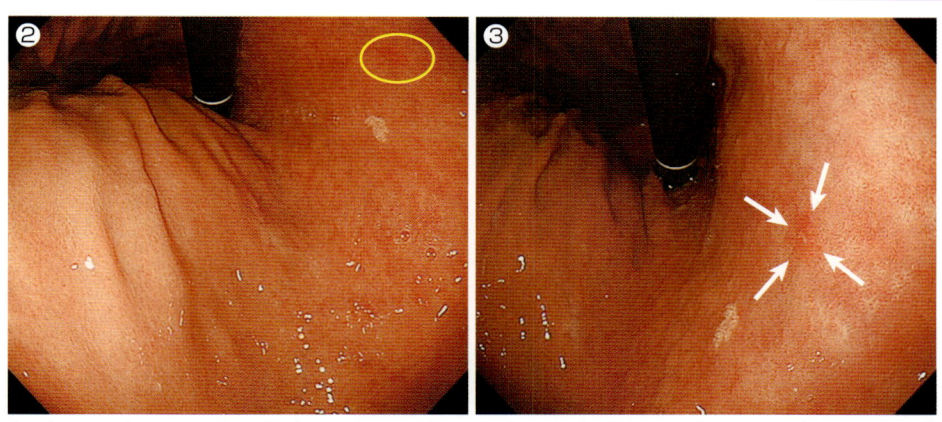

▶ The background mucosa has O–1 atrophy and intestinal metaplasia, as well as conspicuous map-like redness after eradication.
▶ In the lesser curvature of the middle body, xanthoma is present. On the posterior wall of the lesser curvature of the middle body, reddish patches are visible. These are redder than the surrounding map-like redness(indicated by the arrows). Surface irregularities are not clear.

Indigo carmine-sprayed images

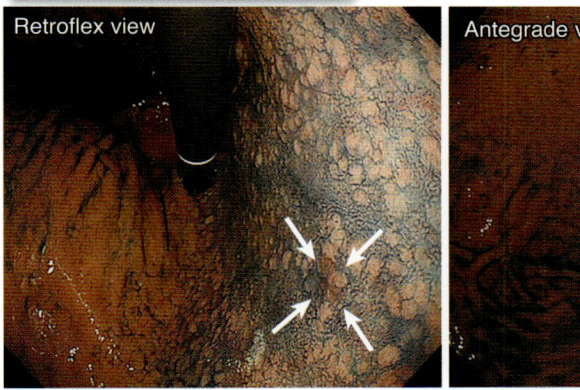
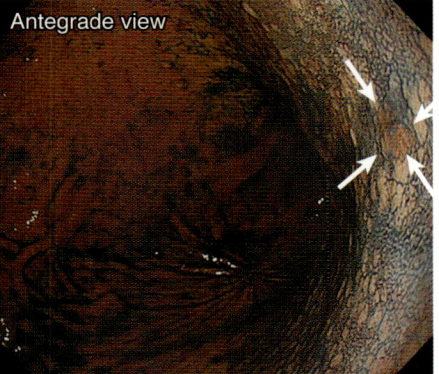

▶ When indigo carmine is sprayed, the redness of the lesion stands out starkly against the blue background of the surrounding mucosa. There are no surface irregularities, indicating that this is a IIb lesion.

Non-magnifying NBI image

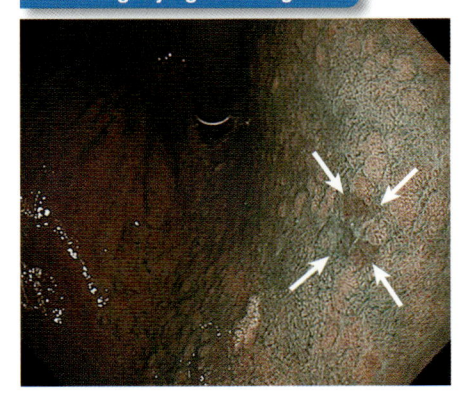

▶ In NBI observation, the lesion looks brownish with clear margins.

Diagnosis Lesser curvature of the middle body, 0–IIb, 4 mm, tub1, T1a (M), UL (−)

Tips

- Look for reddish areas that are redder than the surrounding area.
- Remember that spraying indigo carmine will make the redness of cancer stand out.

What's imaged in the other pictures?

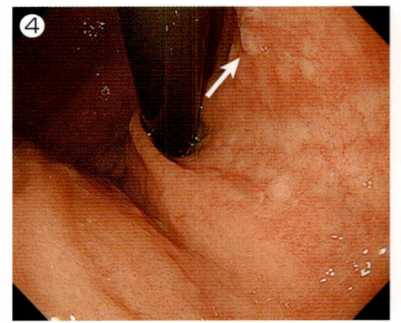
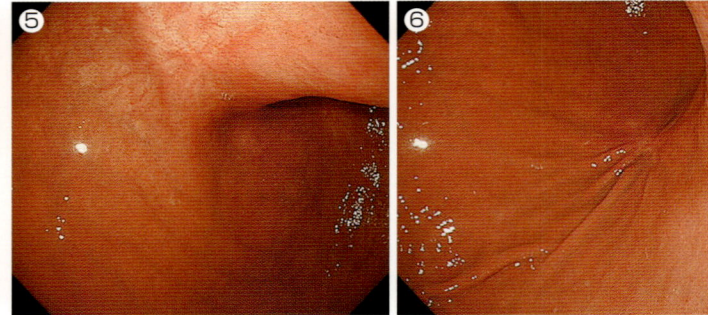

- Multiple white flat elevations are visible. The lesion indicated by the arrow is noticeably elevated, making it difficult to differentiate from adenoma.
- After biopsy, this site was diagnosed as intestinal metaplasia.

- Scars are visible on the anterior wall of the lesser curvature of the lower body and the posterior wall of the greater curvature of the angulus. The folds converge smoothly in the center, and no malignant finding is visible. These are scars from ESD.

Side Note **How to become a proficient endoscopist**

Young doctors sometimes ask me to teach them how to be proficient in endoscopy. Whenever they ask me that, I always tell them to start by undergoing endoscopy themselves. I was a medical student when I first underwent upper GI endoscopy. In our gastrointestinal surgery practice class, one student had to volunteer to serve as an endoscopy subject. To decide who would be the subject, we played rock-paper-scissors and I lost. After the instructing doctor inserted the endoscope, my classmates randomly moved the endoscope around in my stomach. The pain was incredible. I felt like I was being tortured. I found the experience very traumatic. Later on, I started performing endoscopies myself, and my superior told me that I would have to experience endoscopy myself in order to become a skillful endoscopist. So I asked him to perform endoscopy on me. It wasn't quite as bad as the endoscopy I underwent when was in medical school. As it was becoming painful when a strong pharyngeal reflex occurred and the gastric wall was stretched by insufflation, my superior and the assisting nurse told me to relax and stroked my back. I found that very helpful. Unless you experience an endoscopy yourself, you can never fully appreciate just what it feels like and what kind of pain the patient is feeling as you move the endoscope around in different regions. Experiencing it for yourself is the only way to have empathy for the patient. So please, if you really want to be a proficient endoscopist, undergo endoscopy yourself first.

Screening endoscopy after ESD for gastric cancer ④

[Gastric cancer detected after *H. pylori* eradication]

Answer The gastric cancer is imaged in ③ , ④ , ⑤ , and ⑥ .

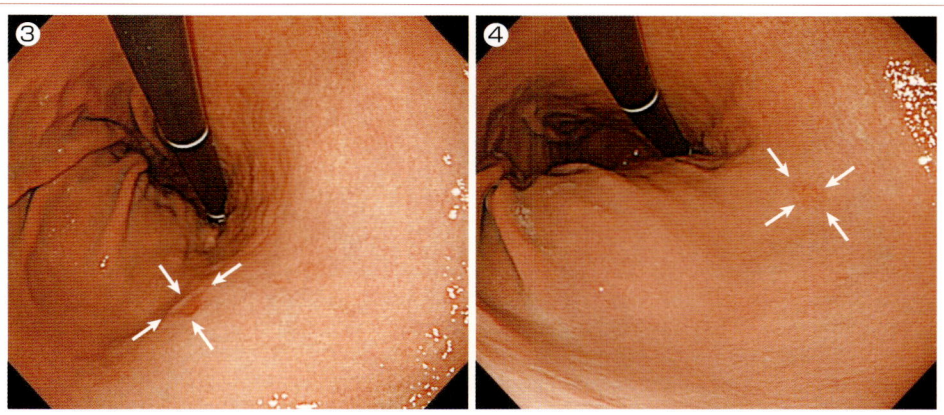

▶ The background mucosa is O–1 atrophy. A reddish depressed lesion is visible on the anterior wall of the middle body. When the lesion is observed in a tangential direction as in ③ , the depression is easy to see, but it is hard to get an overall image of the lesion.

▶ On the other hand, when the lesion is observed from the front as in ④ , you can get an overall image of the lesion , but can no longer tell whether it is depressed or not.

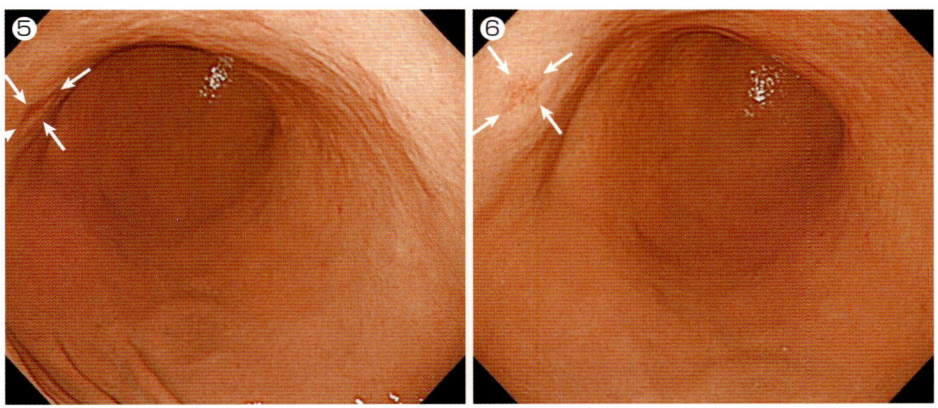

▶ Similarly, in antegrade view, you can clearly see the depression in a tangential direction as in ⑤ but now it is no longer possible to visualize an overall image of the lesion. Conversely, when the endoscope is angulated a little and the lesion is observed from an angle that is closer to a frontal view as in ⑥ , the overall image of the lesion becomes apparent, but the depression becomes indistinct. As there is no similar reddish depression in the surrounding area, it makes it much more likely that this is cancer.

When air is suctioned	Close-up image	Non-magnifying NBI image
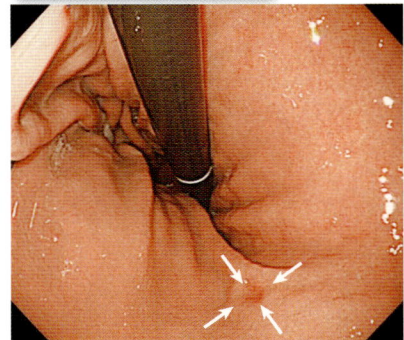	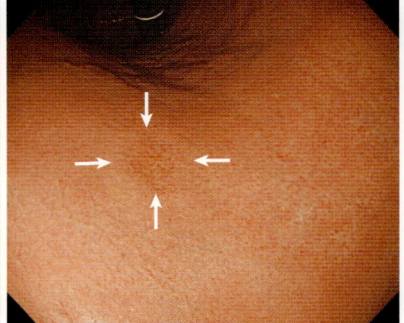	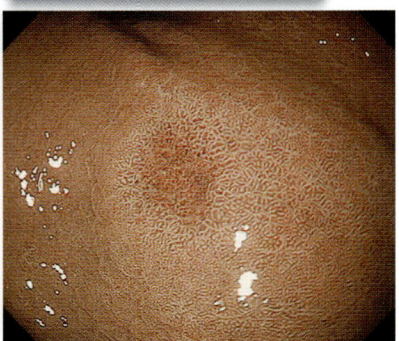
▶ When the amount of air inside the stomach is reduced to adjust for the stretching of the gastric wall, you can see the depression in the lesion more clearly.	▶ In close-up frontal view, it looks like granular reddish mucosa. However, it is not possible to get all the details in conventional endoscopy.	▶ In NBI observation, the lesion looks brownish with clear margins.

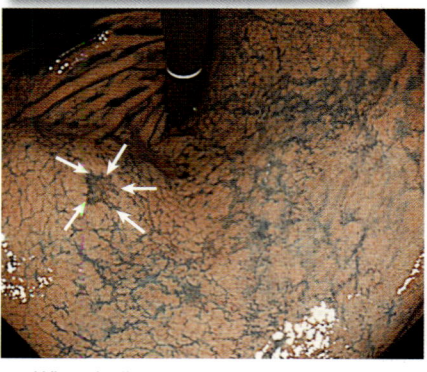 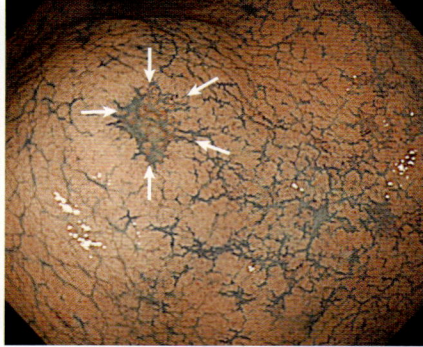

▶ When indigo carmine is sprayed, you can see that the lesion is depressed with clear margins even when viewed from directly in front. You can also see a fine thorn-like encroachment, with a very fine granular mucosal pattern.

▶ The combination of reddish depression, thorn-like encroachment, and fine granular mucosal pattern against a background of atrophy resulted in a diagnosis of differentiated-type gastric cancer.

Diagnosis Anterior wall of the middle body, 0–IIc, 6 mm, tub2, T1a (M), UL (−)

Tips

- Suspect cancer when you see a single depressed lesion.
- Observe a lesion from various angles to capture its characteristics.
- Make a tangential observation to get a better view of the lesion's surface irregularities.
- Observe a lesion from right in front to get a good overall image.
- Reduce air in the stomach to get a clear image of a depression.

Endoscopic image from 1 year previously

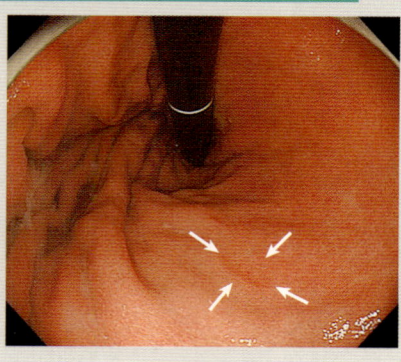

- This picture was taken a year earlier, prior to *H. pylori* eradication. Sticky mucus and diffuse redness are present. When this photo is compared with the post–eradication photo, you can clearly see the difference in the mucosa's color tones.
- The lesion is thought to be present in the area indicated by the arrows. However, it is difficult to identify it in conventional endoscopy. Spraying indigo carmine would probably have made it possible to find the lesion.

Answer   The gastric cancer is imaged in ② .

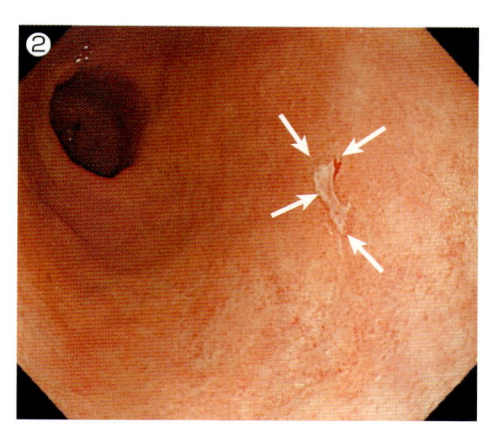

▶ O-3 atrophy is present in the background mucosa. Map-like redness has emerged in the greater curvature of the body. This is a post-eradication change.
▶ A post-ESD scar and residual clip can be seen on the anterior wall of the lower body.
▶ A depressed lesion with mucus attached can be seen on the posterior wall of the antrum. It is also accompanied by bleeding, suggesting a possibility of cancer.

Close-up images

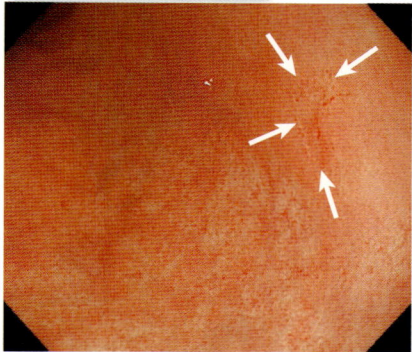
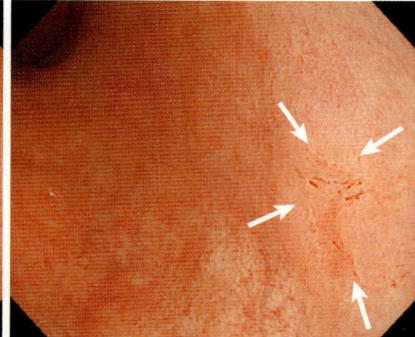

▶ When the site is rinsed with a pronase solution, mucus is removed and the depressed surface becomes clear.
▶ Irrigation clears away any fresh blood attached to the cancer but induces new bleeding. The surface of a cancerous lesion is delicate and tends to bleed easily.
▶ Attachment of mucus is not a finding specific to cancer but may be associated with cancer.

Indigo carmine sprayed image

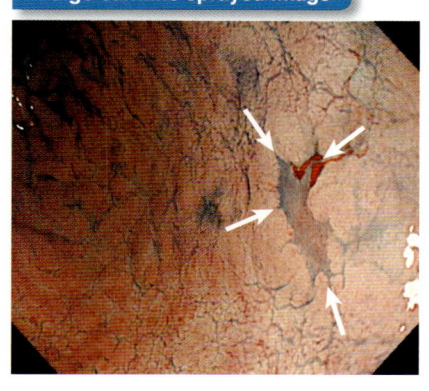

▶ When indigo carmine is sprayed, the depressed surface appears irregular and the edges exhibit fine thorn-like encroachment. This is a typical differentiated-type gastric cancer of the depressed type.

Diagnosis   Posterior wall of the antrum, 0-IIc, 6 mm, tub1, T1a (M), UL (−)

Tips

- Be aware that synchronous multiple lesions are often found after ESD.
- When you see a depression with mucus attached, wash it away with a pronase solution before observing the site.
- Note that there are gastric cancers that can be found by the attachment of mucus.
- Keep in mind that spontaneous bleeding is a finding that brings suspicion of cancer.
- Remember that thorn-like encroachment is a finding of differentiated-type gastric cancer.

case
39

Answer The gastric cancer is imaged in ② and ③ .

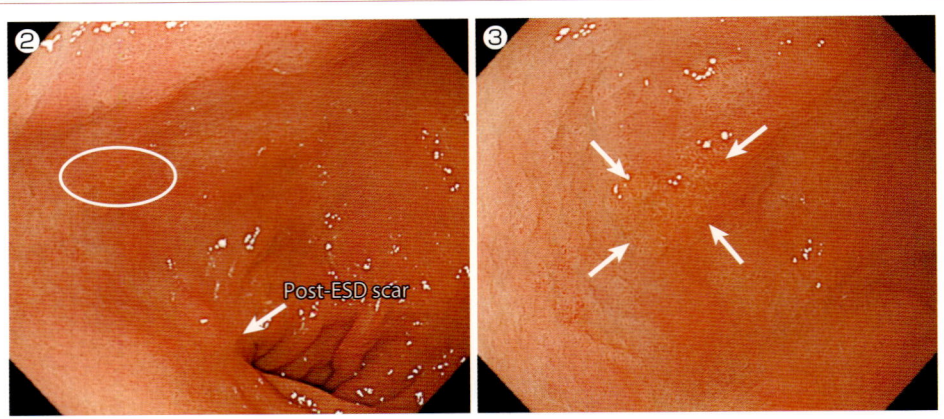

Post-ESD scar

▶ The background mucosa features both atrophy and intestinal metaplasia. Map-like redness — a post-eradication change — can be seen in the antrum and the lesser curvature of the body. Post-ESD scars can be seen on the anterior wall of the antrum and in the lesser curvature of the cardia.
▶ Near the anterior wall of the lesser curvature of the antrum, some mucosa can be seen that is a bit more yellowish than the surrounding mucosa.

Close-up image

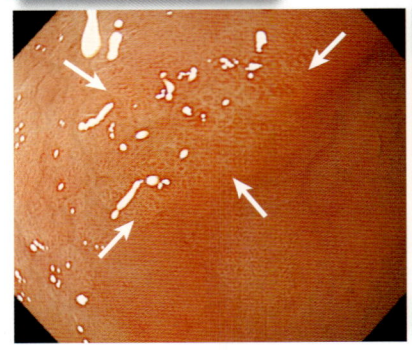

Non-magnifying NBI image

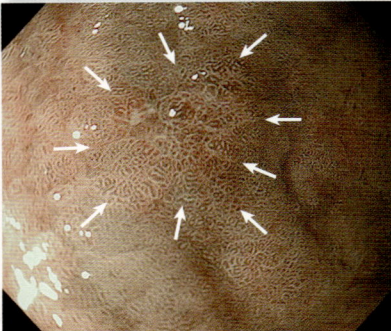

▶ In close-up observation, coarse mucosa that is slightly yellower than the surrounding mucosa can be seen. When mucosa looks yellower than the surrounding mucosa, it may indicate differentiated-type gastric cancer.
▶ In non-magnifying NBI observation, the lesion appears brownish, with a slightly lighter tone than the surrounding area. The margins are a little unclear.

Medium-magnification NBI image

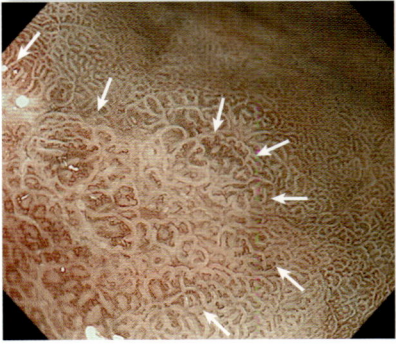

Indigo carmine sprayed image

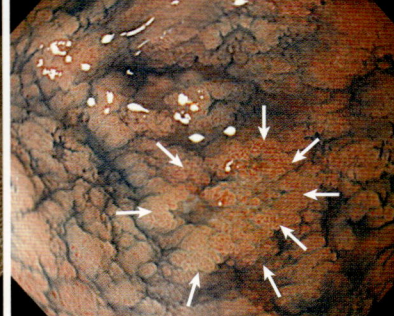

▶ This is a medium-magnification NBI image of the posterior wall side of the lesion. You can see that the surface structure is larger than the surrounding surface structure and varies in size. Dilated, tortuous loop-shaped vessels can be seen inside. The demarcation line is clear, making it possible to diagnose the lesion as cancer.
▶ When indigo carmine is sprayed, granular mucosal patterns are revealed. These vary in size, unlike the areae gastricae pattern in the surrounding area. This made us wonder whether it was 0-IIc or 0-IIc, but we decided on 0-IIb after determining that the lesion did not have a depression deep enough to distinguish it from the other surface irregularities seen in the surrounding mucosa.

Tips

Diagnosis Anterior wall of the lesser curvature of the antrum, 0-IIb, 8 mm, tub1, T1a (M), UL (–)

● When you are observing atrophic mucosa, pay special attention to mucosa that looks yellower than the mucosa around it.

Answer ❶   For the first lesion, pay attention to ⑤ , ⑥ , and ⑨ .

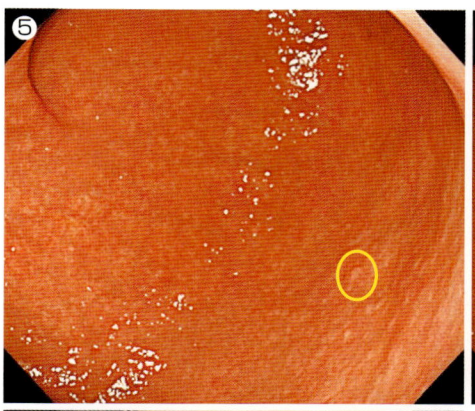

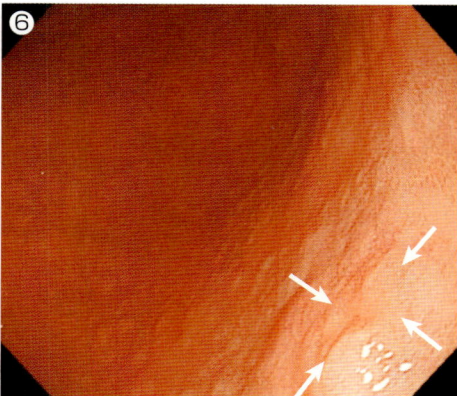

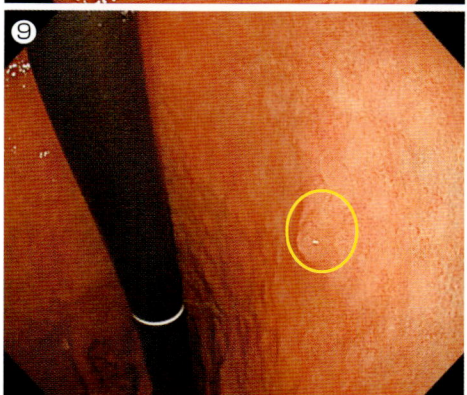

▶ ⑤ : Conspicuous surface irregularities (enclosed in the yellow circle) can be seen near the greater curvature of the posterior wall of the lower body. These are visible from a distance.

▶ ⑥ : In closed-up view, a depressed surface that is slightly yellower than the surroundings can be seen. Elevations are present around the depression.

▶   ⑨ : In retroflex view, it is not possible to obtain a detailed view of the lesion. However, the proximal side of the depression looks elevated when viewed from a distance.

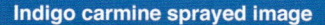

Indigo carmine sprayed image

Medium-magnification NBI image

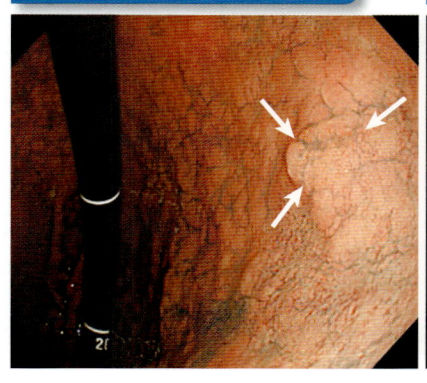

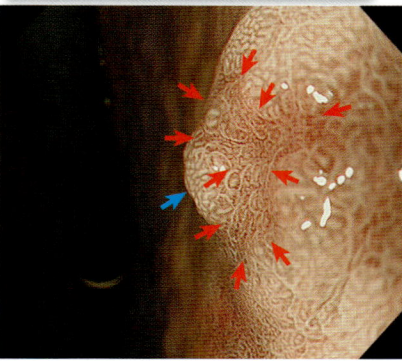

▶ When indigo carmine is sprayed, the distal side of the elevation looks slightly depressed.

▶ In medium-magnification NBI observation, a brownish depressed surface can be seen. The depressed surface is browner than the surrounding region with noticeable blood vessels, while the surface structure is fine and the margins are clear (indicated by the red arrows). As for the elevation on the proximal side, no finding of cancer is seen, and a reactive elevation is suspected (indicated by the blue arrow). Thus, this is an irregular depressed lesion accompanied by marginal elevations, against a background of atrophy, suggesting differentiated-type gastric cancer.

Additional Info   What do stomach conditions pose a high risk of gastric cancer?

- It has been pointed out for quite some time that the incidence rate of gastric cancer increases as atrophy progresses. Inoue et al. reported that the endoscopic detection rates for gastric cancer over a period of 11 years were 0% for C-1, 2.2% for C-2/C-3, 4.4% for O-1/O-2, and 10.3% for O-3[57].
- However, when the background mucosa has severe atrophy, it is difficult to discover small gastric cancer lesions because they are intermingled in the gastritis. In order to find minute gastric cancer lesions, you will need to perform comprehensive observation — for example, bringing the endoscope close to the site and spraying indigo carmine. When you see severe atrophy in the stomach during an endoscopy, look for gastric cancer concealed in the atrophic mucosa.

Histological images of ESD-resected specimen: Lesion 1

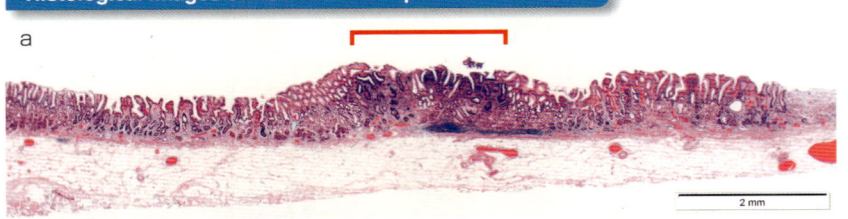

a

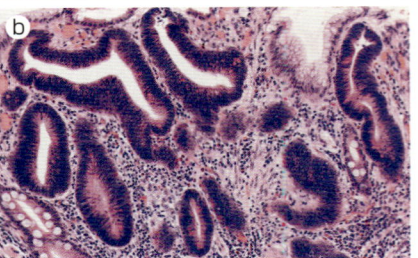

b

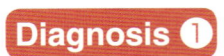

2 mm

a : HE-stained, low-magnification image. A tumor is seen (shown under the red line). The border between the tumor and the non-cancerous mucosa is accompanied by reactive elevations. The lesion shows a shallow depression.

b : HE-stained, high-magnification image of the lesion. A tumor composed of irregular tubular structures can be seen. The nuclei exhibit spindle shapes. Although there are regions that need to be differentiated from intestinal-type tubular adenoma, this is diagnosed as well-differentiated tubular adenocarcinoma (tub1).

Diagnosis ❶ Posterior wall of the middle body, 0–IIc, 3 mm, tub1, T1a (M), UL (−)

Answer ❷ For the second lesion, pay attention to ⑩ and ⑪ .

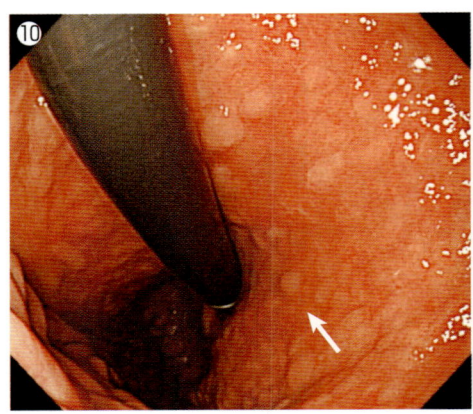

⑩

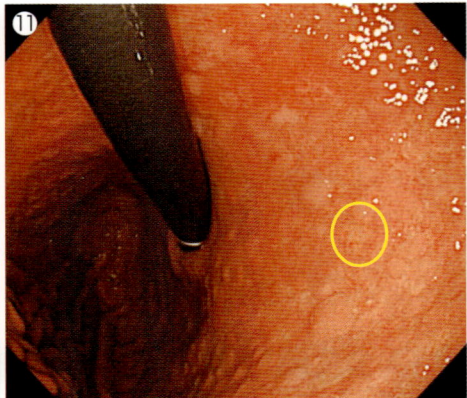

⑪

▶ ⑩ : From a distance, the lesion indicated by the arrow cannot be seen.

▶ ⑪ : Near the posterior wall of the lesser curvature of the middle body, the mucosa appears to be slightly yellower (circled in yellow) than the surrounding mucosa. When you get used to seeing really small lesions, you will be able to notice such subtle differences in color tone and start thinking it is suspicious.

Close-up image	Indigo carmine sprayed image	Medium-magnification NBI image

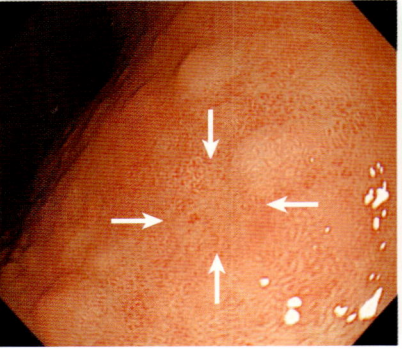

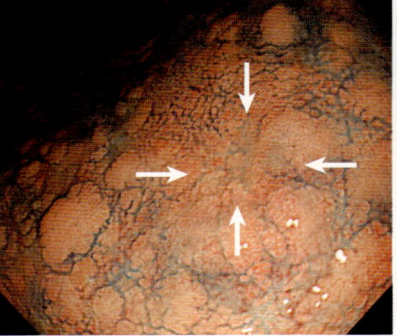

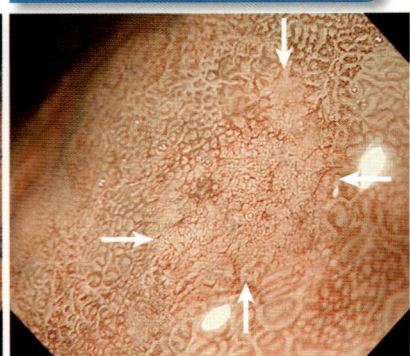

▶ In closed-up view, the mucosal surface looks slightly yellower than the surrounding mucosa.

▶ The margins are a little fuzzy.

▶ When indigo carmine is sprayed, the differences in color tone and mucosal structure become more apparent, making it easier to see the extent of the lesion.

▶ In medium-magnification NBI observation, the lesion looks brownish and a depression is visible. Inside the lesion, the surface structure has disappeared and irregular vessels can be seen, making it possible to diagnose it as cancer. Additionally, the margins are clear.

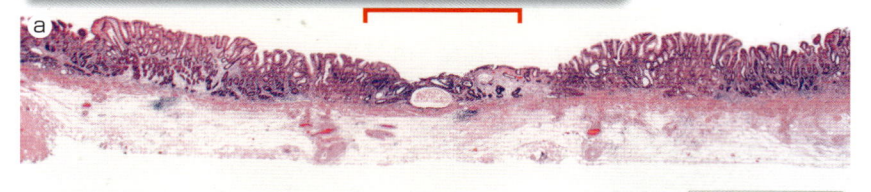

Histological images of ESD-resected specimen: Lesion 2

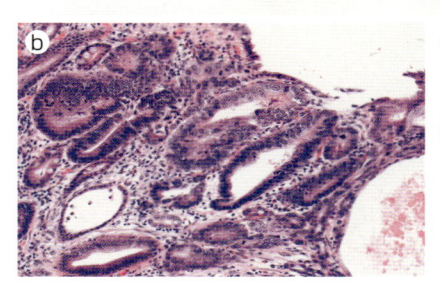

2 mm

a : HE-stained, low-magnification image. A tumor is visible (shown under the red line). The region is more depressed than the surrounding mucosa.

b : HE-stained, high-magnification image of the lesion. A tumor made up of irregular tubular structures in various sizes is shown. The nuclear atypia is high. This is diagnosed as well-differentiated tubular adenocarcinoma (tub1).

Diagnosis ❷ Lesser curvature of the middle body, 0–IIc, 3 mm, tub1, T1a (M), UL (−)

Tips

- Note that a stomach with severe atrophy has a high risk of cancer.
- Keep in mind that a marginal elevation may lead to the discovery of gastric cancer.
- Do not miss subtle changes in color tone.
- Bring the endoscope tip up close or spray indigo carmine to carefully observe anything that looks suspicious.

 What's imaged in the other pictures?

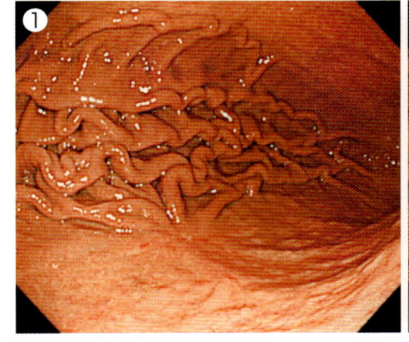 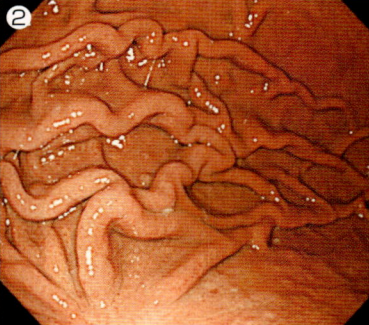

- Atrophy occurs in the entire body except the greater curvature. It is O–3 atrophy.
- The folds converge on the posterior wall of the upper body.
- A post-ESD scar visible.
- The folds converge smoothly in the center.
- There are no interruptions, level differences, or rapid thinning of the folds — which are malignant findings.

Answer   The gastric cancer is imaged in ④ and ⑤ .

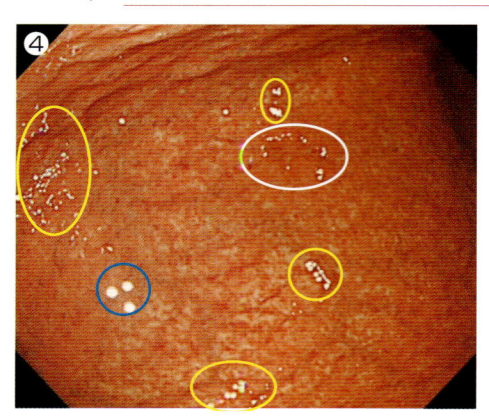

▶ The background mucosa exhibits severe O–3 atrophy. The risk of gastric cancer is high.
▶ Reflection of white light from an endoscope is referred to as halation. This halation is very white. The mucosal structure of the area where this phenomenon occurs is not visible at all. Pointing the illumination from the endoscope tip from directly in front causes catch light to occur when the endoscope is brought too close to the site, there are surface irregularities on the mucosal surface, and fluid is pooled.
▶ The spots circled in yellow are halation produced by surface irregularities in the intestinal metaplasia and vessels. The spot circled in blue is halation caused by pooled fluid left behind after rinsing the greater curvature of the fornix.
▶ In addition, there is an unnaturally oval-shaped halation near the anterior wall of the greater curvature of the upper body, suggesting the existence of an oval depressed lesion (enclosed in the white circle).

Close-up image

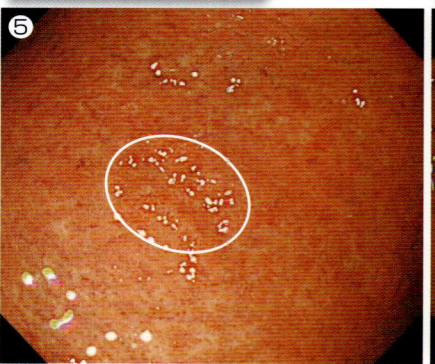

Getting an even closer look

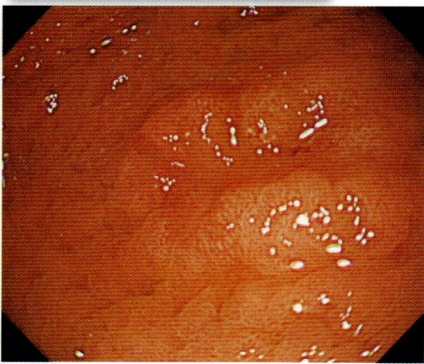

▶ In close-up observation, catch light is visible mainly along the edges of the lesion, suggesting that the margins of the depressed lesion are accompanied by elevations.
▶ When the endoscope is brought even closer and the stomach is suctioned a little, the marginal elevations become more noticeable. Adjusting the amount of air in the stomach can change the lesion's appearance.

Indigo carmine sprayed image

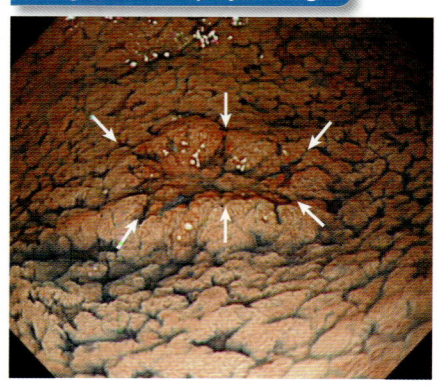

Non-magnifying NBI image

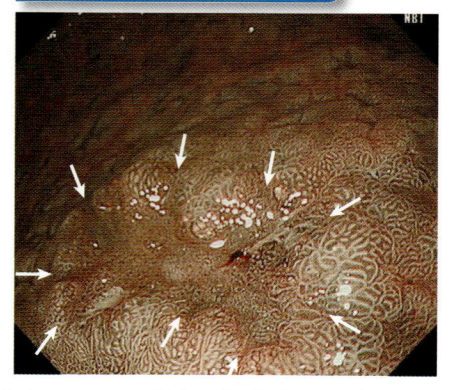

▶ When indigo carmine is sprayed, the margins of the depressed surface are imaged clearly. Encroachment is seen along the edges, suggesting differentiated-type gastric cancer.
▶ With differentiated-type gastric cancer of the depressed type, marginal elevations are reactive elevations. In many instances, cancer does not exist in the elevations.

▶ In non-magnifying NBI observation, substantial differences can be seen between the surface structures of the depressed surface and the marginal elevations, forming clear margins.

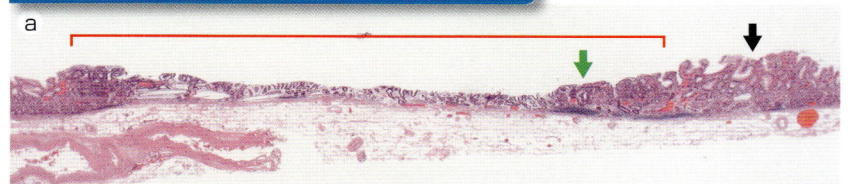

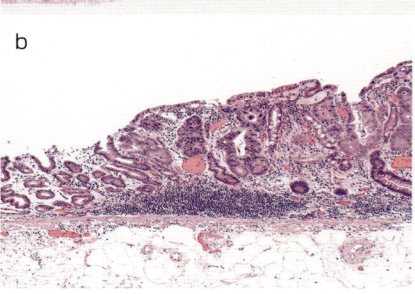
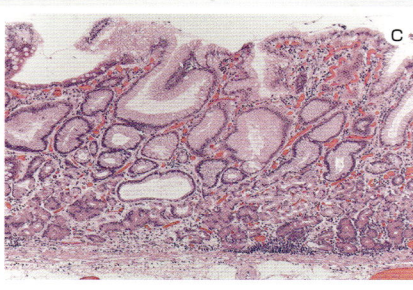

a: HE-stained, low-magnification image. A tumor can be seen extending along the range marked by the red line. In the center of the lesion, the depression is clearer than in the surrounding area.

b: HE-stained, medium-magnification image. This image corresponds to the section indicated by the green arrow in a. A well-differentiated tubular adenocarcinoma (tub1) with an irregular tubular structure is seen in the mucosa.

c: HE-stained, high-magnification image. This image corresponds to the section indicated by the black arrow in a. Hyperplastic changes of the foveolar epithelium are conspicuous in the non-tumorous mucosa in the margins of the lesion. Elevations slightly higher than the surrounding non-tumorous mucosa can be seen. These are so-called reactive elevations. No cancer cells are found here.

Diagnosis Greater curvature of the upper body, 0–IIc, 15 mm, tub1, T1a (M), UL (–)

Tips
- Remember that catch light indicates the presence of surface irregularities.
- Look for a lesion by watching for any abnormal catch light.
- Note that encroachment in the margins suggests differentiated-type gastric cancer.
- Differentiated-type gastric cancer of the depressed type may be accompanied by reactive elevations in the surrounding area.
- No cancer cells exist in the region of a reactive elevation.

What's imaged in the other pictures?

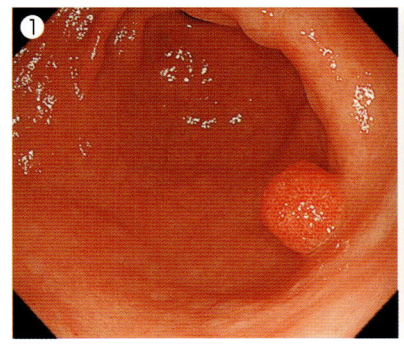
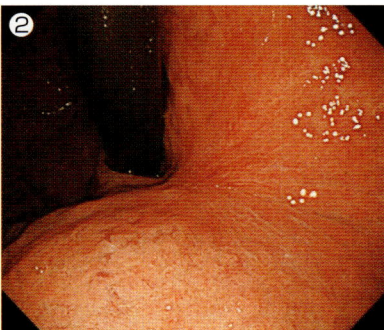

① A reddish Yamada's type II polyp is visible on the posterior wall of the antrum. The surface is smooth and exhibits coarse mucosal patterns, while the margins are clear. This is a typical hyperplastic polyp.

② A post-ESD ulcer scar is visible in the lesser curvature of the cardia. Scars in the lesser curvature of the body are not usually accompanied by converging folds; however, many of the folds show some contraction towards the center of the scar. The contracted region has no surface irregularities and does not have any malignant findings.

Endoscopic images from 4 months previously

- An endoscopy had been performed on this patient 4 months previously. At that time, the lesion was not detected. A fold overlaps the lesion, making it difficult to spot.
- It would have been relatively easy to find the lesion if air had been insufflated to stretch the site sufficiently — as we did when we found the lesion.
- In the greater curvature of the body, lesions can often be missed when observation is conducted from distance. You have to be sure to bring the endoscope up close and observe carefully.

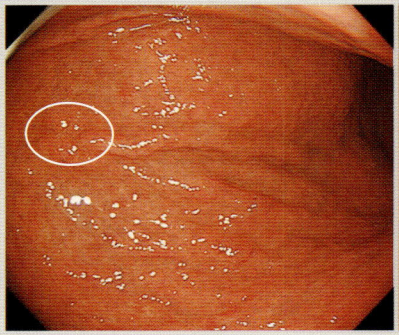
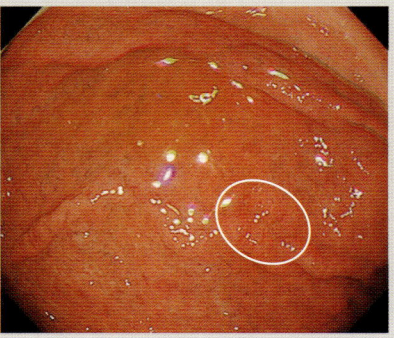

Answer   The gastric cancer is imaged in ③ and ④ .

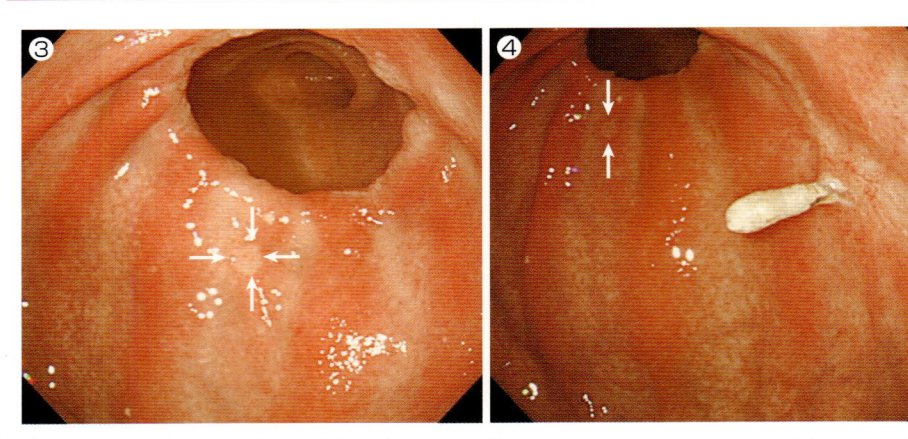

▶ This is a remnant stomach after distal gastrectomy. Atrophy, as well as residual gastritis caused by bile re-flux, can be seen in the background mucosa. On the posterior wall of the body, a post-ESD scar is visible, along with a clip left behind after the treatment. After surgery on undifferentiated-type gastric cancer, the risk of metachronous multiple occurrence of undifferentiated-type gastric cancer is high. When observing this type of stomach, pay special attention to lesions with a faded color tone.

▶ If you take a look at this site while keeping an eye out for faded lesions, you will notice circular fading patterns on the proximal side of the anastomosis even from distance.

Close-up images

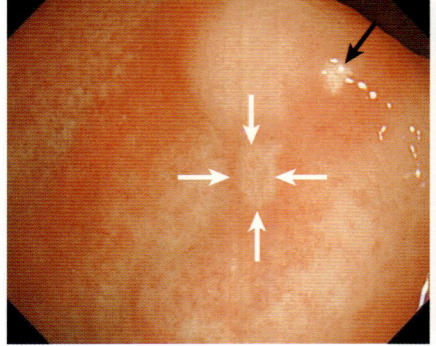
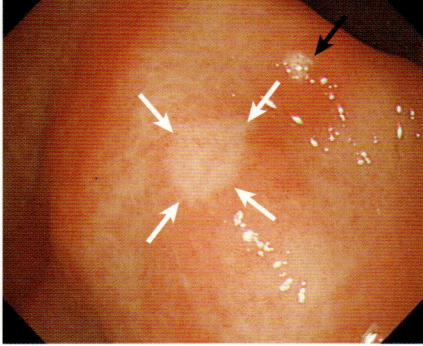

▶ In close-up observation, the lesion is visible as a change of color tone that has clear margins. At this point, undifferentiated-type gastric cancer is strongly suspected.

▶ The yellow patch (indicated by the black arrow) is xanthoma. It is yel-lower than undifferentiated-type gastric cancer.

Indigo carmine sprayed images

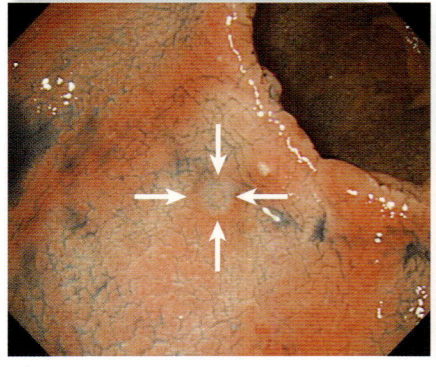
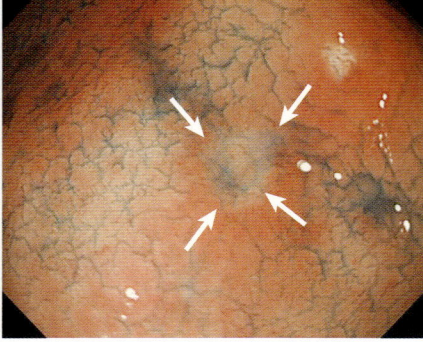

▶ When indigo carmine is sprayed, the lesion shows no changes in sur-face irregularities nor in the areae gastricae patterns on the mucosal surface. In other words, it can be seen that this is a 0–IIb lesion distin-guished only by a change in color tone.

▶ In the initial stage of undifferentiat-ed-type gastric cancer, 0–IIb le-sions with no changes in surface ir-regularities often occur. These cancer lesions are not exposed to the surface; rather, signet ring cell carcinoma is present only in the middle layer of the mucosa.

Diagnosis Greater curvature of the upper body of the remnant stomach, 0–IIb, 3 mm, sig, T1a (M), UL (−)

Tips

- Pay attention to metachronous multiple occurrence of undifferentiated-type gastric cancer when you are observing a remnant stomach after undifferentiated-type gastric cancer surgery.
- Note that undifferentiated-type gastric cancer exhibits faded 0–IIb in its initial stage.

Endoscopic image from 6 months previously

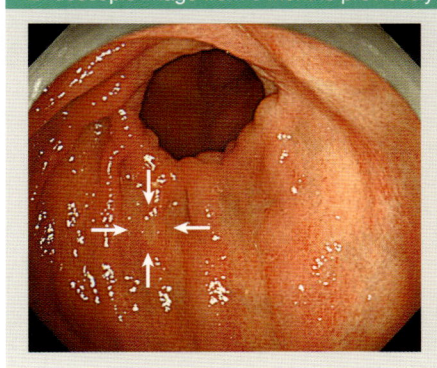

- The lesion was captured in a picture taken 6 months previously, but was not noticed at that time.
- After undifferentiated-type gastric cancer surgery, you can detect minute gastric cancer lesions by keeping an eye out for areas that exhibit fading.

Side Note Should the duodenum be observed first?

Many textbooks say that the duodenum should be observed first, followed by the stomach. But if the duodenum is observed first, the greater curvature of the body and the lesser curvature of the angulus will be grazed by the endoscope. This may make minute lesions unrecognizable. Of course, you could first observe the areas that are likely to be grazed by the endoscope. But that's quite inconvenient. I've started thinking that, instead of taking the trouble to observe those areas first, it would be better to simply observe the stomach first and then move on to the duodenum. When you think about it, there is no advantage of observing the duodenum first. What's more, when you observe the duodenum last, the sedative will have taken full effect and the patient won't feel much discomfort. Now I first observe the stomach thoroughly and then observe the duodenum. However, caution is required. You have to suction air sufficiently from the stomach before moving on to the duodenum; otherwise, the patient will feel discomfort.

Answer The gastric cancer is imaged in ③ and ④ .

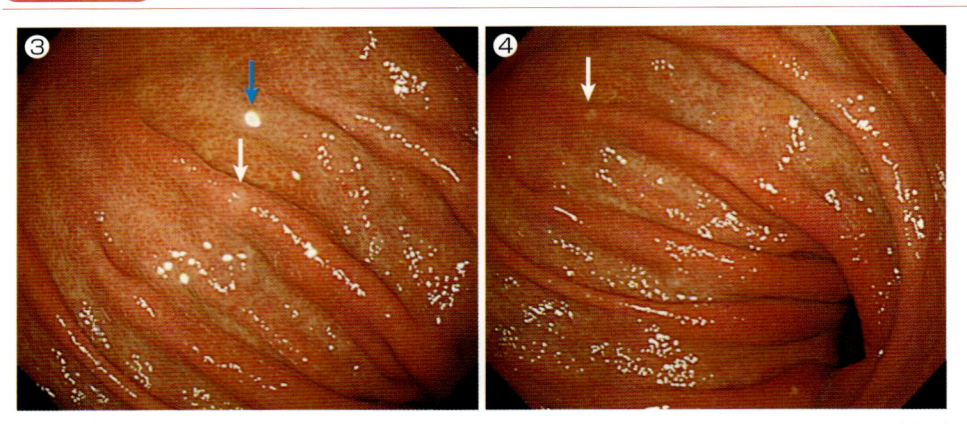

▶ In the background mucosa, atrophy is visible, and the folds are erythematous due to residual gastritis. A small spot (pointed by the white arrow) with faded color tone is visible on the fold in the greater curvature of the upper body of the remnant stomach.

▶ The surrounding area of the lesion is reddish, and the fading is conspicuous even from a distance. There are no surface irregularities. The only finding is a change in color tone.

▶ The blue arrow is reflection (halation) of endoscope illumination.

Histological images of biopsied specimen

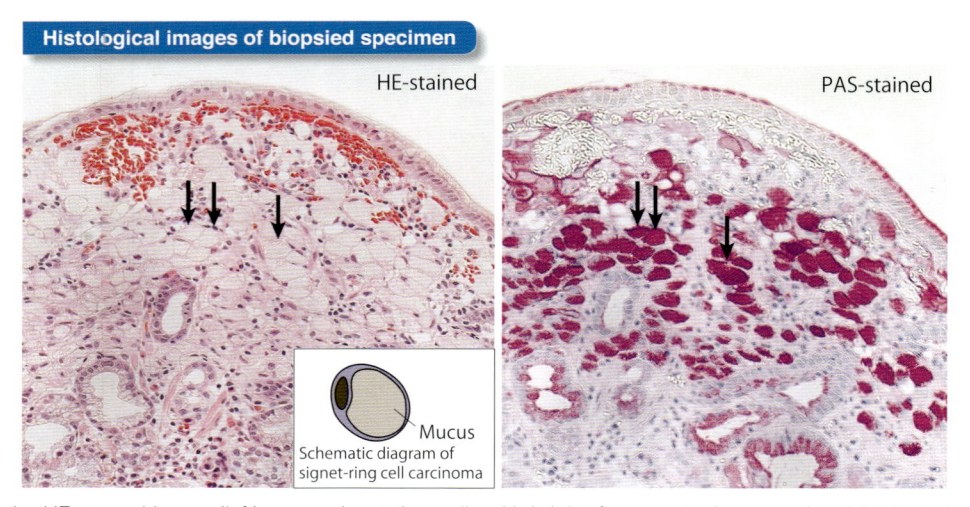

▶ In the HE-stained image (left), many signet-ring cells with bright, foamy cytoplasms and maldistributed nuclei are recognized. The signet-ring cells are dyed reddish-purple in PAS staining (right).

Diagnosis Greater curvature of the body of the remnant stomach, 0–IIb, 2 mm, sig, T1a (M), UL (–)

Tips

- When conducting endoscopy in the remnant stomach after surgery of gastric cancer, pay attention to metachronous cancer.
- Note that undifferentiated-type gastric cancer often occurs in the remnant stomach after surgery of, in particular, undifferentiated-type gastric cancer.
- In its initial stage, undifferentiated-type gastric cancer often exhibits a 0–IIb lesion without surface irregularities without forming a depression.
- Undifferentiated-type gastric cancer exhibits fading.

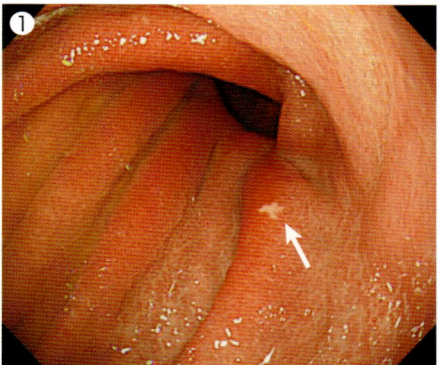

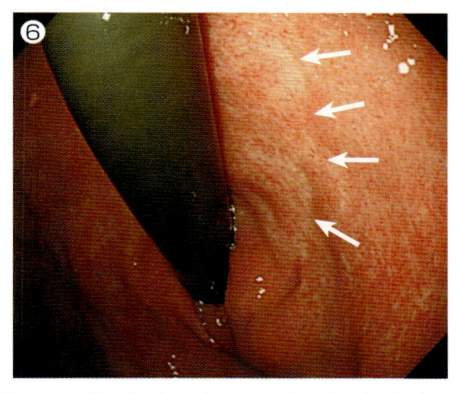

- Indicated by the arrow is xanthoma which is believed to be an accumulation of macrophages after lipid phagocytosis. It has no pathological significance.
- At first glance, xanthoma is likely to be mistaken for fading of the undifferentiated type. However, it is yellower than undifferentiated-type gastric cancer. Once you get used to seeing it, you will be able to diagnose it with endoscopy alone; you will not need to perform a biopsy.

- The scar-like finding that runs longitudinally is a suture from a previous surgery.
- In proximal gastrectomy, a longitudinal suture is often seen on the lesser curvature side.

Previous endoscopies

<2 years previously>   <1 year previously>

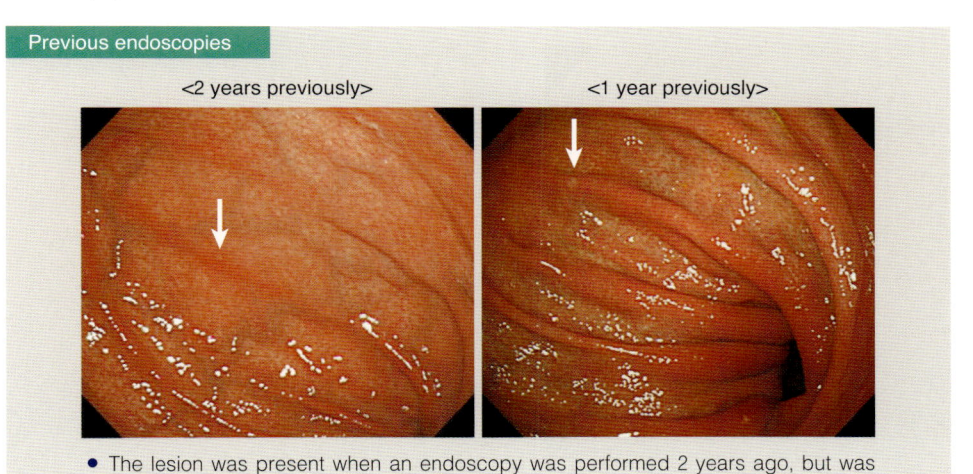

- The lesion was present when an endoscopy was performed 2 years ago, but was not recognized at that time. These pictures show that the lesion showed a tendency to grow gradually.

Side Note Should we use a viscous preparation or spray for pharyngeal anesthesia?

Pharyngeal anesthesia by lidocaine, which is used in preparation for endoscopy, can be administered in two ways: a viscous method where about 5 ml of viscous lidocaine is pooled in the back of the pharynx for a few minutes or a spray method in which lidocaine is sprayed directly on the pharynx and swallowed immediately. Pooling lidocaine in the back of the pharynx causes great discomfort to patients who have a strong gag reflex. When I undergo endoscopy myself, I request the spray method because I find that the viscous method is pretty uncomfortable. A randomized controlled trial on the spray method and the viscous method concluded that the spray method was more acceptable to patients and that the pharyngeal anesthesia effects were almost the same[a].

a) Mizuno Y, Hikichi T, Itabashi M, et al. [A comparative study of the effect and discomfort produced by pharyngeal anesthesia with viscous lidocaine solution and with lidocaine spray in esophagogastroduodenoscopy.] Fukushima J Med Sci. 2011; 61: 12–17. (In Japanese with English abstract.)

case

44

Screening endoscopy before tongue cancer surgery
〔Gastric cancer with active *H. pylori* infection〕

Answer The gastric cancer is imaged in ②, ③ and ⑤.

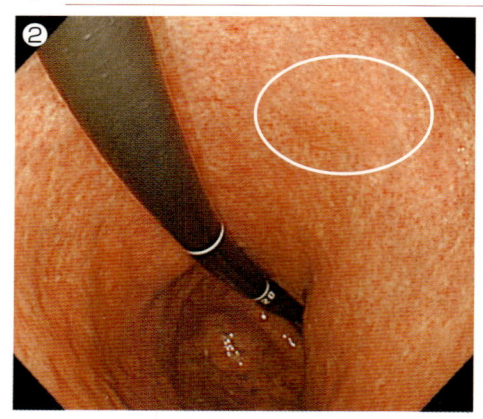

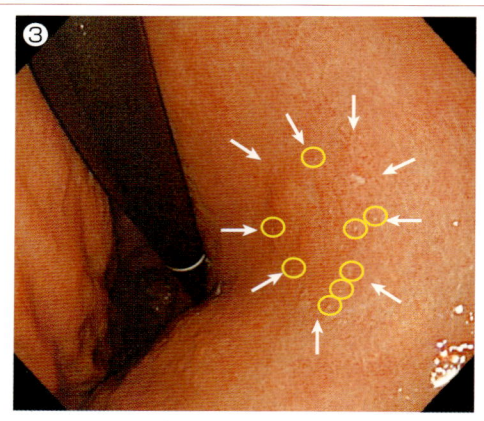

▶ Atrophy and diffuse redness can be seen in the background mucosa. A sticky mucus is attached. These are findings of active *H. pylori* infection.

▶ An area that stands out as being redder than the surrounding mucosa is visible in the lesser curvature of the middle body. The background exhibits patchy fading due to atrophy, but there is no fading present in the erythematous mucosa.

▶ When air is suctioned and the endoscope is brought up close, the erythematous mucosa appears a little thicker than it should be, suggesting 0–IIa. There are multiple small white spots (circled in yellow) in the margins.

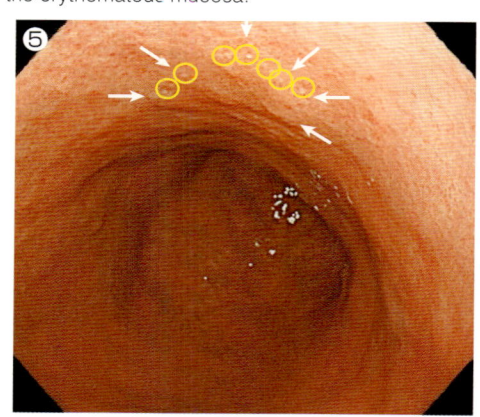

▶ In antegrade view, the margin can be seen on the proximal side (indicated by the arrows). The small white spots (circled in yellow) are present at multiple locations as though outlining the margin.

Indigo carmine sprayed images

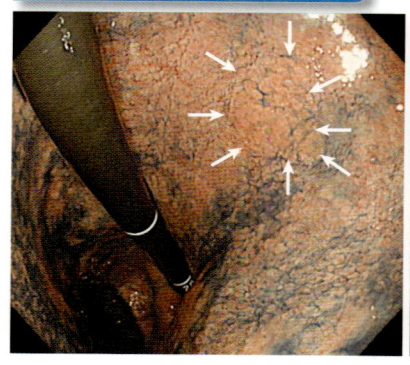
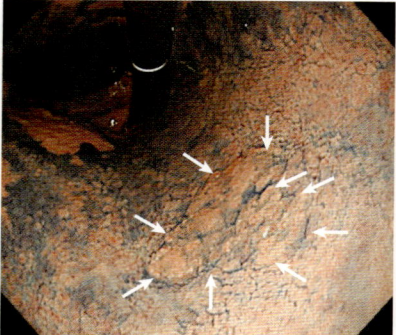
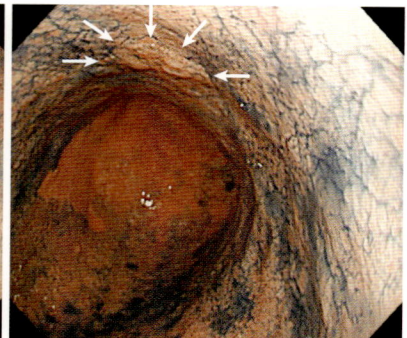

▶ When indigo carmine is sprayed, the areae gastricae pattern inside the lesion looks unclear. Reading the changes in the areae gastricae patterns makes it possible to elucidate the lesion's margins.

▶ Some of the areae gastricae patterns in the background cannot be clearly imaged because they are covered in mucus

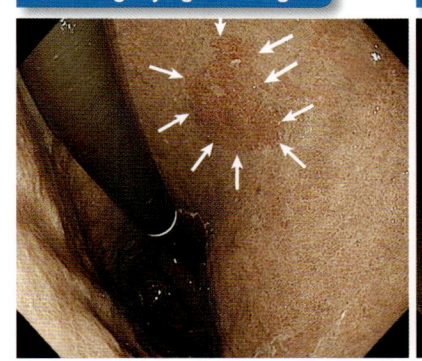

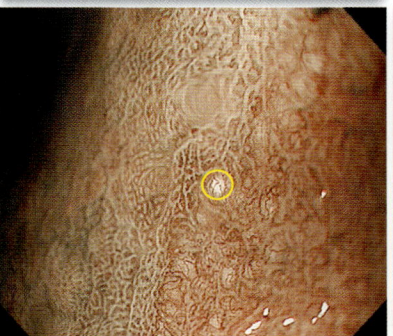
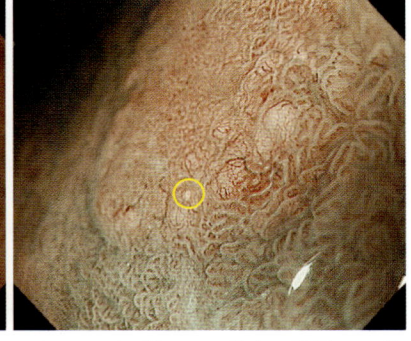

▶ In non-magnifying NBI observation, the lesion looks browner than the surrounding area and the margins look clear.

▶ When the edges of the lesion are observed with magnifying NBI, small white globular objects are recognized. This is a finding specific to cancer called white globe appearance (WGA).

Histological image of WGA

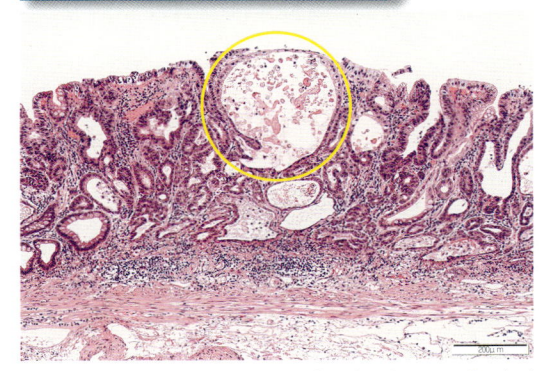

▶ HE-stained, medium-magnification image. Pooled eosinophilic substance (circled in yellow) can be seen in the dilated atypical glands — which contains neoplastic cells that have lapsed into degeneration and necrosis.

Diagnosis Lesser curvature of the middle body, 0–IIa, 18 mm, tub1>tub2, T1a (M), UL (−)

Tips

- Looks for subtle differences in color tone from the background.
- Suction air to get a clear view of the elevation of a lesion.
- Spray indigo carmine to confirm the difference in mucosal patterns.
- Remember that WGA is a finding specific to gastric cancer.
- Note that WGA is useful for detection and extent diagnosis of gastric cancer.

Additional Info White globe appearance (WGA)

- WGA is a small white hemispherical object with a diameter of less than 1 mm that is observed under the epithelium of cancer in magnifying NBI observation. Pathologically speaking, it corresponds to an intraglandular necrotic debris pooled in dilated cancer glands[58, 59].
- Yoshida et al. have reported that WGA is observed in 21.4% of gastric cancers, that the sensitivity for gastric cancer is also 21.4%, and that the specificity is 97.5%[60]. WGA is expected to serve as a novel marker for diagnosis of gastric cancer.
- WGA can be clearly imaged in magnifying NBI endoscopy. However, it can also be confirmed by conventional endoscopy as in this case. It is useful for detection of cancer. Moreover, since WGA exists near the demarcation line on the edge of cancer, it is a finding that supports extent diagnosis of cancer[61].

Answer　The gastric cancer is imaged in ⑤ and ⑥ .

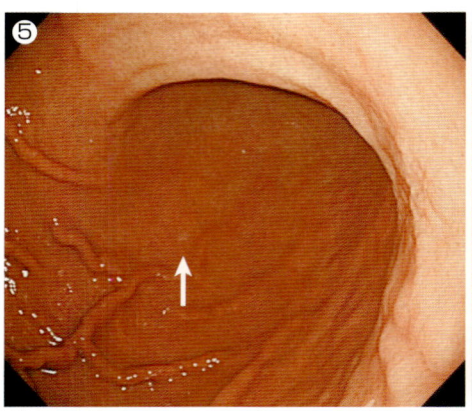

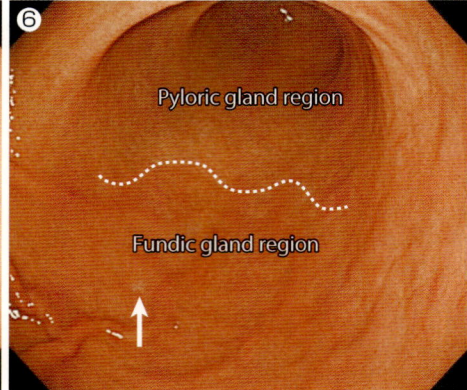

▶ The background mucosa is RAC-positive and is in an *H. pylori*-uninfected condition without atrophy. In normal mucosa, the pyloric gland region is sometimes slightly more yellowish-white than the fundic gland region. This should not be mistaken for atrophy.

▶ In the greater curvature of the angulus, a small area of faded mucosa is visible. The fading in the uniform orange-red in the fundic gland region is conspicuous even from a distance (pointed by the arrow). It is a single fading patch, bringing suspicion of signet-ring cell carcinoma.

Indigo carmine sprayed images

▶ When indigo carmine is sprayed, the lesion appears to be flat and the areae gastricae pattern shows no difference from the surrounding area. It is a finding of signet-ring cell carcinoma that exists only in the middle layer of the mucosa.

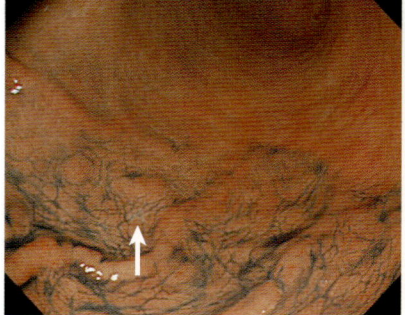

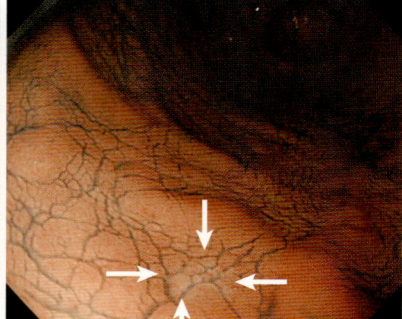

Tips

● Understand the findings of normal pyloric glands.
● Look for faded patches in *H. pylori*-uninfected patients.

Diagnosis　Greater curvature of the lower body, 0–IIb, 2 mm, sig, T1a (M), UL (−)

👓 **What's imaged in the other pictures?**

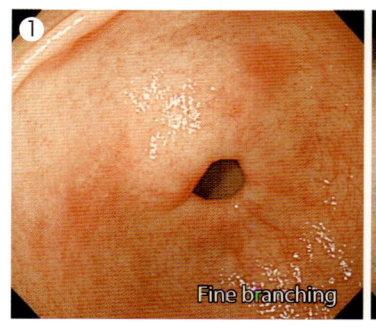

Fine branching

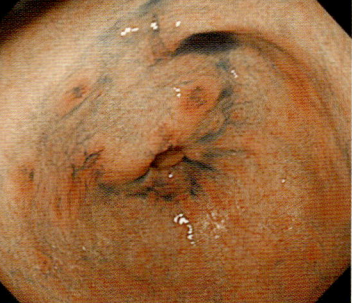

● Multiple erythematous patches have occurred in the antrum. Spraying indigo carmine makes it possible to recognize erosion in the center.

● This is considered to be benign erythematous erosion because the redness in the border gradually decreases as it goes outwards and this gradual decrease of the redness occurs in multiple locations. This is raised erosion, which is a finding often seen in *H. pylori*-uninfected cases. Besides, although the dendritic vessels are conspicuous in the greater curvature of the prepyloric region, it is not a finding of atrophy; rather, it is a finding of a normal pyloric gland region.

46

Screening endoscopy for double cancer after hypopharyngeal cancer surgery

[Gastric cancer detected after *H. pylori* eradication]

Answer The gastric cancer is imaged in ② and ③ .

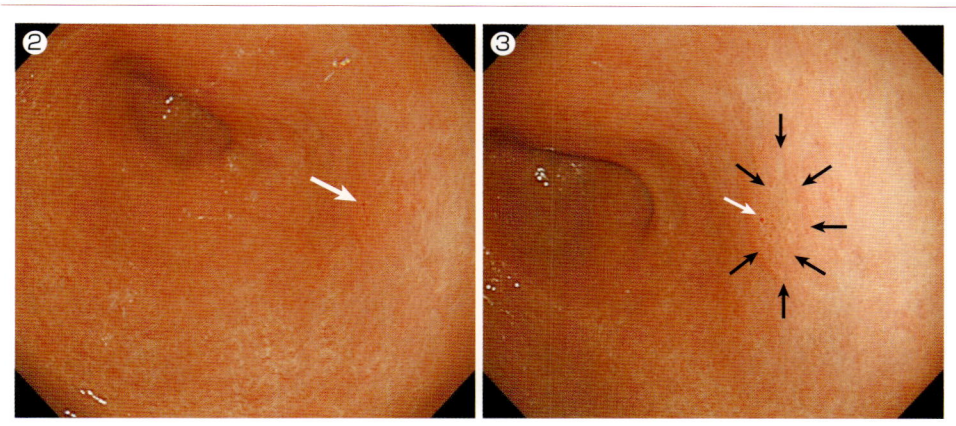

▶ In the background mucosa, O–3 atrophy and intestinal metaplasia are recognized. So the examination is performed while differentiated-type gastric cancer is kept in mind.

▶ A small bleeding point (pointed by the white arrow) is noticed on the posterior wall of the antrum. When this is carefully observed from a close distance, slightly more yellowish-white mucosa (pointed by the black arrows) than the surrounding area is visible.

Indigo carmine sprayed images

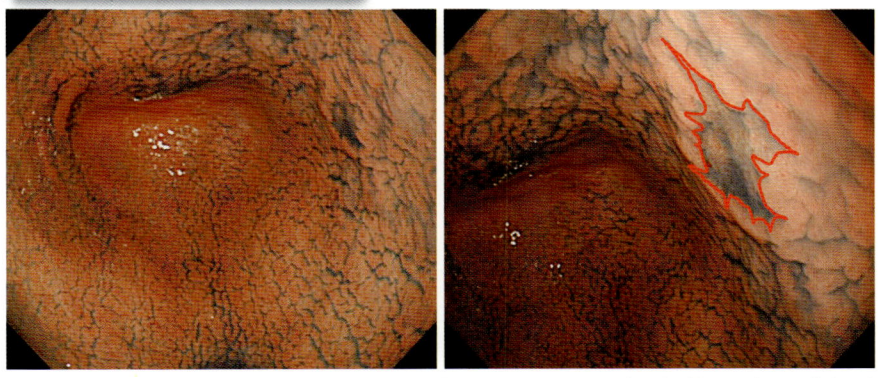

▶ When indigo carmine is sprayed, the depressed surface can be seen clearly. The edges of the depression exhibit encroachment with thorn-like intrusions into the surrounding mucosa, accompanied by a reactive elevation on the distal side.

▶ At this point, it can be endoscopically diagnosed as differentiated-type gastric cancer.

Diagnosis Posterior wall of the antrum, 0–IIc, 5 mm, tub1, T1a (M), UL (–)

Tips

- Suspect differentiated-type gastric cancer when you see mucosa that is slightly more yellowish-white than the surrounding area.
- Spray indigo carmine to clarify the depressed surface.
- Keep in mind that a thorn-like encroachment is a finding that strongly suggests differentiated-type gastric cancer.

Screening endoscopy before surgery for colon cancer ①
〔Gastric cancer with active *H. pylori* infection〕

Answer   The gastric cancer is imaged in ② and ③ .

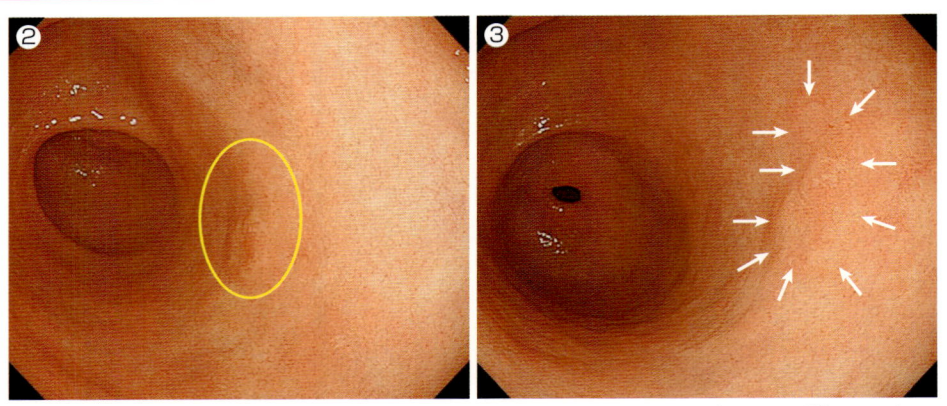

▶ O–2 atrophy is visible in the background mucosa. The non-atrophic mucosa features diffuse redness, indicating an active *H. pylori* infection.
▶ On the posterior wall of the antrum, surface irregularities in some degree are recognized when observed from a distance (②). So observation is proceeded while the existence of cancer is kept in mind.
▶ When the endoscope is brought up close (③), it can be seen that redness caused by the presence of blood vesses is present in the surrounding mucosa. Because there is no redness inside the lesion and the lesion is uniformly skin-colored, the extent of the lesion can be assessed as indicated by the arrows. However, performing extent diagnosis in conventional endoscopy is difficult until you get used to it.

Indigo carmine sprayed images

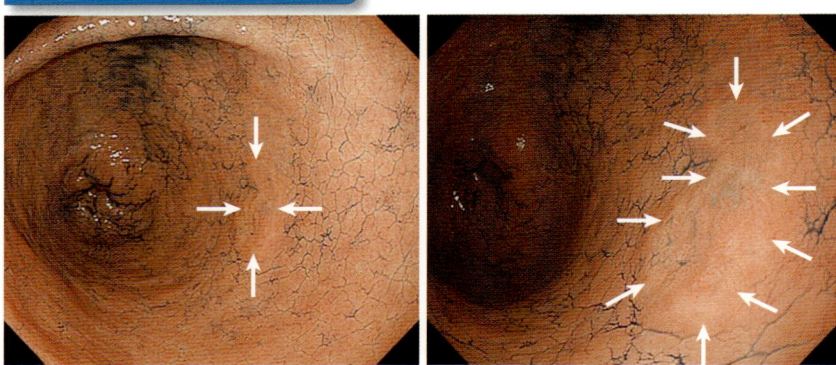

▶ When indigo carmine is sprayed, the dye pools in the grooves of the areae gastricae, making the areae gastricae on the mucosal surface clearly visible. The absence of areae gastricae inside the lesion helps clarify the extent of the lesion.
▶ Ir this way, spraying indigo carmine can improve the visibility of a lesion even when the lesion is difficult to recognize in conventional endoscopy.

Diagnosis   Posterior wall of the antrum, 0–IIc, 15 mm, tub1, T1a (M), UL (–)

Tips

• Look for subtle differences from the background mucosa.
• Always remember that indigo carmine can improve the visibility of a lesion.

Screening endoscopy before surgery for colon cancer ②

〔Gastric cancer detected after *H. pylori* eradication〕

Answer   The gastric cancer is imaged in ③ .

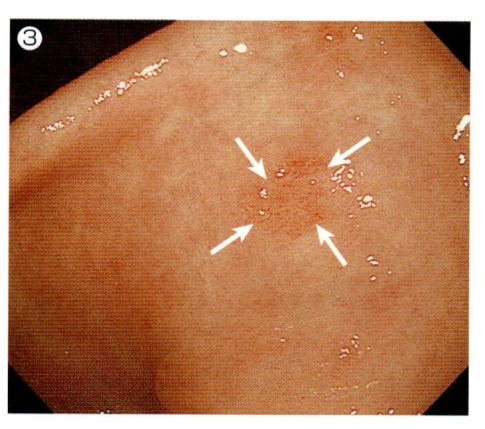

▶ O–2 atrophy and intestinal metaplasia are present in the background mucosa, while map-like redness — which is a post-eradication change — occurs in multiple locations in the body. Erythematous mucosa is visible on the posterior wall of the lesser curvature of the antrum. No similar areas of redness are visible in the surrounding area, which indicates that this spot is unique.

▶ As for color tone, the site is redder than map-like redness. It is necessary to check the lesion carefully while considering the possibility of differentiated-type gastric cancer.

Close-up image

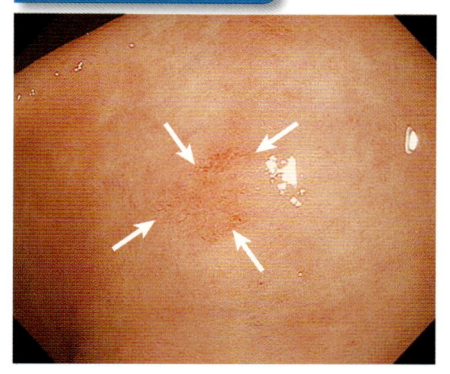

▶ In close up, it looks like a slightly depressed lesion. The reddish surface is not glossy like the surrounding mucosa.

Indigo carmine sprayed image

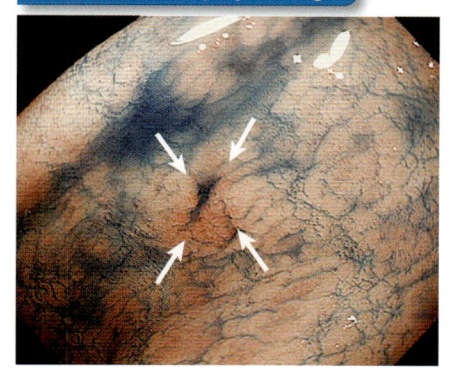

▶ When indigo carmine is sprayed, the depressed surface becomes clear. Compared to the areae gastricae in the surrounding gastritis, the depressed surface has a fine areae gastricae-like pattern.

▶ It is important to look for a lesion by comparing what you are observing with the background mucosa.

Diagnosis   Posterior wall of the lesser curvature of the antrum, 0-IIc, 5 mm, tub1, T1a (M), UL (–)

Tips

- Watch for isolated redness.
- Perform observation while making a comparison with the background gastritis.
- Suspect differentiated-type gastric cancer when you see a reddish depression.

case 49

Answer The gastric cancer is imaged in ③ .

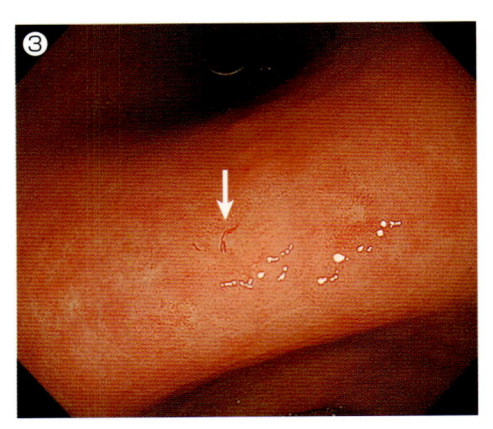

▶ O-2 atrophy, intestinal metaplasia, and diffuse redness are present in the background mucosa, so this case is considered active *H. pylori* infection. Surface irregularities due to chronic gastritis are conspicuous. As for color tone, fading and redness are mixed together. All of this makes it difficult to find gastric cancer in the background mucosa.

▶ Fresh blood is visible in the lesser curvature of the lower body. From this point on, detailed observation was conducted with the awareness that gastric cancer was a strong possibility.

Non-magnifying NBI image

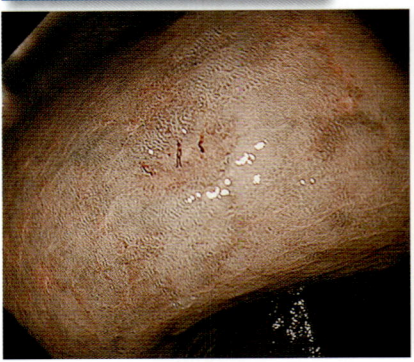

Medium-magnification NBI image

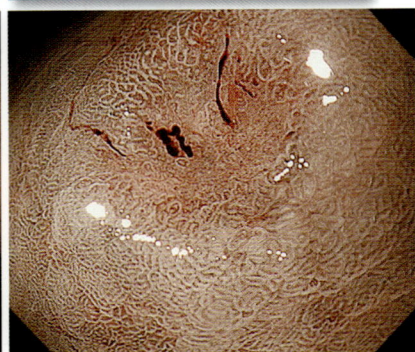

▶ In NBI observation, the lesion is a brownish depression. The depressed surface exhibits papillary surface microstructure while dilated, tortuous looped vessels are seen underneath the surface, making it possible to diagnose this as cancer.

▶ Bleeding caused by irrigation is also observed.

Indigo carmine sprayed image

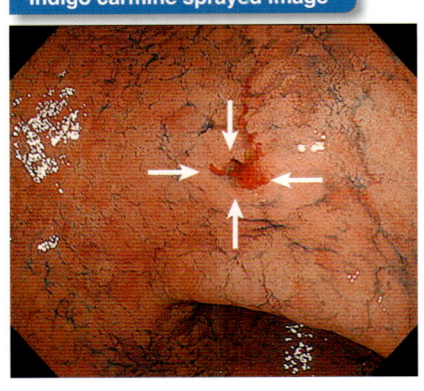

▶ Indigo carmine spraying induced further bleeding. Although detailed observation is not possible due to the bleeding, such delicate mucosa that bleeds easily is a finding that suggests cancer.

Diagnosis Lesser curvature of the lower body, 0-IIc, 4 mm, tub1, T1a (M), UL (−)

Tips

● Be aware that gastric cancer may be hidden behind spontaneous bleeding.

Screening endoscopy before surgery for colon cancer ④

〔Gastric cancer with active *H. pylori* infection〕

Answer   The gastric cancer is imaged in ③ .

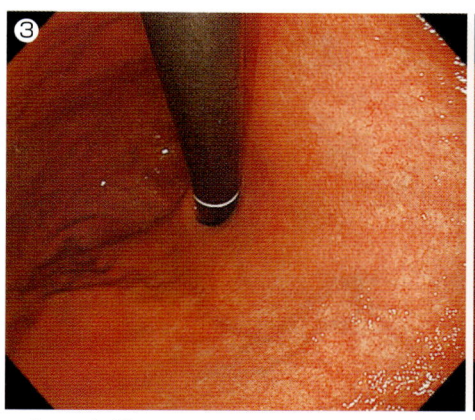
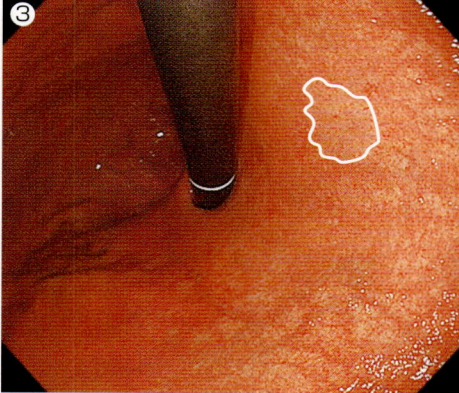

▶ O–2 atrophy and diffuse redness are present in the background mucosa, indicating active *H. pylori* infection. When you see background mucosa that looks like this, look for adenoma and differentiated-type gastric cancer.

▶ Near the posterior wall of the lesser curvature of the upper body, a patch of slightly whitish mucosa with a diameter of about 5 mm is visible. Unlike the surrounding atrophy, vessels are not visible inside the lesion (absence of a vascular pattern).

▶ When you see a flat lesion with a whitish color tone like this, include adenoma and very well-differentiated adenocarcinoma in any differential diagnosis.

Indigo carmine sprayed image

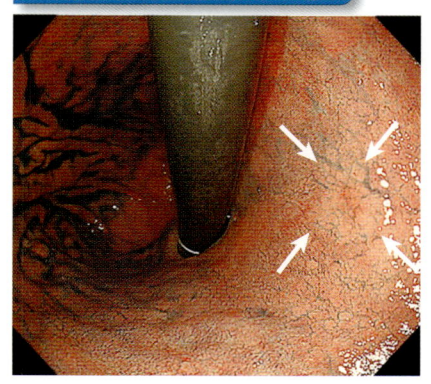

▶ When indigo carmine is sprayed, it can be seen that the lesion is a 0–IIb lesion without surface irregularities. The areae gastricae pattern is larger than the patterns in the surrounding area and looks somewhat unclear.

Medium-magnification NBI image

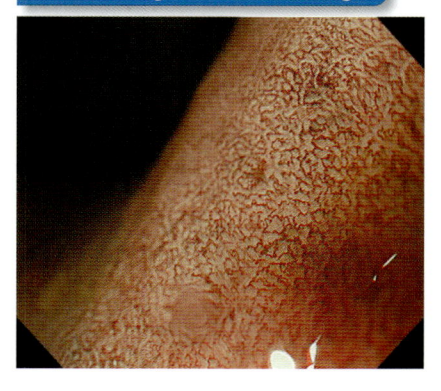

Non-magnifying NBI image

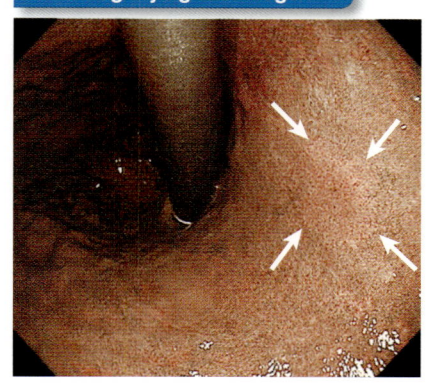

▶ In non-magnifying NBI observation, the lesion is visible as a brownish lesion with clear margins. The visibility of this lesion is better under non-magnifying NBI than under WLI.

▶ Olympus's EVIS LUCERA ELITE system is brighter than conventional systems and enables screening observation even in non-magnifying NBI. Non-magnifying NBI often shows cancer in a brownish color tone and is a useful tool for finding cancer, especially when there are no conspicuous surface irregularities.

▶ Under magnification, blood vessels can be seen that form a complete mesh pattern, suggesting differentiated-type gastric cancer.

Histologic image of biopsy specimen

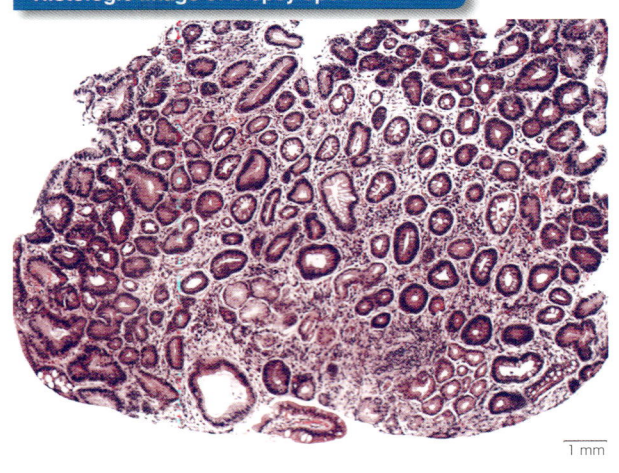

1 mm

▶ HE-stained, medium-magnification image. Tubular adenocarcinoma is seen. The cellular atypia is not so severe.Glandular size is small and density is high.

▶ Differentiated-type gastric cancer with low-grade cellular atypia is occasionally called very well-differentiated adenocarcinoma. Sometimes the problem is how to differentiate it from intestinal tubular adenoma that shows severe atypia.

▶ This case falls under tub1 according to the *Japanese Classification of Gastric Cancer* (15th edition)[29].

Diagnosis

Lesser curvature of the upper body, 0–IIb, 5 mm,

tub1 (so-called very well-differentiated adenocarcinoma), T1a (M), UL (−)

Tips

- In cases where severe atrophy is visible in the background mucosa, perform observation while watching for any changes in color tone (white, reddish, etc.) and for the absence of vascular patterns.
- So-called very well-differentiated adenocarcinoma (differentiated-type gastric cancer with low-grade celluler atypia) often exhibits a color tone ranging from normal to white. Differentiating this from adenoma can be a problem.
- In screening endoscopy under non-magnifying NBI, watch for changes in the brownish color tone.

Side Note Examination time and gastric cancer detection rate

Studies have found a correlation in colonoscopy between the examination time and the adenoma detection rate, concluding that observation should be conducted while withdrawing the colonoscope over a period of at least 8 minutes[a]. Does this have any relevance to the detection rate of gastric cancer? Of course, the examination time varies depending on the background mucosa. For example, if there is no atrophy in the gastric mucosa, a relatively simple observation would suffice. But in cases where atrophy or severe intestinal metaplasia is present in the gastric mucosa, more careful and detailed observation is required. And that means taking more time. According to one study, doctors who spend more than 7 minutes observing the stomach have a gastric cancer detection rate cancer that's 3 times as high as that of the doctors who spend less time on observation[b].

a) Barclay RL, Vicari JJ, Greenlaw RL. Effect of a time–dependent colonoscopic withdrawal protocol on adenoma detection during screening colonoscopy. Clin Gastroenterol Hepatol. 2008; 6: 1091–1098.
b) Teh JL, Tan JR, Hau LJ, et al. Long examination time improves detection of gastric cancer during diagnostic upper gastrointestinal endoscopy. Clin Gastroenterol Hepatol. 2015; 13: 480–487.

Answer The gastric tumor is imaged in ⑥ .

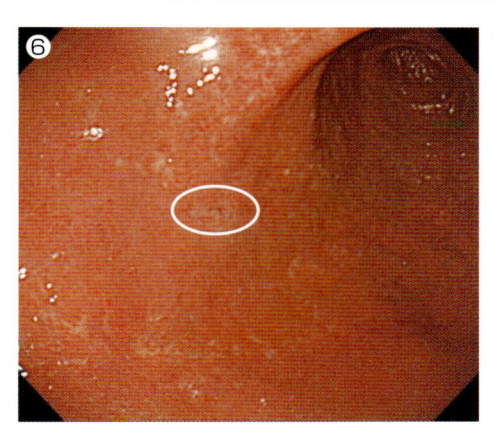

▶ O–1 atrophy is visible in the background mucosa. Diffuse redness is present in the non-atrophic region. These findings indicate an active *H. pylori* infection.
▶ Faded depressions caused by atrophy are present in multiple locations on the anterior wall of the lower body. Conspicuous among these is a depression with a dull, faded color tone. When observing, you have to compare what you see with the surrounding mucosa.

Indigo carmine sprayed images

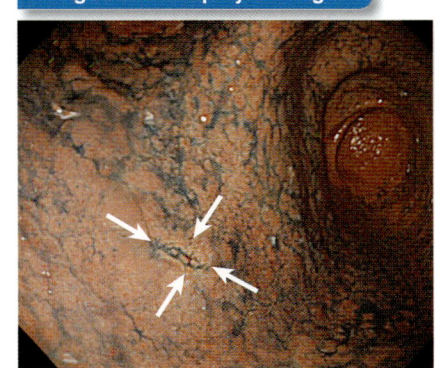
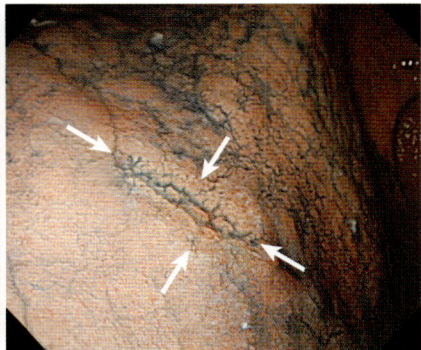

▶ Indigo carmine spraying makes the difference in color tone stand out.
▶ The depressed surface has a granular texture with granules of various sizes.

 **Diagnosis** Anterior wall of the lower body, 0–II-like lesion, 5 mm, tubular adenoma with moderate atypia

Tips • Look for subtle differences in color tone from the surrounding area.

Side Note Post-biopsy bleeding

Although post-biopsy bleeding is rare, you have to be careful to try and avoid it as major hemorrhaging can sometimes occur, dramatically lowering blood pressure. According to Cancer Institute Hospital of JFCR data, bleeding that required emergency endoscopy for hemostasis occurred in 0.03% of biopsy cases[a]. The risk factors were administration of anti-thrombotics and implementation of multiple biopsies. Many of the bleeding points were located in the lesser curvature of the middle and upper body, and severe atrophy was recognized in the background mucosa. In areas where the mucosa is thinned like this, a biopsy is likely to penetrate the submucosa which contains many blood vessels, making bleeding more likely. Therefore, it is recommended that biopsy forceps with small cup diameters (forceps designed for slim endoscopes) be used for patients and sites that have a high risk of bleeding.

a) Suganuma T, Hirasawa T, Shimizu T, et al. [Risk of bleeding after endoscopic biopsy with screening esophagogastroduodenoscopy.] Jpn Gastroenterol. 2012; 55: 588–593. (In Japanese with English abstract.)

References

1) Yagi K, Nakamura A, Sekine A. Characteristic endoscopic and magnified endoscopic findings in the normal stomach without *Helicobacter pylori* infection. J Gastroenterol Hepatol. 2002; 17: 39–45.

2) Yagi K, Ajioka Y. [Magnification Endoscopic Diagnosis of the Stomach (2nd edition).] Tokyo: Igaku Shoin, 2014. (In Japanese.)

3) Dobashi Y, Fujita T. [Vascular Structure.] Kawai K ed [Stomach — Morphology and Its Functions.] Tokyo: Igaku Shoin, 1975, 54–61. (In Japanese.)

4) Yagi K, Tsuboi K, Nakamura A, et al. [Features of *Helicobacter pylori* positive and negative gastric mucosal findings: diagnosis by magnifying endoscopy.] I to Cho (Stomach Intest). 2006; 41: 1017–1024. (In Japanese.)

5) Yagi K, Nakamura A, Sekine A, et al. [Endoscopic features of the normal gastric mucosa without *Helicobacter pylori* infection.] Gastroenterol Endosc. 2000; 42: 1977–1987. (In Japanese.)

6) Ono S, Kato M, Suzuki M, et al. [Differentiation of benignancy and malignancy of gastric erosion and redness seen after *H. pylori* eradication.] Endosc Dig. 2011; 23: 1761–1766. (In Japanese.)

7) Matsuhisa T, Kusakabe S, Maeda S, et al. [Observation of esophageal, gastric and duodenal lesions after *Helicobacter pylori* eradication.] Therap Res. 2001; 22: 1872–1874. (In Japanese.)

8) Okazaki Y, Takeo S. [Red streaks (Kammrötung).] I to Cho (Stomach Intest). 2012; 47 ([Extra issue. Atlas: I to Cho Glossary of Terms 2012.]): 691. (In Japanese.)

9) Takeo S. [Relationship between red streaks on gastric mucosa and *H. pylori* infection.] Jpn Med J. 2013; 4655: 63–64. (In Japanese.)

10) Haruma K (supv ed). Kyoto Classification of Gastritis. Tokyo: Nihon Medical Center, 2014.(Englsh edition : Tokyo : Nihon Medical Center,2017)

11) Kato T, Yagi N, Kamada T, et al. [Diagnosis of *Helicobacter pylori* infection in gastric mucosa by endoscopic features: a multicenter prospective study.] Gastroenterol Endosc. 2014: 56: 1813–1824. (In Japanese.)

12) Kimura K, Takemoto T. An endoscopic recognition of atrophic border and its significance in chronic gastritis. Endoscopy. 1969; 1: 87–97.

13) Sakaki N, Kato H, Arakawa T, et al. [Endoscopic diagnosis of glandular regions and *Helicobacter pylori*] I to Cho (Stomach Intest). 1997; 32: 1571–1580. (In Japanese.)

14) Kaminishi M, Yamaguchi H, Nomura S, et al. Endoscopic classification of chronic gastritis based on a pilot study by the Research Society for Gastritis. Dig Endosc. 2002; 14: 138–151.

15) Fukuta N, Ida K, Kato T, et al. [Endoscopic diagnosis of gastric intestinal metaplasia: a prospective multicenter study.] Gastrol Endosc. 2015; 57: 1219–1229. (In Japanese.)

16) Uedo N, Ishihara R, Iishi H, et al. A new method of diagnosing gastric intestinal metaplasia: narrow band imaging with magnifying endoscopy. Endoscopy. 2006; 38: 819–824.

17) Kamada T, Haruma K, Inoue K, et al. [*Helicobacter pylori* infection and endoscopic gastritis — Kyoto Classification of Gastritis.] Jpn J Gastrroentrol. 2015; 112: 982–993. (In Japanese.)

18) Nomura S, Terao S, Adachi K, et al. Endoscopic diagnosis of gastric mucosal activity and inflammation. Dig Endosc. 2013; 25: 136–146.

19) Kato M, Terao S, Adachi K, et al. Changes in endoscopic findings of gastritis after cure of *H. pylori* infection: multicenter prospective trial. Dig Endosc. 2013; 25: 264–273.

20) Ida K, Matsumoto N, Uchiyama K, et al. [Changes in endoscopic images of the gastric mucosa before and after *Helicobacter pylori* eradication: short-term follow-up cases] I to Cho (Stomach Intest). 1998; 33: 1115–1121. (In Japanese.)

21) Terao S, Nisizawa A, Tamura I, et al. [Assessment of endoscopic images of gastritis after *H. pylori* eradication in cases under observation for a period of 10 years following eradication and comparison of magnifying NBI images immediately after eradication and 10 years later (changes in endoscopic images over the course of long-term follow-up after *H. pylori* eradicaticn.] Gastroenterol. 2013; 57: 111–118. (In Japanese.)

22) Ohkusa T, Takashimizu I, Fujiki K, et al. Disappearance of hyperplastic polyps in the stomach after eradication of *Helicobacter pylori*: a randomized, clinical trial. Ann Intern Med. 1998; 129: 712–715.

23) Imano M, Muraoka S. [Features of *Helicobacter pylori* gastritis in children.] Helicobacter Res. 1999; 3: 32–37. (In Japanese.)

24) Kamada T, Haruma K, Sugiu K, et al. Case of early gastric cancer with nodular gastritis. Dig Endosc. 2004; 16: 39–43.

25） Nagata N, Shimbo T, Akiyama J, et al. Predictability of gastric intestinal metaplasia by mottled patchy erythema seen on endoscopy. Gastroenterol Res. 2011; 4: 203–209.

26） Terao S, Yamashiro K,Nishizawa A,et al. [Changes in diffuse redness before and after *Helicobacter pylori* eradication: including map-like redness manifesting after eradication.] Helicobacter Res. 2015; 19: 343–348. (In Japanese.)

27） Yagi K, Ajioka Y. [Endoscopic Diagnosis of Gastric Cancer Discovered after *H. pylori* Eradication.] Tokyo: Igaku Shoin, 2016. (In Japanese.)

28） Hirasawa T. [Gastric Carcinoid (application part 19).] Watanabe M, Fujishiro M, ed. [Gastrointestinal diseases found with images, vol. 1, upper gastrointestinal tract.] Tokyo: Igaku Shuppan, 2013: 144–147. (In Japanese.)

29） Japanese Gastric Cancer Association ed. [Japanese Classification of Gastric Cancer (15th edition).] Tokyo: Kanehara Shuppan, 2017. (In Japanese.)(3rd English edition : Gastric Cancer.2011 ; 14: 101–112)

30） Nakamura K. [Structure of Gastric Cancer (3rd edition).] Tokyo: Igaku Shoin, 2005. (In Japanese.)

31） Fujino T, Maehata T, Matsuo Y, et al. [Factors determining lesion color tone and morphology and factors that make endoscopic diagnosis difficult.] Endosc Dig. 2014; 26: 917–933. (In Japanese.)

32） Nakashima H, Ohkura Y. [Histologic types and macroscopic images of early gastric cancer.] Endosc Dig. 2014; 26: 1097–1105. (In Japanese.)

33） Hirasawa T, Fujisaki J, Yamamoto Y. [Utility of magnifying NBI endoscopy findings in ESD cases of early undifferentiated-type gastric cancer.] Gastroenterol Endosc. 2009; 51 (Suppl): 743. (In Japanese.)

34） Okada K, Fujisaki J, Kasuga A, et al. Diagnosis of undifferentiated type early gastric cancers by magnification endoscopy with narrow-band imaging. J Gastroenterol Hepatol. 2011; 26: 1262–1269.

35） Horiuchi Y, Fujisaki J, Yamamoto N, et al. Accuracy of diagnostic demarcation of undifferentiated-type early gastric cancers for magnifying encoscopy with narrow-band imaging: endoscopic submucosal dissection cases. Gastric Cancer. 2016; 19: 515–523.

36） Aikawa K, Iwafuchi M, Watanabe H, et al. [Pathology of pure type IIb early gastric cancer] I to Cho (Stomach Intest). 1986; 21: 371–378. (In Japanese.)

37） Hirasawa T, Osumi H, Morishige K, et al. [Tips on detection of early gastric cancer — focusing on conventional endoscopy.] Endosc Dig. 2013; 25: 1681–1688. (In Japanese.)

38） Kakugawa Y, Kusano C, Otake Y, et al. [Endoscopic diagnosis of gastric cancer that resembles gastritis.] Endosc Dig. 2010; 22: 63–67. (In Japanese.)

39） Hirasawa T, Yamamoto Y, Fujisaki J, et al. [Clinical characteristics of the undifferentiated-type early gastric cancers satisfying the expanded criteria for endoscopic resection.] Gastroenterol Endosc. 2013; 55: 1625–1632. (In Japanese.)

40） Haruma K, Shiotani A, Kamada T, et al. [Adverse effects induced by long-term use of proton pump inhibitor: development of gastric polyp.] Gastroenterol. 2013; 56: 190–193. (In Japanese.)

41） Ueyama H, Yao T, Nakashima Y, et al. Gastric adenocarcinoma of fundic gland type (chief cell predominant type): proposal for a new entity of gastric adenocarcinoma. Am J Surg Pathol. 2010; 34: 609–619.

42） Yao T, Ueyama H, Kushima R, et al. [A new type of gastric cancer: fundic gland type gastric cancer — clinical pathological characteristics, growth and development patterns, and malignancies.] I to Cho (Stomach Intest). 2010; 45: 1192–1202. (In Japanese.)

43） Ueyama H, Matsumoto K, Nagahara A, et al. Gastric adenocarcinoma of the fundic gland type (chief cell predominant type). Endoscopy. 2014; 46: 153–157.

44） Nonaka K, Ishikawa K, Shimizu M, et al. Gastrointestinal: gastric mucosa-associated lymphoma presented with unique vascular features on magnified endoscopy combined with narrow-band imaging. J Gastroenterol Hepatol. 2009; 24: 1697.

45） Kamada T, Tanaka A, Yamanaka Y, et al. Nodular gastritis with *Helicobacter pylori* infection is strongly associated with diffuse-type gastric cancer in young patients. Dig Endosc. 2007; 19: 180–184.

46） Kushima R. [Gastric and duodenal lesions in young people.] I to Cho (Stomach Intest). 2011; 46: 1305–1307. (In Japanese.)

47） Japan Esophageal Society ed. Japanese Classification of Esophageal Cancer (11th edition). Tokyo: Kanehara Shuppan,

2015.

48） Omae M, Fujisaki J, Shimizu T, et al. [How to diagnose Barrett's esophageal adenocarcinoma: problems and solutions — diagnosis of the degree of advance.] Jpn Clin Gastroenterol. 2011; 14: 466–472. (In Japanese.)

49） Omae M, Fujisaki J, Shimizu T, et al. [Significance of acid reflux in patients with Barrett's adenocarcinoma.] Jpn Clin Surg. 2013; 68: 406–412. (In Japanese.)

50） Bosman FT, Carneiro F, Hruban RH, et al. (eds). WHO Classification of Tumors of Digestive System, 4th ed. Lyon: IARC Press, 2010.

51） Delle Fave G, O'Toole D, Sundin A, et al. ENETS consensus guidelines update for gastroduodenal neoplasms. Neuroendocrinology. 2016; 103: 119–124.

52） Japanese Neuroendocrine Tumor Society ed. [Guideline for Pancreatic and Gastroenteric Neuroendocrine Tumor.] Tokyo: Kanehara Shuppan, 2015. (In Japanese.)

53） NCCN Clinical Practice Guidelines in Oncology. Neuroendocrine tumors version 2. Available at: https://www.nccn.org/professionals/physician_gls/PDF/neuroendocrine.pdf. Accessed 2016.

54） Rindi G, Luinetti O, Cornaggia M, et al. Three subtypes of gastric argyrophil carcinoids and gastric neuroendocrine carcinoma: a cliniccpathological study. Gastroenterology. 1993; 104: 994–1006.

55） Yao K, Iwashita A, Tanabe H, et al. White opaque substance within superficial elevated gastric neoplasia as visualized by magnification endoscopy with narrow-band imaging: a new optical sign for differentiating between adenoma and carcinoma. Gastrointest Endosc. 2008; 68: 574–580.

56） Ueo T, Yonemasu H, Yada N, et al. White opaque substance represents an intracytoplasmic accumulation of lipid droplets: immunohistochemical and immunoelectron microscopic investigation of 26 cases. Dig Endosc. 2013; 25: 147–155.

57） Inoue K, Fujisawa T, Chinuki D, et al. [Background mucosa where gastric cancer originates — endoscopic investigations in general medical examinations.] I to Cho (Stomach Intest). 2009; 44: 1367–1373. (In Japanese.)

58） Doyama H, Yoshida N, Tsuyama S, et al. The "white globe appearance" (WGA): a novel marker for a correct diagnosis of early gastric cancer by magnifying endoscopy with narrow-band imaging (M-NBI). Endosc Int Open. 2015; 3: E120–124.

59） Watanabe Y, Shimizu M, Itoh T, et al. Intraglandular necrotic debris in gastric biopsy and surgical specimens. Ann Diagn Pathol. 2001; 5: 141–147.

60） Yoshida N, Doyama H, Nakanishi H, et al. White globe appearance is a novel specific endoscopic marker for gastric cancer: a prospective study. Dig Endosc. 2016; 28: 59–66.

61） Doyama H. [WGA (white globe appearance).] Clin Gastroenterol. 2016; 31: 1162–1166. (In Japanese.)

Afterword

In the 1990s, a children's book titled *Where's Wally?* was very popular. It was a picture book that was like a game in which the reader tried to find the protagonist whose name was Wally. Wally wore a distinctive red-and-white-striped shirt and the reader had to try and pick him out of the crowd. I was a senior high student at that time. I remember my friends and I often competed to see who would find Wally first. Trying to find early gastric cancer (which looks a lot like gastritis) in a stomach afflicted with gastritis is a lot like trying to find Wally. However, unlike *Where's Wally?* you can't find gastric cancer just by luck. What you need are an understanding of gastritis and gastric cancer including histopathological findings, sufficient skill in endoscopy to minimize the chances that you will miss a lesion, and actual experience of seeing many gastric cancers.

Having already gained some experience in endoscopy before I joined the Cancer Institute Hospital of JFCR, I was under the misapprehension that upper GI endoscopy was easy. At the Cancer Institute Hospital of JFCR, however, I saw lesions I had never seen before — such as gastritis-resembling cancer, minute gastric cancer, and 0-IIb lesions — being detected one after the other. I was astonished by the difference between my competence and that of the doctors at the Institute. When asked one of them what the secret to finding gastric cancer was, he said that the lesion looked luminous. At first, I didn't understand what he meant. But once I had looked at enough lesions to get used to them, lesions started jumping out at me. And I understood it was what he meant when he said the lesion looked luminous.

Eventually, I became a staff doctor and started instructing newcomers. I thought a lot about what would be the best way to teach someone how to efficiently find gastric cancer. In order to get people used to what lesions looked like by seeing a lot of them, I came up with the idea of starting a mailing list in which quizzes with endoscopic pictures were sent out periodically to young doctors. When Dr. Masahiro Igarashi, then Director of the Gastroenterological Medicine Department of the Cancer Institute Hospital of JFCR, saw these quizzes with endoscopic pictures, he recommended that I write a series of articles for *Clinical Gastroenterology* with the idea of eventually turning them into a book. Ultimately, that led to the publication of this book. Without Dr. Igarashi, this book would never have come into being. So I am deeply indebted to him and would like to express my utmost gratitude for his efforts.

While preparing this book, I referred to a wide range of medical literature and textbooks. But there were still some things I didn't understand, so I asked leading doctors and they were kind enough to help me. Here I would like to thank Dr. Kazuyoshi Yagi of Uonuma Kikan Hospital, Dr. Noriya Uedo of Osaka International Cancer Institute, and Dr. Hisashi Doyma of Ishikawa Prefectural Central Hospital.

Also I would like to thank Dr. Junko Fujisaki, who is the current Director of the Gastroenterological Medicine Department, for supervising this book, Dr. Hiroshi Kawachi, who wrote pathological sections for this book despite his enormous workload, and all my senior and junior colleagues who provided me with questions based on the many gastric cancers they found.

I hope that this book — which began four years ago as a series of simple quizzes with endoscopic pictures for intra-hospital use — will prove useful to doctors engaged in endoscopic diagnosis. Nothing would make me happier.

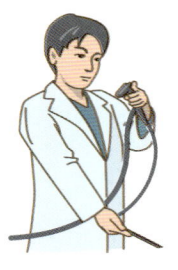

Toshiaki Hirasawa
October 2016

Index

0–I 38
0–IIa 38
0–IIb 38, 64, 149, 150, 167
0–III 39

Author Profiles

Toshiaki Hirasawa   Head, Upper GI Medicine Department, Cancer Institute Hospital of JFCR

Born in 1974, Dr. Hirasawa graduated from Kochi Medical School in 1999. He spent all his time playing soccer from elementary school to college. For three years after graduation, he underwent junior residency training at St. Luke's International Hospital centering around internal medicine. In 2002, he joined the staff of the Chiba University Hospital's First Internal Medicine Department and underwent residency training in gastroenterology. He subsequently pursued his career as a gastroenterologist at National Yokohama Higashi Hospital and Kimitsu Chuo Hospital. In 2004, he moved to Tokatsutsujinaka Hospital, where he focused on colonoscopy, while also studying colonoscopy at Matsushima Clinic and National Cancer Center Hospital East. Since 2006, he has been working at the Cancer Institute Hospital of JFCR and conducting clinical practice and studies focusing on diagnosis and endoscopic treatment of gastric cancer. Today, he is a board certified gastroenterologist of the Japanese Society of Gastroenterology and a board certified fellow/trainer of the Japan Gastroenterological Endoscopy Society. He is also a committee member of the compilation of the Endoscopic Guidelines for Diagnosis of Early Gastric Cancer. He received the Nishi Memorial Award in Gastric Cancer for a paper on undifferentiated-type gastric cancer and also the Distinguished Paper Award of the Japan Gastroenterological Endoscopy Society for a paper on LECS for cardiac SMTs. He has recently been concentrating on gastroscopy check-ups and gastric cancer detection.

Hiroshi Kawachi   Head, Department of Pathology, Cancer Institute Hospital of JFCR

Born in Omuta, Fukuoka Prefecture in 1972, Dr. Kawachi graduated from Tokyo Medical and Dental University Faculty of Medicine. He belonged to a volleyball club at the university. After graduation, he continued his study of pathological diagnosis at Tokyo Medical and Dental University Graduate School. After finishing graduate school, he underwent clinical training in gastroenterology at Showa University Northern Yokohama Hospital Digestive Disease Center and then went on to pursue his study of histopathological diagnostics — particularly gastrointestinal pathology — at the Pathology Department, Tokyo Metropolitan Cancer and Infectious Diseases Center Komagome Hospital. In 2006, he joined the Pathology Department at the Tokyo Medical and Dental University Hospital. Starting 2012, he was posted for three years to Santiago, Chile, where TMDU's overseas collaborative research center is located, and participated in Chile's and Ecuador's national colonoscopy check-up projects while practicing as a visiting pathologist. He has been working at his present position since returning to Japan in March 2015. He is engaged in pathological diagnosis concentrating on lesions in the esophagus, stomach, and colon. He is now a pathologist/pathology instructor and cytologist. As of 2016, he is a member of the Committee for Guidelines for Clinical and Pathologic Studies of the Japan Esophageal Society, a member of the Pathology Committee of the Japanese Society for Cancer of the Colon and Rectum, and a member of the Editorial Committee of *Digestive Endoscopy*.